Fundamentals of
Nursing Models, Theories and Practice

Fundamentals of
Nursing Models, Theories and Practice

THIRD EDITION

Hugh P. McKenna

Ulster University
UK

Majda Pajnkihar

University of Maribor
Slovenia

Dominika Vrbnjak

University of Maribor
Slovenia

WILEY Blackwell

Registered Offices
John Wiley & Sons, Inc., 111 River Street, Hoboken, NJ 07030, USA
John Wiley & Sons Ltd, New Era House, 8 Oldlands Way, Bognor Regis, West Sussex, PO22 9NQ, UK

For details of our global editorial offices, customer services, and more information about Wiley products visit us at www.wiley.com.

The manufacturer's authorized representative according to the EU General Product Safety Regulation is Wiley-VCH GmbH, Boschstr. 12, 69469 Weinheim, Germany, e-mail: Product_Safety@wiley.com.

Wiley also publishes its books in a variety of electronic formats and by print-on-demand. Some content that appears in standard print versions of this book may not be available in other formats.

Library of Congress Cataloging-in-Publication Data applied for

Paperback ISBN: 9781394192755

Cover Design: Wiley
Cover Image: © imtmphoto/Shutterstock

Set in 9.5/12.5pt Source Sans Pro by Straive, Pondicherry, India
SKY10100377_031825

Contents

Preface

It is often the case that once you write a book, you have nothing more to say on the topic. However, due to positive feedback, we were persuaded to write a second edition, which was published in 2014. It was also translated into Slovenian. Now, a decade later, we have been encouraged to write a third edition. This was based on the strong suggestion from Wiley, the publisher. Apparently, the feedback from the second edition was fulsome in its praise. The other stimulus was that sales were good and, in particular, the book was well received in Europe and the United States. However, we are busy academics and producing a new edition simply because previous ones were well received was not seen by us as a good enough reason for spending months writing the various chapters.

We are passionate about nursing theory and were aware that much had been written in the past decade on the topic. We also spoke to university professors who had used the second edition in their teaching. They gave us some good advice on how a new edition could be enhanced. This enthused us to write this book and once we completed the updated chapters, we gave some thought to this preface. It is the last section that writers write and the first section that readers read. Normally, it should set out how the new edition differs from the previous one. Let us share these with you.

First, and significantly, we have a new co-author Dr Dominika Vrbnjak, who is an associate professor in nursing at the University of Maribor in Slovenia. She teaches and researches nursing theory and is motivated by how it improves the quality and safety of nursing care. She brings many new and welcome perspectives to the team.

It will not surprise readers to hear that a great deal of new research and publications have been produced in the past ten years. We have updated the literature, but without losing the essence of the previous edition. Readers will also see that we have included new key concept boxes, reflective exercises, multiple choice questions, true/false questions, additional reading sources and relevant websites.

Therefore, for these reasons and many others, we believe that this edition is a considerable improvement on the previous one. It still takes the reader on a theory-generating journey, from identifying phenomena in clinical practice to forming concepts and propositions and constructing a new theory. We also show how the theory can be tested to help nurses describe, explain, predict and prescribe care for patients, families and communities. Like all professions, nursing requires a body of knowledge pertaining to its craft. Therefore, we demonstrate how theory and research lead to nursing science. As a backdrop to this, we outline the different ways that nurses know and impart knowledge.

Nursing theories are of little use unless they are used by clinicians to guide and improve patient care. In fact, they have been criticised over the years as being simply academic exercises. However, to use a theory in practice, nurses must select an appropriate one. To do otherwise would place the nurse and the patient in theoretical straitjackets. Grand theories, which are sometimes called nursing models, have often been implemented in an uncritical top-down fashion because a nurse manager or a nurse educator saw them in use elsewhere. The book criticises this approach to choosing a theory that is the best fit for different types of nursing practice. We discuss 12 different criteria that can be used to help readers select such a theory.

There are now over 50 grand theories of nursing, and these tend to be broad conceptualisations from theorists such as Dorothea Orem, Virginia Henderson, Nancy Roper and Callista Roy, and not always based on research. We differentiate the often controversial relationship between these grand theories and nursing models. In contrast, mid-range and practice theories are more focused and precise, often developed as a result of research and more acceptable to clinical nurses. There are over 60 mid-range theories, and we describe how some have been used and their advantages and limitations.

We outline the relationship between theory and research and argue that research does two main things – it generates or tests theory. We guide readers through the different methodological approaches used to do this. This also provides insight into how researchers use theory to frame their research.

Finally, we highlight how the worth of a theory is ascertained through rigorous and systematic analysis and evaluation. Criteria are identified to help readers assess theories to show that they are valid and reliable. We also guide readers on how theories are refuted and altered as a result of refutation.

We have structured this book in such a way that the readers can dip in and out and put it down and lift it without losing continuity. We believe that nursing theories are going through a renaissance where their importance to practice, research and education is being rediscovered. Therefore, we believe that this publication is timely and relevant. Regardless of whether you are a student, a registered clinical nurse, a nurse educator or a nurse manager, we hope you enjoy reading this book as much as we enjoyed writing it.

Hugh P. McKenna
Majda Pajnkihar
Dominika Vrbnjak

Acknowledgements and Dedications

This book is dedicated to all the patients, families and communities who have taught us so much over the years. It is also dedicated to those theorists and students who have shaped our thinking.

In addition, we wish to acknowledge the patience and fortitude of our friends and families, specifically Tricia, Gowain and Saoirse McKenna, Boris Kac, Grega and Jasna Pajnkihar, Daria Pak, lovely grandchildren Lev and Aurora and Matej, Živa and Zoja Vrbnjak.

Hugh P. McKenna
Majda Pajnkihar
Dominika Vrbnjak

Features contained within your textbook

Every chapter begins with
an **outline** of the chapter
and an introduction to the topic.

Outline of Content

This chapter covers the following: the case for theory; the argument that all intentional and rational actions, including nursing actions, by definition, must have an underlying theory; an initial definition of theory; and how theory and practice become integrated into nursing *praxis*.

Learning Outcomes

At the end of this chapter, you should be able to:

1. Understand what nursing theory is
2. Define theory
3. Understand the construction/development of a theory
4. Discuss the relationship between nursing theory and science
5. Evaluate the relationship between nursing theory and practice
6. Know the limitations of nursing theory
7. Understand the importance of nursing theory for contemporary nursing

Learning outcome boxes give a summary of
the topics covered in a chapter.

Key Concept boxes give
definitions of theories.

Key Concepts 1.2

Paradigm: a discipline's 'world view'. What is important to that discipline underpins the discipline's beliefs, behaviours and mission.

Metaparadigm: The central elements that are important to a discipline or profession. For nursing, it has been composed of person, health, nursing and environment. Therefore, all nursing theories should say something about these four essential elements – otherwise, it may not be considered a nursing theory. Different theories deal with these four elements differently (see Appendix A).

Reflective Exercise 1.1

Theory

Write down or discuss with other people two different theories for one of the following:

- origins of the COVID-19 outbreak
- the rise of TikTok as a social media phenomenon
- climate change
- newborn babies smiling when spoken to

Consider if there is a basis of truth in any of these theories.

Reflective Exercises provide ways to put
theories into practice.

Each chapter ends with a list of **Revision
Points** to summarize important topics.

Revision Points

- Theory is a body of knowledge.
- Theory is a core part of science, wherein we formulate statements about phenomena (theories) and then test these empirically (research).
- Theory needs to be aligned to the real world and a means by which we can explain systematically things done and things observed.
- Theory is always something seen and/or thought about from a particular perspective, and thus by definition, a partial and (to some extent) subjective view of the world or the phenomena within it.
- Nursing theories can contribute to new knowledge in contemporary nursing.

Your textbook is full of **illustrations and tables**.

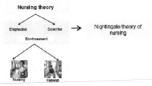

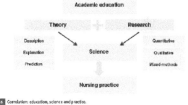

 The website icon indicates that you can find accompanying resources on the book's companion website.

About the Companion Website

Don't forget to visit the companion website for this book:

www.wiley.com/go/nursingmodels3e

There you will find valuable material designed to enhance your learning, including:

- Interactive multiple-choice questions
- Interactive true/false questions
- Case studies to test your knowledge
- Additional reflective questions to give a deeper understanding of topics
- Revision points from the book to consolidate learning

CHAPTER 1

The Case for Nursing Theory

Outline of Content

This chapter covers the following: the case for theory; the argument that all intentional and rational actions, including nursing actions, by definition, must have an underlying theory; an initial definition of theory; and how theory and practice become integrated into nursing *praxis*.

Learning Outcomes

At the end of this chapter, you should be able to:

1. Understand what nursing theory is

2. Define theory

3. Understand the construction/development of a theory

4. Discuss the relationship between nursing theory and science

5. Evaluate the relationship between nursing theory and practice

6. Know the limitations of nursing theory

7. Understand the importance of nursing theory for contemporary nursing

Introduction

In the realm of nursing, understanding and defining the construction and function, as well as limitations, of nursing theory is crucial for both education and practice. Before nursing students and registered nurses recognise the content and function of theory, they often ask themselves questions such as the following. What are nursing theories?

Fundamentals of Nursing Models, Theories and Practice, Third Edition. Hugh P. McKenna, Majda Pajnkihar and Dominika Vrbnjak.
© 2025 John Wiley & Sons Ltd. Published 2025 by John Wiley & Sons Ltd.
Companion website: www.wiley.com/go/nursingmodels3e

Why study them? What has this got to do with nursing? How can something so theoretical and abstract be valuable to a practical field like nursing? Nursing theories provide a structured framework that guides clinical decision-making, patient care and educational curriculums. Theory presents a description of the practice of nursing in mental images. However, recognising the limitations of these theories is essential to adapt and apply them effectively in diverse healthcare settings.

This book will help to answer these questions. Theories exist everywhere in society. There are numerous theories of the family, of the spread of fake news on social media, of how electric vehicles impact the environment, of how cancer cells multiply, of potential effects of artificial intelligence on the job market and of theories about climate change. And perhaps what you, as a student, are familiar with, because you encounter and experience the educational process on a daily basis, are theories about education. The world is full of theories, some tested as accurate, some untested and some speculative. It is no surprise, then, that there are theories of nursing. But what do theories do? In essence, they are simply used to describe, explain or predict phenomena (see Reflective Exercise 1.1). This will be explored in detail later.

Reflective Exercise 1.1

Theory

Write down or discuss with other people two different theories for one of the following:

- origins of the COVID-19 outbreak
- the rise of TikTok as a social media phenomenon
- climate change
- newborn babies smiling when spoken to

Consider if there is a basis of truth in any of these theories.

Now, none of the theories that you outlined for any of the topics in Reflective Exercise 1.1 may be true. In fact, they may be erroneous or downright preposterous. The point is that we all use theories to explain what goes on in our lives or in the world. But if you wanted to, you could probably test or find out whether your theories are true. Later on in this chapter, we will outline what theories are made of and how they are formed.

In many ways, theories are like maps. Maps are used to give us directions or to help us find our way in a complicated landscape or terrain. Maps often make simple what is a very complex picture. At their best, nursing theories also give us directions, instructions and information on how to design integrated care as to how to best care for patients or give us a broad picture of nursing care. But why have we got so many nursing theories? If you take any large city, there are many maps. For instance, in London, there are street maps, underground maps, electricity supply maps, Ordinance Survey maps and so on. Consider the London Underground or Paris Metro maps – they are simple and easy to follow but they do not look anything like the complex reality of the underground networks they represent. In other words, they make a complex system understandable.

Similarly, nursing can be highly complex, and we need different theories to help us understand what is going on. A theory that can be used in emergency care may not be of much use in mental health care, and a theory that can be used to help nurses in a busy surgical ward may be of little use in community care. In addition, the different theories attempt to highlight different phenomena that occur in practice and thus emphasise approaches to patient care such as equal partner-like relationships, caring, adaptation or self-care.

Nursing theories can provide frameworks for practice, and in many clinical settings, they have been used in the assessment of patients' needs. For instance, one of the most popular nursing theories in the United Kingdom was designed by three nurses who worked at Edinburgh University – Nancy Roper, Winifred Logan and Alison Tierney. They based their theory on the work of an American nurse called Virginia Henderson. Her theory outlined how nurses should be focused on encouraging patients to be independent in certain activities of daily living (ADLs), such as sleeping, eating and mobilising. Roper et al. (1983) took this a step further by identifying 12 ADLs. They stressed that the nurses' role was to prevent people from having problems with these ADLs. If this could not be achieved, nurses should help the patients be independent in the ADLs. If this was not possible, then nurses should give the patient and/or the patient's family the knowledge and skills to cope with their dependence on the ADLs. Many clinical nurses use the ADL theory to assess patients. They simply see how independent the patient is for each ADL and then focus their care on those for which the patient is dependent.

Therefore, theory can help us to carry out an individual patient's care and can contribute to better observations and recognition of specific patient needs, be they physical, psychosocial, emotional or spiritual. Nursing theories are often derived from practice. In other words, nursing theorists have constructed their theories based on what they have experienced when working with patients and their families, and by observing and describing phenomena in practice. Understanding the basic elements of a theory and its role and taking a critical view of it can help develop a body of knowledge that nurses need for everyday practice, education and research.

In this book, we want to highlight the need for and use of nursing theory and its function. This first chapter will introduce you to new words and ideas. You can read it in short bursts instead of tackling it all in one go. However, once you have mastered this first chapter, the rest of the book will be relatively easy to understand and, believe it or not, enjoyable and intellectually engaging. Several aspects of nursing theory are discussed in later chapters, and when reading those, dipping back into this first chapter will be helpful. Have a look at Reflective Exercise 1.2.

Reflective Exercise 1.2

Terminology

When you get involved in a new subject, you often have to learn new words to understand the topic. If you are a nursing student, you have had to learn many new anatomical or psychological words and phrases. Also, think of all the new words you would have to learn to take on any of the following hobbies:

- streaming
- gaming
- music
- fitness/wellness

See how many more you can think of. People accept learning new terms as part of understanding something in which they have an interest. The same is true in nursing theory.

The Necessity and Meaning of Theory

While it is true that some may argue that theories in nursing are only of concern to nursing academics and not always applicable in the practical world, we firmly stand by a different perspective. We believe there is no such thing as nursing without theory because there is no such thing as atheoretical nursing. Nursing is theory in action and every nursing act finds its basis in some theory. Thus, the theory is not abstract and reserved for academics but an integral part of the very essence of nursing. For instance, if a nurse is talking to a patient, they may be using communication theory. At its simplest, a communication theory would include a speaker, a listener, a message and understanding between the speaker and the listener. Similarly, if the nurse is putting a dressing on a patient, they may be using a theory of asepsis from the field of microbiology. Nurses might not always think about these theories by name or even say they are not using them. But behind what they do, there is usually a purpose or a reason, which often links back to a theory. Fawcett (2022) explained that theories are typically thought of as formulations that are not relevant for practice, which is the source of the so-called theory–practice gap.

When providing care to a patient, we are doing something in a *purposeful* manner – every action we take has a purpose. While doing it, we seek to understand, uncover meaning and determine how we should act based on our understanding. This process is essentially what we mean by 'theorising' or 'theory construction'. In this sense, theory is not some fancy concept for academics alone; it is a practical tool every nurse uses multiple times daily to provide the best care possible. Whether or not nurses use a particular theory in practice, it can be observed that they use the terminology or terminologies of different theories to describe what they want to emphasise when working with patients. Very often, the terminology of self-care, caring, equal partner-like relationships and basic living activities is used in describing the desired patient's treatment.

From the moment we start to think about something intentionally, we are constructing a theory. When we speak of construction, we are referring to how something is built or how the parts are put together to form a whole structure. Frequently, we are referring to a building that has been constructed, such as a house or a bridge. When we bring *thoughts* together to form some understanding, we are also constructing. In this instance, we are producing a mental building with a sense of wholeness that can be explained and shared with others through language.

This draws attention to another significant aspect of this process: when we think, we do so in language. A set of symbols that label the mental images are constructed, made up of our thoughts and the connections we make between them. In daily life too, people use different words and symbols to express meaning. In the same way, all theorists constructing their own theory use their own language and symbols to express and describe the theory.

For example, the highly recognised, respected and distinguished American nurse theorist Watson (1979) developed a theory that differentiates nursing from medicine and advocates a moral stance on caring and nursing as a service driven by specific value systems regarding human caring. According to this theory, the purpose of nursing is to preserve the dignity of clients. The theory describes the core essence of nursing since the development of modern nursing but uses new language and symbols.

Similarly, another American theorist, Orem (1991), began to see that most people are self-caring, e.g. they feed themselves, get themselves out of bed and wash themselves. This is a normal way of living for most of the population. Orem saw that self-care is very important for the preservation of dignity and independence. How would you feel if someone started feeding you or helping you to walk when you could do these things very well yourself? Her theory focused on encouraging patients and helping them towards as much self-care as possible (Pajnkihar 2003). Orem also uses language and symbols that are typical of self-care theory. So, both Watson and Orem use different terminology and, of course, construct their theories differently.

Therefore, theory involves thinking (describing) and seeking meanings and connections (explaining) and often leads to actions (predicting). Such knowledge included in different nursing theories can help not only to describe and explain what is significant about patient care but also to assist with the prediction of what would work with different patients' problems (Pajnkihar 2003; Alligood 2018, 2022). As we outlined earlier, there are many nursing theories to help us describe, explain or predict nursing practices. However, we need to be selective in the use of theories, and this will be dealt with in a later chapter. We can adopt, adapt or develop our own theories, but many of the existing ones have been researched and found to be useful guides for practice and so might be more useful than simply constructing our own. But as with the map analogy discussed earlier, we need to consider them as guides that inform our actions (Meleis 1997, 2007, 2018). It has been said that there is nothing as practical as a good theory. In essence, theories hold value when they can be applied in practice. A theory is a description of practice and the actual treatment of patients.

Theory Defined

The question of what theory actually *is* will be revisited throughout this and the following chapters. There are almost as many definitions of theory as there are nursing theories. Multiple definitions are presented here to illustrate the diversity in describing and defining nursing theories.

To best understand the various definitions of theory, it would be useful to describe the components that make up a theory – essential building blocks. We have already mentioned some aspects. For example, theories describe, explain or predict phenomena. But what, you may ask, are phenomena? Put simply, phenomena are things we witness through our senses (hearing, seeing, touching, smelling and tasting). So, a patient falling is a phenomenon, a wet floor is a phenomenon, a dog barking is a phenomenon and wound healing is a phenomenon.

When we put a name to a phenomenon, it becomes a concept. The examples discussed earlier of a patient falling, a dog barking, a wet floor and an assassination are all concepts. They tend to encapsulate what the phenomenon is. If we can define the concepts, they help clarify our view of the phenomena. So, concepts are the building blocks of a theory.

When two or more concepts are linked, this is called a proposition. The obvious proposition from one of the concepts introduced earlier would be the link between a wet floor (concept a) and a patient falling (concept b). So, a proposition would be that the patient fell because of the wet floor. This would be termed a causal proposition. There are different types of propositions and, as you will see in the following, they can be seen as the cement or mortar that binds the concepts (bricks) together to form the structure (a theory). Propositions bind and explain the concepts into the overall structure and function of the theory.

Another term that you will find when you study nursing theory is 'assumption'. You accept an assumption as true even though it has not been tested. For instance, I think readers can assume that people are composed of biological, psychological and social dimensions. If you take the example of a car crash, you may assume that the driver did not want to crash. Or if you look at Roy's Adaptation Theory, you will find that she identified three types of assumptions that she believed to be true (see Key Concepts 1.1).

Key Concepts 1.1

Phenomenon: something that you experience through your senses

Concept: a name given to a phenomenon

Proposition: a statement that explains and links concepts together in different types of relationships

Assumption: something that you take for granted even though it has not been proven or tested

From these exercises, you will hopefully be able to understand some of the definitions that exist to explain nursing theory. For example, Dickoff and James (1968: 105) defined nursing theory as a 'conceptual system or framework that is invented to serve some purpose', emphasising the importance of testing and confirmation as well as the theory having a purpose (Chinn, Kramer & Sitzman 2022). Chinn and Jacobs (1978: 2) saw theory as 'an internally consistent body of relational statements about phenomena which is useful for prediction and control'. Chinn and Jacobs (1987) later developed the definition further as: 'a set of concepts, definitions and propositions that project a systematic view of phenomena by designating specific interrelationships among concepts for the purpose of describing, explaining, predicting or controlling the phenomenon'. The definition highlights the theory's content, context and function, pointing to the construction of a theory (concepts, definitions and propositions) and the interrelationships between theory elements and functions of a theory (describing, explaining and predicting).

Another definition, this time by Meleis (1997: 11; Im & Meleis 2021: 13), drew attention to a theory as something that is purposefully structured: 'theory means an organised, coherent, and systematic articulation of a set of statements related to significant questions in a discipline that are communicated in a meaningful whole to describe or explain a phenomenon or a set of phenomena'. This clearly states that the theory represents a body of nursing knowledge and answers questions that interest nursing.

According to Chinn, Kramer and Sitzman (2022: 155), theory is defined as 'a creative and rigorous structuring of ideas that project a tentative, purposeful, and systematic view of phenomena'. This definition highlights theory's purposeful and dynamic nature and its specific characteristics. The development of theory also relies on the creativity of the theorist, and theoretic statements are always open to revision as new evidence and insights emerge. Furthermore, the concepts within a theory should be precisely defined and logically connected to establish a coherent pattern. Earlier in this chapter, we wrote that theories may reflect fact or, indeed, be totally untrue. When a theory is tested many times and stands up to that test, it is beginning to take on the shape of a law in theoretical language.

For example, let us say a theory of skin integrity led nurses to turn bed-bound patients once every two hours to prevent pressure ulcers. If this was consistently tested through research and found to be true, then the theory could be taking on law-like properties.

According to McEwen and Wills (2019: 53), nursing theory is summarised as: 'set of logically interrelated concepts, statements, propositions, and definitions, which have been derived from philosophical beliefs of scientific data and from which questions or hypotheses can be deduced, tested, and verified. A theory purports to account for or characterise some phenomenon'. Additionally, Wills (2019) emphasised that nursing theory clarifies the role of nursing and its purpose, differentiating it from other caring professions and establishing professional boundaries.

Lately, Fawcett emphasises the use of theory as evidence in advanced nursing practice, or what she prefers to call advanced practice nursology, and calls the discipline of nursing a discipline of nursingology (Fawcett 2018, 2022).

Butts and Rich (2018, 2022) claim people have difficulty understanding precisely what a theory is, what it can do to guide research and how to decide which theory to use. However, according to various definitions above, a nursing theory is constructed out of specific phenomena represented as concepts, definitions, assumptions and propositions that help describe, explain or predict how nursing may support and help patients, families or society. It is therefore a mental theoretical formulation of describing, explaining and predicting the outcomes of the practice of nursing, or how the theoretician would guide us to treat patients and their families.

We hope these definitions have not confused readers. They can all be encapsulated in the following sentence: A theory is composed of a number of concepts and propositions that help nurses describe or explain nursing or enable them to predict how patients will respond to nursing care.

In synthesising these definitions, it becomes evident that nursing theories are foundational tools in education and practice. They offer a structured approach to understanding nursing phenomena, guiding research and improving patient care. However, recognising the limitations and evolving nature of these theories is essential for their effective application in diverse and ever-changing healthcare environments.

Reflective Exercise 1.3

Defining Theory

Using your learning and library resources, look up the definitions for phenomena, concepts, definitions, propositions, description, explanation and predictions. See if you can find six different definitions of a theory. They do not have to be from the nursing literature. You should find that most of the definitions are composed of the words in the list.

To summarise, the definitions point out that:

- Theory consists of an organised and coherent set of concepts (two or more), definitions and propositions (two or more) that encapsulate specific phenomena in a purposeful and systematic way.
- The proposition(s) must claim a relationship or relationships between the concepts contained in the statement.
- It is a purposeful process and demands creative and rigorous structuring and tentative description of phenomena.
- The purpose of a theory is to describe, explain and/or predict.
- Theories use specific language, ideas or sometimes symbols to give answers to practice-based nursing problems.
- Theories are made up of mental building blocks and they can be explained and shared with others through language.

Some of the definitions proposed here are rather complex. While they aim to be thorough, there is a risk that they might become challenging to grasp. Therefore, it is essential to take some time to reflect on these definitions and the terminology employed. Bear in your mind that however each definition of theory is presented, the intention in all definitions is that the theory should present, in a simple, systematic and structured way, the theoretical core of knowledge that is of interest to the discipline and profession of nursing and nurses.

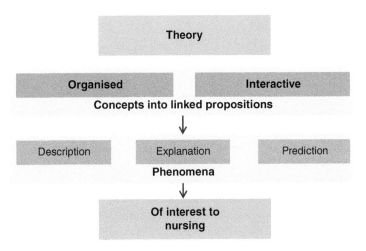

FIGURE 1.1 The links between theory and practice.

Reflection on the Definition

Theory often means different things to different people. For example, we have emphasised in our definition above the notion that theory requires concepts (two or more) linked by propositions (one or more) (Figure 1.1). However, it is worth noting that not everyone shares this perspective. As you have likely discovered in Reflective Exercise 1.1, there is a multitude of varying definitions. It is important for us to acknowledge these differences and recognise the diverse ways in which people use the term 'theory'.

Rodgers (2022: 97) emphasised the significant efforts made to define nursing theory's core concepts and advance research that fosters theory-based nursing practice. Alligood (2018: 8) stated that theory-based research enhances evidence-based practice by grounding empirical findings in theoretical frameworks. This type of research supports and informs evidence, reinforcing the practical application of nursing theories. Additionally, there is a global appreciation for the diverse values encapsulated within nursing theories, illustrating the rich theoretical landscape of the field. Butts & Rich (2022) articulated that scientific theories are instrumental in interpreting reality by providing descriptions, explanations and predictions of phenomena, thereby contributing profoundly to the understanding and development of nursing practice.

Theory or Model

There is also some confusion about the terms *theory* and *model*. These are often used interchangeably. Some authors, such as Fawcett (2005), see them as very different, whereas others, like Meleis (1997, 2021a), see them all as theories, with models simply being a theory at an earlier stage of development or not as advanced – but a theory nonetheless. Therefore, the differences between a theory and a model lie in the level of abstractedness and the level of development. Models are more abstract and are associated with notions of something practical that illustrate real situations. You may prefer the term 'model' because it accompanies us through life and illustrates the models we associate and see in everyday life. For example, toys (cars), anatomical models (bodies), simulators in a simulation clinical environment, nursing practice simulators and diagrammatic representations are all models. This difference will be explained in more detail in Chapter 5.

Key Concepts 1.2

Paradigm: a discipline's 'world view'. What is important to that discipline underpins the discipline's beliefs, behaviours and mission.

Metaparadigm: The central elements that are important to a discipline or profession. For nursing, it has been composed of person, health, nursing and environment. Therefore, all nursing theories should say something about these four essential elements – otherwise, it may not be considered a nursing theory. Different theories deal with these four elements differently (see Appendix A).

Construction of Theory

As we saw earlier, theory consists of *concepts* linked by statements that propose particular types of connections that join and explain these concepts together (*propositions*). Put simply, concepts are connected by statements that reveal their relationships. To expand on the idea of theory as a construct, you can think of it as a structure with concepts (like bricks) held together by statements (like mortar or cement).

The concepts (bricks) may be of different forms and levels of abstraction, from concrete to abstract (of different shapes and sizes and made of different materials). They may be 'people' bricks, 'object' bricks or even bricks consisting of more abstract concepts such as 'love' or 'care'. They may be joined together to make descriptive, explanatory or predictive propositional statements (mortar/cement). Additional concepts (bricks) may be added, but they must not look out of place and must adhere in a meaningful way to the propositions (mortar/cement). All concepts are inter-linked with the propositions. The basic concepts in the theory, such as caring, and the metaparadigm concepts (person, environment, nursing and health) are inter-linked with each other. The metaparadigm and its concepts are the global consensus within the nursing discipline and clearly present the core of a nursing theory. Another way of looking at it is that the metaparadigm forms the essence of a theory, illustrating how the theorist views nursing, health, the human being and the environment (see Appendix A).

We can also see in the following definition that the concepts of the metaparadigm are interconnected by propositions. Fawcett (2023: 2) stated:

> *the metaparadigm as the global concept that identify the phenomena of central interest to a discipline, the global non-relational propositions that define and describe the concepts, and the global relational propositions that state the relations between the concepts. This definition refers to the metaparadigm concepts as of* central *interest, specifies* non-relational and relational propositions *and* adds the word, define, as well as describe, to the non-relational propositions of the metaparadigm.

In the discussion of nursology, Fawcett also brings the global aspect to the concepts of metaparadigm and changes the term 'person' to 'human being'.

Further insights into the metaparadigm will be explored in Chapter 5.

The journey to theoretical understanding starts with seeing and trying to interpret phenomena. Some examples of directly observing and describing a phenomenon in practice are seen to underpin the theories of Florence Nightingale (1859/1980) and Hildegard Peplau (1952). Nightingale described her time in the Scutari's Barrack Hospital during the Crimean War: she saw the unsanitary environment as the main cause of soldiers dying unnecessarily. The old barracks across the Bosphorus from Constantinople had been redesigned as a military hospital; it had poor ventilation and a dead horse was found in the water supply. It is not surprising that most of the soldiers died from infections rather than from the wounds of battle. Nightingale believed that such infections were caused by a 'miasma' that travelled through the air. Therefore, the phenomena she saw in her physical environment were related to better cleanliness and better ventilation. Her theory, not surprisingly, focuses mainly on the environmental element of the metaparadigm (Figure 1.2). She wrote that

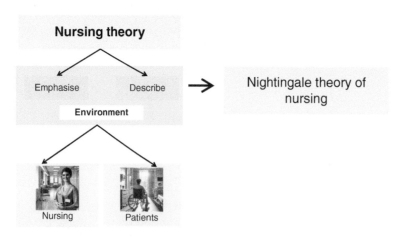

FIGURE 1.2   Nightingale theory of nursing.

the nurse's role was to place the patients in the best position to let nature cure them (Nightingale 1859/1980). She emphasised the importance of the physical environment in the health and treatment of patients. In her theory, she stressed the importance of improving the physical environment because it has a negative impact on patients' health and recovery. She ensured that the corridors and rooms of the hospital were scrubbed clean and the windows opened to get rid of the 'miasma'. She also sent her 'nurses' into Constantinople market to buy materials for bedsheets and dressings. It may not surprise readers to know that the doctors in the hospital were against most of these interventions. However, under her approach, the levels of infection decreased and more patients recovered than previously. Her emphasis on the environment remains relevant today, particularly concerning hospital-acquired infections and the effects of global warming on health.

Peplau's (1952) theory was constructed from the years she spent working as a nurse in psychiatric hospitals in the United States. She began to be convinced that the leading cause of mental illness was the lack of interpersonal communication. Therefore, Peplau's theory is mainly centred on how nurses should establish and sustain interpersonal relations with patients. Peplau's theory continues to have a significant impact today because it provides a theoretical core of interpersonal relationships relevant to practice and daily life.

Roper et al. (1983) observed how patients often lost independence in some of their ADLs (e.g. walking, eating or sleeping). Their theory provides nurses with knowledge on how to change dependence to independence in ADLs (see Reflective Exercise 1.4).

Reflective Exercise 1.4

Building Theory

A cancer nurse notices that patients often become sick when a nurse is giving them chemotherapy. This is a phenomenon that the nurse observes. Nurses' conceptual name for this phenomenon is 'chemotherapy-induced nausea'. The proposition is the link between the two concepts of nausea and chemotherapy. The theory that describes this phenomenon is that every time the patient received chemotherapy, they became nauseated. Think about your work in practice, choose one event and discuss what the phenomenon is and identify the related concepts and propositions.

Theory and Science of Nursing

In this section, the relationship between the theory and science of nursing is described (Figure 1.3). The starting point is that a theory represents knowledge developed by a systematic process, with the purpose of being useful and helping to

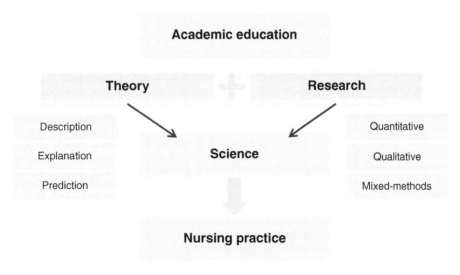

FIGURE 1.3 Correlation: education, science and practice.

improve practice. This is new knowledge, which still has to be tested (Pajnkihar 2003). The theory is best tested by research, and once this has been undertaken, the theory becomes part of nursing science.

$$\text{Science} = \text{Theory} + \text{Research}$$

Therefore, theory represents knowledge and research refers to the methods used to develop and test the theory (Boyd et al. 1991 in Polifroni 2022: 45). Science, which comes from the Latin word scientia, meaning 'knowledge', traditionally refers both to processes and to the outcomes of the processes, such as general laws and observations. Rodgers (2022) added that science is a general term used for the core knowledge of a discipline that has been developed rigorously and systematically throughout history and is the term that refers to credible knowledge.

Popper (1989) famously said the theory was like a paper boat that you placed into a pond to see if it floats or sinks. If it continued to float under different circumstances (e.g. wind or waves), then you could be confident that it was a good paper boat (theory). However, if it sank after many successes, then there was a question over the soundness of the design. This can also be seen in nursing theory. If nurses were to research a new theory of oral hygiene for cancer patients and find it effective every time, then such a theory would enter nursing science and become standardised practice. However, if, at a later date, some researchers found that it did not work or was not effective with people who had a particular form of cancer, then the theory would have failed, and its position in nursing science would have to be re-evaluated.

From this explanation of what science is and what theory is, we can assert the following: when a nursing **theory** is developed, it forms a body of knowledge that describes, explains and/or predicts phenomena from practice and that gives nursing professional meaning and relevance. Once research shows that theory does what it should do and does so consistently – the end product contributes to nursing **science**.

Meleis (2012, 2018) defined science as a unified body of knowledge based on agreed-upon evidence, addressing disciplinary and central questions within the discipline. She views nursing science as the systematic study of nursing practices, experiences and outcomes, emphasising the integration of theoretical and practical knowledge to improve patient care.

Previously, Keck (1998) viewed science as a unified body of knowledge focused on specific subject matter, encompassing the skills and methodologies needed to acquire such knowledge. Jacox (1974) distinguished between science as a process involving methods for developing and testing knowledge and science as a product, which refers to an accumulated body of knowledge describing selected aspects of the universe. Jacox described nursing science as a body of knowledge developed through research and logical analysis, focusing on improving nursing practice and patient outcomes. Nursing science therefore can be described as a body of knowledge, developed by different methods and approaches that nurses can use to describe, explain and/or predict phenomena. When described as a product, it means a theory; when described as a process, it means the way (research methods used and research process) in which a theory is developed (Pajnkihar 2003).

Therefore, nursing science is simply nursing theory that has been tested. How nurses practice and how they use this knowledge in their practice to treat patients can be said to be the art of nursing. It is obvious that nursing as a science and as an art are both related to nursing research. The purpose of the science of nursing is to develop knowledge that is applicable and useful in nursing practice (Pajnkihar 2003).

Undoubtedly, reliable scientific knowledge is essential for nursing practice. Hinshaw (1989) emphasised nursing's duty to create a relevant, accurate and reliable knowledge base to guide practice. This knowledge must remain pertinent and precise, as societal needs evolve. With nursing care developing over time, theories may require ongoing adjustments to be relevant to practical application (Pajnkihar 2003).

Theory provides practitioners with a foundation for informed decision-making rooted in thoughtful judgement. As nurses gain clinical experience, they can integrate theoretical and practical knowledge along with critical thinking to enhance their clinical decision-making and, consequently, improve their practice. Another definition of nursing science is a systematic body of knowledge that supports the practice and education of nursing, incorporating theories, research and practical application (McEwen & Wills 2019). Theories provide the basis for understanding and recognising nursing as a scientific discipline because they provide a core of knowledge that differentiates nursing from other health disciplines.

Rodgers (2022) described the term science as referring to the body of knowledge of a discipline, e.g. nursing, that has been rigorously and systematically developed. He maintained that nursing science is a dynamic and evolving discipline, integrating research, theory and practice to address the complexities of health and illness.

Together, these definitions emphasise the integration of theoretical, empirical and practical knowledge to advance the field of nursing and improve patient care. As Alligood (2018) pointed out, theory-based research is essential for the advancement of evidence-based practice in nursing. Nursing theory-based research informs evidence and enriches nursing values globally through diverse models and theories. As more nurses adopt theory-based practice, the theoretical works in nursing literature become clearer.

The relationships between research and theory are explained more fully in Chapter 8.

Other Interpretations of Theory

For some people, theory is simply a term that differentiates thinking (theorising) from doing (practice). This has a parallel in some people believing that poetry or art have little to do with the practicalities of the real world. When nurses say that theory is of no relevance to their work, it is often the term 'theory' that they are rejecting. An important extension of this meaning is where theory is used as a synonym for the entire body of knowledge that underpins nursing. More precisely, when we speak of a discipline's *theory*, we are referring to its *body of knowledge*, whether or not this is linked to any practical value.

At the outset of this chapter, we emphasised that nursing practice is based on theories, but not everyone agrees on this. Some people assert that theory has no relevance to practice and therefore to nursing. Marrs and Lowry (2006) maintained that, on the one hand, there are nursing theorists who emphasise 'knowing' and, on the other, practising nurses who focus on 'doing' and deny that theories are useful to them in their everyday practice. In essence, this is separating the 'what' and 'why' of nursing from the 'how' of nursing. We would not subscribe to this view; rather, we take a similar stance to Khairulnissa and Moez (2011), who argued that theory is not relevant if it cannot be directly applied and used in nursing practice.

The idea that theory is separate from practice is problematic in nursing; if theory has no relevance to practice, by definition, it can have no relevance to nursing. Those who reject such a premise nevertheless recognise the problem of turning theory into practice. Theories that are used in education or research and are not applied and used in practice do not serve their purpose. This is referred to as the *theory–practice gap* (see Reflective Exercise 1.5).

11

Reflective Exercise 1.5

The Theory–Practice Gap

Produce a brief one-page (300 words) account of the theory–practice gap. Reflect carefully on whether this is a bad thing or a good thing in any discipline. After all, the research findings in any profession are almost always ahead of the findings being disseminated and introduced into practice. Therefore, perhaps there will always be a theory–practice gap and it is a good thing. However, you can argue the contrary to this view. Finally, consider ways in which this problem of the gap may be overcome.

As this matter is taken up again in Chapter 3, you should retain the results of this exercise.

Jacobs and Huether (1978: 66) deny nursing the status of science on the terms outlined earlier. Rather, they favour the development of nursing practice based on a strong body of theoretical knowledge, believing that without this, nursing lacks cohesiveness. To improve this, they, along with Schwirian (1998: 37), suggested that nursing should develop scientifically, thus helping to close or minimise the gap between practice and theory.

Main Paradigms and Philosophies and Their Influence on the Development of Nursing Science

The term 'paradigm' is closely associated with Thomas Kuhn (1970). He introduced the word to the scientific community to explain how disciplines develop their knowledge (Meleis 2012, 2018; McEwen & Wills 2019). The simplest definition of a paradigm is that it is the way in which we view the world. A nursing paradigm is considered to offer a perspective on what nursing is, and it is influenced not just by different scientific traditions but by the problems of the nursing discipline that require different perspectives for understanding (Kim 1989: 169).

Nurses practice within a particular world view, which has significant implications for the profession and patients (Nagle & Mitchell 1991). Let us look at two contradictory nursing paradigms:

- **Paradigm 1.** All patients are dependent and the nurse's role is to carry out all those activities that the patients cannot do themselves.
- **Paradigm 2.** All patients need to be as independent as possible and the nurse's role is to encourage patients to do as much as they can for themselves.

These two world views or paradigms of nursing can influence how we nurse, how we teach nursing and how we manage nursing. Kuhn (1970) argued that science without theory is pre-paradigmatic; that is, it is haphazard, has no guiding principles and, in fact, is not science at all (see Reflective Exercise 1.6).

Reflective Exercise 1.6

The Theory–Paradigm Relationship

Each discipline or science has a particular paradigm – a conceptual orientation or way of seeing the world. The development of nursing theories will also be influenced by the prevailing paradigm within nursing. Consider the two paradigms outlined earlier. How would theories differ if the nursing profession adopted one rather than the other?

It will not surprise you to learn that there are numerous paradigms in nursing. We can classify theories into one of four influential paradigms: systems, interactional, behavioural and developmental. In later chapters, you will see that some theories are affiliated to one or other of these paradigms. Certainly, we might argue that one or other paradigm is the best source of truth for nursing. The counter-argument is that none can be a 'best source' and that they are looking at different things or at the same things from different angles. This relates to one of the earlier understandings of theory we addressed in this chapter – the idea of theory as a spectacle or a view from a particular perspective. If we take the view that nursing by definition must look to the needs of the whole person within a whole physical and social world, and that its dominant orientation is *holistic*, then paradigms that fragment the whole person into parts are counterproductive. In this argument, nursing theories that are based on the paradigms from other disciplines (psychological, biological, socio-logical, etc.) may not be good for nursing. It could also be argued that for nurses to research these paradigms would be a case of developing those disciplines rather than nursing. This debate on borrowed theory versus home-grown theory will be returned to in Chapter 7 when we discuss how to select a suitable theory for practice.

One American theorist, Rosemary Parse (1987), has written that nursing is based on two distinct paradigms. In recognis-ing how parts are integral to the whole person and that the whole person is greater than the sum of his or her parts, she coined the term 'simultaneity paradigm'. In contrast to this, she identified the 'totality paradigm', where the parts are more important than the whole person. In the simultaneity position, the person is seen as an irreducible whole, while in the total-ity paradigm, the person is seen as greater than the sum of his or her parts. This is relevant in nursing, where we deal not with simple anatomical parts but with complex persons. Nurses work in the complex world of human beings where looking at the whole person is preferable to looking only at parts, such as the heart, personality and emotion. To summarise, Fawcett's model of nursing paradigms highlights the three main world views: reaction, reciprocal interaction and simultaneous action. She described how these paradigms view human beings and their interactions with the environment, noting the progression from viewing humans as sums of their parts to understanding them as participants in an unpredictable and complex pro-cess. She emphasised the impact of these paradigms on the development of nursing theories and their coexistence within the field of nursing as it evolves (Fawcett 2000). In contrast, Hardin (2018) explained how definitions (describe concepts) and relational statements (describe relationships between and among concepts) form the basis of nursing theory.

One way of explaining the difference between the simultaneity and totality paradigms is through the analogy of a birthday cake. Suppose we had a birthday cake with 'Happy Birthday to Mary' written in the icing. When you slice the cake, you get a number of separate parts. To Mary, the cake is greater than simply all the separate slices. It represents celebration, a happy occasion, a milestone in her life. This reflects the simultaneity paradigm, where the whole person is more than just a collection of biological, psychological and social parts. Consider the opposite view, where the slices of the cake simply make up the cake and when you look at one slice the birthday message is lost. This reflects the totality paradigm where we focus on individuals' diseases or pathologies rather than on the whole person. To a proponent of this paradigm, a coronary patient is simply that – pathology. That the presenting patient is a chief executive, has seven children and also has some financial problems are not matters worthy of consideration.

This is a perfect description of the biomedical model favoured for many years by physicians. Patients were perceived as a collection of anatomical parts and physiological systems. When these went wrong, the doctor had to diagnose and treat the pathology. In the past, nurses were taught through the biomedical model, but today, it has limited value for nurses or doctors.

Earlier, the case was made for the value of theory and also the need to keep such theory under constant review (e.g. the paper boat sinking). Kuhn (1970) has argued that a discipline without a body of theory is unscientific. There is an element of common sense in synthesising both arguments. If we *do* need a theory that is sound, tested and up-to-date, by definition, we are speaking of a growing body of theory in the sense that Kuhn proposed. Yet, in taking this position, we must also be cognizant of the nature of such theory and its limitations. As you saw in Reflective Exercise 1.7, theories tend to be specific within a particular paradigm or world view, and as such, may provide only a partial view of the real situation.

One approach for the nursing profession is to devise all-encompassing frameworks that show not only the elements that make up the totality of the body of knowledge but also the relations and differences between these elements. This may be seen as particularly important in nursing, where knowledge is being drawn from many different disciplines and paradigms. We call a body of knowledge so structured a *taxonomy* (from the Ancient Greek words *taxis* meaning arrangement and *nomie* meaning method). Similarly, Carper (1978), in the nursing context, speaks of *ways* of knowing in nursing as encompassing empirics, ethics, personal knowing and aesthetic knowing (see Chapter 2). In this context, it can be said that nursing theories can be derived from one or more paradigms, depending on how the theorist chooses to present the theory. Theories bring a complex core of knowledge to help inform and guide nursing practice. The types of knowledge that nurses might use in their practice are dealt with in Chapter 2 (see also Reflective Exercise 1.7).

Reflective Exercise 1.7

The Place of Theory in Science

Review your literature, this time looking up the terms science, research, world view and paradigm. What you should seek are further commentaries on how theory might influence science and how science (or a particular science's world view) might influence how its practitioners construct and use theory.

Make brief notes for later reference when we expand on some of these issues in Chapter 2.

Kääriäinen et al. (2011) claimed that we need tested theories to develop nursing science because they give more valid information about the concepts and their usefulness. The interaction between developing, testing and applying theory to practice is a never-ending circle, which is linked to research to ensure a solid core of knowledge. Without testing, we cannot and should not take theory into practice, especially if we have taken it from another discipline. How to select a suitable model or theory and a more detailed explanation of the advantages and disadvantages of borrowed theories are given in Chapter 7.

Theory and Practice of Nursing

Education and research foster the conditions for knowledge development in nursing. Any theory that supports everyday nursing actions and decision-making by nurses for the benefit of clients has to emanate from practice and return to inform practice. Johnson (1959: 212) emphasised that for any profession to thrive, it must explicitly establish its

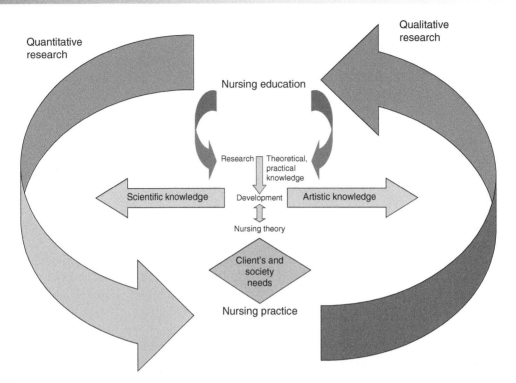

FIGURE 1.4   Basic structure of nursing. Reproduced from Pajnkihar (2003) Theory Development for Nursing in Slovenia.

theoretical foundations, and nursing is no exception. To assert itself as a profession, nursing requires a unique body of knowledge, and theories constitute a significant component of this knowledge, contributing to the evolution of nursing (Pajnkihar 2003, 2011).

McKenna et al. (2014) stated that nothing is more practical than nursing theory and that 'there is no such thing as nursing without theory'. A theory has to be 'alive' in order to inform practice. Nursing theory helps us to focus on the essential elements that give nursing its unique structure, character, presence and strength (Gorman 2009) and also helps us to define the unique role of nurses in the healthcare service (Colley 2003; Bultemeier 2012). They serve as the cornerstone for evidence-based nursing (Fawcett 2012) and provide the guidelines for decision-making, problem-solving and intervention development (Selanders 2010). Furthermore, nursing theory provides a framework for research, fostering the development of more refined theories (Figure 1.4).

Parker (2006) stressed that both practice and theory in nursing should mutually contribute to each other, guided by their intrinsic values and beliefs. However, no single theory can comprehensively explain the entirety of nursing. Instead, theories shed light on the various facets and meanings within the field (Colley 2003).

Because many nursing theories exist, they need to be reviewed, compared, analysed, evaluated and tested before being used in a care setting. Unfortunately, nurses have at times selected theories uncritically, neglecting robust criteria for theory selection, analysis and evaluation, often lacking a basis in scientific evidence (Pajnkihar 2003). 'Adaptation' of a theory in practice needs to be done on the basis of what patients need for the best care (Pajnkihar 2009, 2011). Further insights into theory analysis, testing and evaluation can be found in Chapter 9.

Do We Really Need Theory?

Because we need 'a reliable body of knowledge', in a constantly changing healthcare context there needs to be a *growing* body of knowledge that has to be constantly *updated* and *modified*, and continually subjected to *tests of refutation* (remember the paper boat). However, the argument here is two-fold: because we *do* need the 'tested theory', we also need to continue to 'produce' theory. As such, theory is always open to question. We are *always* testing the theory in the live situation and each situation is to some extent unique. We have to 'fit' the theory to the situation, adapt it and look for alternatives if it is not readily applicable. In so doing, we are questioning, analysing, synthesising and seeking patterns in the specific clinical situation, formulating propositional explanations and trying them out. Nurses who do this have been described as 'knowledgeable doers'. Benner (1999) had spoken of 'clinical wisdom'. In our context, we might describe it as the thoughtful, reflective, analytical, insightful, critical practice of nursing being a process of theorising in practice (which we refer to as *praxis* meaning 'living theory'). On this basis, every competent nurse is a theorist.

Nursing Theories Today

It could be argued that the first nursing theory was developed by Florence Nightingale and described in her book *Notes on Nursing* (Nightingale 1859/1980). For some reason, there was a hiatus in any further development of nursing theory for over 100 years. Then, in 1952, Hildegard Peplau published her theory on interpersonal relationships in nursing (Peplau 1952). This marked the start of a further 30 years of theory development – mostly in the United States of America. This was due to a range of professional, social and political factors. Alligood (2018) describes the history and significance of nursing theory through different eras: pioneer Nightingale, the curriculum, research, graduate education and the theory and theory utilisation era. The impact of undergraduate and postgraduate education on the expansion of research and the development of knowledge can be seen everywhere in the world. Awareness of the development and application of nursing theories for use in practice and to support education and research depends on the level of education and knowledge in the discipline.

Below you can find a brief overview of how nursing theories are accepted by nurses in the United States and the United Kingdom.

Nursing Theories in the United States

Most of the existing nursing theories emanated from the United States. As stated previously, it started with Peplau in 1952 and continued through the 1960s, 1970s and 1980s. During this time, about 40 theories were constructed. At one time, it appeared that there was a race among American academic nurses to come up with the ultimate nursing theory. Their emergence had a lot to do with the move of nurse education into the university system and a disenchantment with the biomedical model, which, as alluded to above, sees the patient as a collection of signs and symptoms, diseases and pathologies. Nursing theorists were treated like rock stars and many had their own literature and conference circuits. They even had their own followers – for example, those who supported Roger's (1980) theory were called Rogerians and those who supported Parse's (1981) theory were called Parsarians! Today, there is less hype about nursing theories in the United States, but some of the more meaningful ones have stood the test of time. We would include in this the theories of Parse, Orem, Roy and Watson (see Reference list). The main reason for their longevity and popularity is the research that has been undertaken to test and verify them.

Nursing Theories in the United Kingdom

In the United Kingdom, the entrance of nursing education to universities began in the 1970s, and McKenna (1997) noted that nurse teachers began to search for unique knowledge for the discipline. For these reasons, in the 1980s and 1990s, British nurses began to develop theories. Today, the most widely used nursing theory in the United Kingdom is that constructed by Roper, Logan and Tierney (RLT) (1980, 1985, 1990). It is interesting to note that the unquestioned and uncritical imposition of nursing theories in the 1980s on busy clinical nurses in the United Kingdom did theoretical nursing more harm than good. In the past, they tended to be introduced by nurse academics, nurse teachers or nurse managers. Rather, clinical nurses did not see them as helpful, perceiving them as getting in the way of care. This was the result of each theory generating a large volume of nursing paperwork. There is some evidence that there is a renewal of interest in nursing theories in the United Kingdom, with clinicians seeing them as helpful rather than a hindrance. The history of nursing theory development will be dealt with in greater detail in a later chapter.

Level of Education and Knowledge Development

Nurse education in the United States has a much longer tradition compared to education in Europe. Nurses in Central and Eastern Europe still have to work very hard to introduce developments that are taken for granted elsewhere, such as doctoral education in nursing, education in advanced nursing practice (ANP) or a doctorate in nursing practice (DNP).

The shortage of nurse educators with postgraduate academic qualifications is therefore still a big concern in some countries. A major problem is the lack of knowledge about alternative theories in nursing and the fact that there is almost no research on the choice or application of theories. Encouraging and facilitating nurse education is key to understanding the core of nursing knowledge. The development and application of mid-range theories is a key goal of DNP education, according to Chism and McLain (2022). They asserted that it is crucial for DNP graduates to have an understanding of mid-range theories and, most importantly, to have the knowledge and skills to apply and to apply them to practice.

Nursing Theories in Contemporary Nursing

The growing interest of nurses in applying nursing theories has also stimulated the development of new theories. The development of mid-range theories from existing grand theories (e.g. Peplau and Orem) has begun, resulting in an increased level of ease of use and a lower level of new abstraction of the theories, as well as congruence with the phenomena in practice, limited specificity of the nursing population (the scope of the theory is narrowed) and appropriateness to the level of nursing knowledge (Im & Meleis 2021). In addition, Meleis (2021b) claimed that fifth-generation theorists develop theories at different levels of abstraction and are not limited to developing only one type of theory. She also introduced the development of nursing situation-specific theories (SSTs). The main difference between grand and middle-range SSTs lies in abstraction, scope, generalisation and diversities. SSTs (sometimes called 'practice theories') can be developed based on the synthesis and integration of research findings and clinical cases on a specific situation or population and are designed to understand the specific situation of a group of clients. Chinn (2021) pointed out that SSTs are a good response to today's nursing knowledge development needs because they deal directly with everyday experiences and the different contextual circumstances that shape these experiences. You will be able to read more on SSTs in Chapter 3.

Today, people demand improved safety, quality, productivity, effectiveness and efficiency to maintain or improve patients' rights and equality. Due to financial and economic crises, there are fewer resources and fewer nurses available in healthcare systems. There is a danger that individual person-centred nursing care may disappear. Nonetheless, there is an increasing requirement for holistic, compassionate, person-centred and individualised care. Despite the criticism of nursing theories, they can help us to achieve these requirements. For example, as seen earlier, empowering patient self-care and autonomy is congruent with the theory of self-care developed by Orem (1980, 1991). Similarly, supporting patients towards independence in their ADLs is core to Roper et al.'s theory. Roy (1980) emphasised the need for patients to adapt to their environment and to their own abilities. Therefore, if used appropriately, these nursing theories and others can demonstrate cost-effectiveness by reducing dependency, encouraging self-care, and helping in the early detection of patients' problems.

Caring theories could significantly advance nurses' knowledge about their own and clients' personal values and beliefs in order to protect human dignity and respect and value individuality. Research carried out in Slovenia into Jean Watsons's 'carative factors' – 'processes' of nursing care – showed that nurses believed that they were especially caring when they assisted patients in fulfilling their basic human needs and in giving hope (Pajnkihar 2013).

Theories can provide a systematic basis for assessing, planning, implementing and evaluating care and offer a way to 'revitalise' the nursing process. New frameworks for our work for more holistic and individualised care can be established. In times of crisis, we can preserve or return to the fundamental values that are increasingly demanded nowadays.

However, in order to do that, we first need some basic theoretical knowledge, and hopefully, this book will provide you with the grounding to realise the importance of nursing theory.

In the pursuit of excellence in nursing education, it is imperative to delve into the theoretical underpinnings that shape the discipline. Theories in nursing serve as the foundation upon which the practice is built, offering insights into the multifaceted roles nurses embody and the distinct phenomena encountered within the field. As Meleis (2021a) articulated, the exploration of theories is vital in delineating the unique essence and substance of nursing from other disciplines. This differentiation not only elucidates what nurses do but also aims to evaluate the outcomes of their actions, emphasising the creation of mental models that mirror the real-world perspective of theorists (Chinn 2021).

The dynamic, cyclic nature of theory development underscores the need for a continual embrace of change and openness to the growth of theoretical nursing. This adaptability is crucial for enhancing nursing care outcomes, as highlighted by Im (2021). The unique focus of nursing knowledge development distinguishes it from other fields, directing inquiry and expanding the discipline (Smith 2018). Understanding the structure and organisation of nursing knowledge is essential for both learners and scholars within the discipline, as it guides practice through a theory-guided, evidence-informed approach. The development and application of nursing theories facilitate a systematic view of phenomena of concern, providing a structured way of understanding and acting within the discipline (Smith 2018).

Furthermore, the philosophical underpinnings and empirical generalisations that define nursing also delineate its process of reasoning. The language used to describe the essence of ideas, the specification of concepts at different levels of abstraction and the understanding of these concepts within the theoretical discourse are pivotal in grasping the theoretical landscape of nursing (Smith & Liehr 2018).

The international perspective on the development of nursing theories underscores the dynamic and interconnected nature of healthcare across borders. As nursing continues to evolve as a globally recognised profession, the exchange of ideas, practices and theoretical frameworks becomes increasingly vital. From the pioneering works of Florence Nightingale to contemporary scholars worldwide, the evolution of nursing theories reflects diverse cultural contexts, healthcare systems and societal needs. Embracing this international viewpoint not only enriches the theoretical landscape of nursing but also fosters collaboration and innovation in addressing the complex challenges of modern healthcare. Moving forward, nurturing a global dialogue among nurses and scholars will be essential in shaping inclusive and effective theoretical frameworks that resonate across diverse contexts and contribute to the advancement of nursing practice, education and research on a global scale.

In summary, the journey through nursing theories not only equips students with the analytical tools necessary for practice but also instils a deep appreciation for the theoretical foundations that distinguish nursing as a unique, dynamic discipline. By embracing the evolving nature of nursing theories and evaluating their applicability and value in practice, nursing education can foster a profound understanding of the discipline, guiding future nurses towards achieving professional excellence.

Conclusion

Praxis is understood as knowledge in action. We are constantly being called to 'base' or 'inform' our practice on sound evidence. In praxis, theory and theorising become integral parts of our practice, and our practice is in turn the living enactment of our theory and theorising. This chapter makes the argument that practice must be informed by theory and that theory is in turn informed by practice.

We have argued that theory is necessary in nursing. We have defined it as a means by which we can describe, explain and predict phenomena of importance to nursing care. In so doing, we have recognised the problems that exist. There are different views about what theory actually is. There are vastly different positions ranging from the view that theory is mere conjecture and of no value at all, to the view that it is essential to the construction of knowledge and our application of this in practice. We have, nevertheless, also recognised that theory is always a view from a particular perspective and always a tentative description, explanation or prediction of reality. We are, it was argued, always called on to challenge theory and to recognise that it must be adapted to each unique patient, rather than having the patient adapt to the theory.

In one sense, this opening chapter has raised many questions about nursing theory, but by doing so, it has arguably met one of its main aims: the recognition that theory *is* an important issue that must be addressed in nursing. In the remaining chapters, we will describe and discuss the related issues in greater depth.

Revision Points

- Theory is a body of knowledge.

- Theory is a core part of science, wherein we formulate statements about phenomena (theories) and then test these empirically (research).

- Theory needs to be aligned to the real world and a means by which we can explain systematically things done and things observed.

- Theory is always something seen and/or thought about from a particular perspective, and thus by definition, a partial and (to some extent) subjective view of the world or the phenomena within it.

- Nursing theories can contribute to new knowledge in contemporary nursing.

Additional Reading

Fawcett J. (2019) Nursology revisited and revived. *Journal of Advanced Nursing*, **75**(5), 919–920.

Hansen B.S. & Dysvik E. (2022) Expanding the theoretical understanding in advanced practice nursing: framing the future. *Nursing Forum*, **57**(6), 1593–1598.

Pajnkihar M., McKenna H.P., Štiglic G. & Vrbnjak D. (2017) Fit for practice: analysis and evaluation of Watson's theory of human caring. *Nursing Science Quarterly*, **30**(3), 243–252.

References

Alligood M.R. (2018) Introduction to nursing theory: its history and significance. In Alligood M.R. (ed.) *Nursing Theorists and Their Work*, 9th edition, pp. 2–10. St. Louis, MO: Elsevier.

Alligood M.R. (2022) *Nursing Theorists and Their Work*, 10th edition. St. Louis, MO: Elsevier.

Benner P. (1999) Nursing leadership for the new millennium. Claiming the wisdom & worth of clinical practice. *Nursing and Health Care Perspectives*, **20**(6), 312–319.

Boyd R., Gasper P. & Trout J.D. (1991) *The Philosophy of Science*. Cambridge, MA: MIT Press.

Bultemeier K.I. (2012) Nursing in Malawi: nursing theory in the movement to professionalize nursing. *Nursing Science Quarterly*, **25**(2), 184–186.

Butts J.M. & Rich K.L. (eds) (2018) *Philosophies and Theories for Advanced Nursing Practice*, 3rd edition. Burlington: Jones & Bartlett Learning.

Butts J.M. & Rich K.L. (eds) (2022) *Philosophies and Theories for Advanced Nursing Practice*, 4th edition. Burlington: Jones & Bartlett Learning.

Carper B.A. (1978) Fundamental patterns of knowing in nursing. *Advances in Nursing Science*, **1**(1), 13–23.

Chinn P.L. & Jacobs M.K. (1978) A model for theory development in nursing. *Advances in Nursing Science*, **1**(1), 1–12.

Chinn P.L. & Jacobs M.K. (1987) Theory and Nursing; A Systematic Approach. St Louis: CV Mosby.

Chinn P.L. (2021) Equity and social justice in developing theories. In Im E.O. & Meleis A.I. (eds) *Situation Specific Theories: Development, Utilization, and Evaluation in Nursing*, pp. 29–37. Cham: Springer.

Chinn P.L., Kramer M.K. & Sitzman K. (2022) *Knowledge Development In Nursing: Theory and Process*, 10th edition. St. Louis: Elsevier.

Chism L.A. & McLain N. (2022) The essentials of the doctor of nursing practice: a philosophical perspective. In Butts J.M. & Rich K.L. (eds) *Philosophies and Theories for Advanced Nursing Practice*, 3rd edition. Burlington: Jones & Bartlett Learning.

Colley S. (2003) Nursing theory: its importance to practice. *Nursing Standard*, **17**(4), 33–37.

Dickoff J. & James P. (1968) A theory of theories: a position paper. *Nursing Research*, **17**(3), 197–203.

Fawcett J. (2000) *Analysis and Evaluation of Contemporary Nursing Knowledge: Nursing Models and Theories*. Philadelphia, PA: F.A. Davis.

Fawcett J. (2005) *Contemporary Nursing Knowledge: Analysis and Evaluation of Nursing Models and Theories*, 2nd edition. Philadelphia, PA: F.A. Davis.

Fawcett J. (2012) Thoughts about evidence-based nursing practice. *Nursing Science Quarterly*, **25**(2), 199–200.

Fawcett, J. (2018) Our name: Why nursology? Why.net? Blog. https://nursology.net/2018/09/24/our-name-why-nursology-why-net/

Fawcett J. (2022) Using theory in evidence based advanced nursology practice. In Butts J.M. & Rich K.L. (eds) *Philosophies and Theories for Advanced Nursing Practice*, 3rd edition. Burlington: Jones & Bartlett Learning.

Fawcett, J. (2023). Evolution of one version of our disciplinary metaparadigm. Blog. https://nursology.net/2023/01/17/evolution-of-one-version-of-our-disciplinary-metaparadigm/

Gorman C. (2009) At work with Malawi's nurses: clinic and hospital nurses in a country with one of the world's worst nursing shortages. *The American Journal of Nursing*, **109**(6), 26–30.

Hardin S.S. (2018) Theory development process. In Alligood M.R. (ed.) *Nursing Theorists and Their Work*, 9th edition, pp. 35–43. St. Louis, MO: Elsevier.

Hinshaw A.S. (1989) Nursing science: the challenge to develop knowledge. *Nursing Science Quarterly*, **2**(4), 162–171.

Im E.O. (2021) Development of situation-specific theories: an integrative approach. In Im E.O. & Meleis A.I. (eds) *Situation Specific Theories: Development, Utilization, and Evaluation in Nursing*, pp. 49–70. Cham: Springer.

Im E.O. & Meleis A.I. (2021) *Situation Specific Theories: Development, Utilization, and Evaluation in Nursing*. Cham: Springer.

Jacobs M.K. & Huether S.E. (1978) Nursing science: the theory practice linkage. *Advances in Nursing Science*, **1**, 63–78.

Jacox A.K. (1974) Theory construction in nursing: an overview. *Nursing Research*, **23**(1), 4–13.

Johnson D.E. (1959) The nature of a science of nursing. *Nursing Outlook*, **7**, 291–294.

Kääriäinen M., Kanste O., Elo S., Pölkki T., Miettunen J. & Kyngäs H. (2011) Testing and verifying nursing theory by confirmatory factor analysis. *Journal of Advanced Nursing*, **67**(5), 1163–1172.

Keck J.F. (1998) Terminology of theory development. In Tomey A.M. & Alligood M.R. (eds) *Nursing Theorists and their Work*, 4th edition. St Louis: Mosby.

Khairulnissa A. & Moez S. (2011) Gap between knowledge and practice in nursing. *Procedia – Social and Behavioral Sciences*, **15**, 3927–3931.

Kim H.S. (1989) Theoretical thinking in nursing: problems and prospects. In Nicoll L.H. (ed.) *Perspectives on Nursing Theory*, 3rd edition. Philadelphia, PA: J.B. Lippincott.

Kuhn T.S. (1970) *The Structure of Scientific Revolutions*, 2nd edition. Chicago: University of Chicago Press.

Marrs J.A. & Lowry L.W. (2006) Nursing theory and practice: connecting the dots. *Nursing Science Quarterly*, **19**(1), 44–50.

McEwen M. & Wills E.M. (2019) *Theoretical Basis for Nursing*, 5th edition. Philadelphia, PA: Wolters Kluwer.

McKenna H.P. (1997) *Nursing Theories and Models*. London: Routledge.

McKenna H.P., Pajnkihar M. & Murphy F.A. (2014) *Fundamentals of Nursing Models Theories and Practice*. London: Wiley Blackwell.

Meleis A.I. (1997) *Theoretical Nursing: Development and Progress*, 3rd edition. Philadelphia, PA: Lippincott.

Meleis A.I. (2007) *Theoretical Nursing: Development and Progress*, 4th edition. Philadelphia, PA: Lippincott Williams & Wilkins.

Meleis A.I. (ed.) (2012) *Theoretical Nursing: Development and Progress*, 5th edition, pp. 179–228. Philadelphia, PA: Wolters Kluwer/Lippincott Williams & Wilkins.

Meleis A.I. (2018) *Theoretical Nursing: Development and Progress*, 6th edition. Philadelphia, PA: Wolters Kluwer/Lippincott Williams & Wilkins.

Meleis A.I. (2021a) Historical background for theories: revisiting the past to create the future. In Im E.O. & Meleis A.I. (eds) *Situation Specific Theories: Development, Utilization, and Evaluation in Nursing*. Cham: Springer.

Meleis A.I. (2021b) Development of situation-specific theories: an integrative approach. In Im E.O. & Meleis A.I. (eds) *Situation Specific Theories: Development, Utilization, and Evaluation in Nursing*, pp. 49–65. Cham: Springer.

Nagle L.M. & Mitchell G.J. (1991) Theoretical diversity: evolving paradigmatic issues in research and practice. *Advances in Nursing Practice*, **14**(1), 17–25.

Nightingale F. (1859/1980) *Notes on Nursing: What It Is and What It Is Not*. Edinburgh: Churchill Livingstone.

Orem D.E. (1980) *Nursing Concepts of Practice*, 2nd edition. New York: McGraw Hill.

Orem D.E. (1991) *Nursing Concepts of Practice*, 4th edition. St. Louis: Mosby.

19

Pajnkihar M. (2013) Caring and interpersonal relationships in nursing care. In Pajnkihar M. & Lorber M. (eds) International Conference Knowledge Brings Development and Health, May 2013. Faculty of Health Sciences, University of Maribor (in Slovene).

Pajnkihar M. (2003) Theory Development for Nursing in Slovenia. PhD thesis. Manchester: University of Manchester, Faculty of Medicine, Dentistry, Nursing and Pharmacy.

Pajnkihar M. (2009) Nurses' (un)partner-like relationships with clients. *Nursing Ethics*, **16**(1), 43–56.

Pajnkihar M. (2011) Teorija v praksi zdravstvene nege. Theory in nursing practice. *Utrip*, **19**(2), 4–5. (in Slovene)

Parker M.E. (2006) Studying nursing theory: choosing, analyzing, evaluating. In Parker M.E. (ed.) *Nursing Theories and Nursing Practice*, 2nd edition, pp. 14–35. Philadelphia, PA: F.A. Davis.

Parse R.R. (1981) *Man-Living-Health: A Theory of Nursing*. New York: John Wiley & Sons.

Parse R.R. (1987) *Nursing Science: Major Paradigms, Theories, and Critiques*. Philadelphia, PA: Saunders.

Peplau E.H. (1952) *Interpersonal Relations in Nursing: A Conceptual Frame of Reference for Psychodynamic Nursing*. New York: G.P. Putnam & Sons.

Polifroni E.C. (2022) Philosophy of science: an introduction and a grounding for your practice. In Butts J.M. & Rich K.L. (eds) *Philosophies and Theories for Advanced Nursing Practice*, 4th edition. Burlington: Jones & Bartlett Learning.

Popper K. (1989) *Conjectures and Refutations: The Growth of Scientific Knowledge*, revised edition. London: Routledge.

Rodgers B.L. (2022) The evolution of nursing science. In Butts J.M. & Rich K.L. (eds) *Philosophies and Theories for Advanced Nursing Practice*, 4th edition. Jones & Bartlett Learning: Burlington.

Rogers M.E. (1980) *An Introduction to a Theoretical Basis of Nursing*, 2nd edition. Philadelphia, PA: F.A. Davis & Co.

Roper N., Logan N. & Tierney A. (1980) *Elements of Nursing*, 1st, edition. Edinburgh: Churchill Livingstone.

Roper N., Logan N. & Tierney A. (1983) *Using a Model for Nursing*. Edinburgh: Churchill Livingstone.

Roper N., Logan N. & Tierney A. (1985) *Elements of Nursing*, 2nd edition. Edinburgh: Churchill Livingstone.

Roper N., Logan N. & Tierney A. (1990) *Elements of Nursing*, 3rd edition. Edinburgh: Churchill Livingstone.

Roy C. (1980) The Roy adaptation model. In Riehl J.P. & Roy C. (eds) *Conceptual Models for Nursing Practice*. New York: Appleton-Century-Crofts.

Schwirian P.M. (1998) *Professionalization of Nursing*, 3rd edition. Philadelphia and New York: Lippincott.

Selanders L.C. (2010) The power of environmental adaptation: Florence Nightingale's original theory for nursing practice. *Journal of Holistic Nursing*, **28**(1), 81–88.

Smith M.C. (2018) Disciplinary perspectives linked to middle range theory. In Smith M.J. & Liehr P.R. (eds) *Middle Range Theory for Nursing*, 4th edition. New York: Springer Publications.

Smith M.J. & Liehr P.R. (2018) *Middle Range Theory for Nursing*, 4th edition. New York: Springer Publications.

Watson J. (1979) *A Model of Caring: An Alternative Health Care Model for Nursing Practice and Research*. American Nurses Association.

CHAPTER 2

Knowing in Nursing and Nursing Knowledge

Outline of Content

At the conclusion of this chapter, readers will be able to define knowing and knowledge as they relate to nursing and how both are developed. They will be taken on a journey down the centuries, exploring how knowledge was understood and analysed by proponents of, what were termed, rationalism, empiricism and historicism. Within these philosophies of science, readers will be introduced to the influences of positivism, logical positivism, post-positivism, critical theory and constructivism. Their impact on nursing knowledge and nursing theory will be discussed. The four patterns of knowing in nursing as described by Carper will be highlighted, and we will show how these have been expanded upon since the 2014 edition of this book.

Learning Outcomes

At the end of this chapter, readers will be able to:

1. Define 'knowing' and 'knowledge' and why they are important for nursing

2. Understand three key stages in the philosophy of knowledge development

3. Discuss the differences between 'know how', 'know that' and 'know why' knowledge, giving updated examples from nursing practice

4. Analyse and give updates on Carper's (1978) 'ways of knowing' and Kerlinger's (1986) 'categories of knowledge' and give examples from and for practice

5. Identify existing and emerging strategies to develop nursing knowledge

Fundamentals of Nursing Models, Theories and Practice, Third Edition. Hugh P. McKenna, Majda Pajnkihar and Dominika Vrbnjak.
© 2025 John Wiley & Sons Ltd. Published 2025 by John Wiley & Sons Ltd.
Companion website: www.wiley.com/go/nursingmodels3e

Introduction

How theory was related to nursing practice was outlined in Chapter 1, as was the importance of recognising how knowledge contributes to theory development in nursing. In this chapter, the focus will be more concerned with knowing in nursing and the types of knowledge that nurses might use in clinical settings. First, we will share with you a short history of what is referred to as epistemology – the philosophy of knowledge. This will entail the following:

- exploring three stages of knowledge development that has had an influence on nursing – rationalism, empiricism and historicism;
- examining what different types of knowledge nurses might use in their practice and whether some are more valued than others;
- investigating the differences between 'know how', 'know that' and 'know why' knowledge and how each relates to nursing;
- analysing and giving updates on how Carper (1978) and Kerlinger (1986) described patterns and categories of knowing in nursing;
- exploring approaches that nurses might use to produce knowledge for their practice.

Definitions of Knowing and Knowledge

As with most of the concepts presented in this book, defining knowing and knowledge is not as straightforward as it may appear (see Key Concepts 2.1). Suffice to say that there are distinct differences between knowing and knowledge. According to Chinn et al. (2022: 3), 'knowing is a particular and unique awareness that ground and expresses the being and doing of a person'. We 'know' through our experiences, through reading, through listening, through thinking and a range of other ways. This implies that knowing is always changing. As we learn new things and are exposed to new experiences, our knowing develops. There is a more esoteric view of knowing from the Jewish *Talmud* (cited in McKenna et al. 2014):

> the child in the womb of his mother looks from one end of the world to the other and knows all the teaching, but the instant he comes in contact with the air of earth an angel strikes him on the mouth and he forgets everything.

This suggests that once we are born, we forget all the knowing that we had beforehand. But not all is forgotten; children are born with instincts such as blinking, sucking and retina dilatation. These could be termed instinctive knowing.

In contrast, 'knowledge refers to ideas that are expressed in a form that can be communicated with others in a spiepr DHYPlanguage that is taught and communicated in different forms' (Chinn et al. 2022: 3).

Key Concepts 2.1

Knowing: an awareness of the self, others and the world in ways that can be brought to some level of conscious awareness.

Knowledge: knowing that we can share or communicate with others.

This definition of knowledge implies that there may be knowledge that we will not share or cannot communicate to others, and so, this is not knowledge! Therefore, people know more than they will ever share as knowledge. If you were sworn to secrecy about something, what you learned contributed to your knowing but because you never share this knowing, by this definition, it is not knowledge.

However, if you share or communicate your knowing with others, this 'knowledge' becomes part of their store of knowing (see Reflective Exercise 2.1). Similarly, if people share knowledge with us, it becomes part of our store of knowing. In Chapter 1, you learned that we experience phenomena through our five senses: hearing, seeing, touching, smelling and tasting. Similarly, we know through these five senses.

Nursing knowledge is that which is of importance to our discipline. It forms the 'essence' of what nursing is. In nursing, we share knowledge in many different ways, such as through speaking, use of the written word and through our behaviour.

Reflective Exercise 2.1

Shared Knowledge

Think about a lecture or a conference that you attended. How was the knowledge shared with attendees or delegates?

Philosophies of Knowledge

There are three philosophical positions that help explain how knowing and knowledge have developed in the world:

- rationalism
- empiricism
- historicism

An overview of these is presented in Table 2.1.

Rationalism

Rationalism has its stem in *ratio,* the Latin word for 'reason'. Rationalism was seen as an advancement in knowledge development because before that, religion and God's word were the main sources of knowledge for most of humankind. Rationalists believed that knowledge developed through trying to understand why something happened and identifying the best possible reason for its occurrence.

TABLE 2.1   **Philosophies of knowledge.**

	Key concepts	Key writers and movements
Rationalism	Reason	René Descartes – 'I think, therefore I am' Cartesian dualism
Empiricism	Sensory experience	John Locke – *tabula rasa* (blank slate) Auguste Comte – Positivism The Vienna Circle – logical positivism Karl Popper – principle of falsification (post-positivist empiricism)
Historicism	Interpretative-constructionist	Thomas Kuhn – paradigm shifts The influence of phenomenology – Edmund Husserl and Martin Heidegger Critical science – the Frankfurt School (enlightenment, empowerment, emancipation) Postmodernism

Therefore, rationalism is founded on the idea that theorists, without access to data obtained through the senses, can generate theory through mental reasoning. In Chapter 1, readers were introduced to the term 'proposition'. Put simply, this is a relationship between two or more individual concepts. Rationalists formulate propositions through theorising how one concept could be related to others. For example, it is reasonable to believe that cruelty to animals is wrong. Here, there are two concepts, cruelty and animals, and they have been joined together in a relationship to form a proposition. Rationalists did not go out to survey people to find that cruelty to animals is wrong. Rather, they rationalise it. This 'arm-chair theorising' has been criticised, mainly because of the absence of hard data. Nonetheless, the absence of data has not stopped people taking such theories seriously. For example, Freud used rationalism to develop his theories of psychoanalysis; he had very little data to support his theories on the Oedipus complex, or the id, ego and superego (Freud 1949).

In essence, rationalists theorise without data and then experiments can be conducted in the real world to see if they were correct and if the theory can be corroborated (Fieser 2020). This is best described as the 'theory then research' approach (McKenna et al. 2014) because the theory comes before the research to test it. This is also called deductive or *a priori* reasoning. In terms of knowledge, it is seen as arising before experience or, perhaps more accurately, without the necessity of experience. In other words, it precedes experience or the need for it. Knowledge in this form is said to be independent of any need for supporting evidence. Even if a person was locked in solitary confinement with no access to any data, they could come up with (through reason) some theories about their surroundings or even some basic mathematics. There is evidence that Einstein used rationalism in his mathematical calculations, and it was many years before the technology existed to test some of his theories. It is one of the best-known examples of the development of such knowledge.

Einstein's general theory of relativity was formulated in 1916 but required the development of the global positioning system (GPS) in 1973 for its value to be realised. Similarly, lasers were invented in the 1960s, using ideas that Einstein had developed 40 years earlier. Laser inventors could not have foreseen that, in a further 60 years, lasers would have an impact in eye surgery and in DVD technology.

Charles Darwin (1809–1882) stated that of all the faculties of the human mind, reason stands at the summit (Barnhart & Barnhart 1976). His theory of evolution was proposed before there was reliable data to confirm it. His theory challenged divine beliefs on the development of humanity. In fact, because of his lack of data to support his theory, he was castigated by the church for suggesting that people evolved from monkeys. Copernicus (1473–1543) was also criticised by the church because he reasoned that the Sun, not the Earth, was the centre of the universe. Therefore, throughout history, the rationalist way of developing knowledge was often seen as a threat to the status quo. The accusations focused on how could rationalists possibly know these things in the absence of research data?

René Descartes

Rationalism as a formal approach to knowledge development can be traced to René Descartes (1596–1650), the 17th-century French philosopher and mathematician. He spent most of his adult life in Holland and influenced other famous rationalists such as Antoine Arnauld (1612–1694), Benedict de Spinoza (1632–1677) and Gottfried von Leibniz (1646–1716). Nine years before his death, Descartes published a book entitled *Meditations on First Philosophy* (1641). This was to influence the development of knowledge for the next 300 years. Perhaps the best word to signify his contribution to rationalism is the word 'doubt'. He realised that to arrive at new knowledge, you must put former opinions, experiences and data in doubt. When we do this, we can build knowledge from basic principles, without undue influence from other sources.

Descartes suggested that the senses can play tricks on us. For example, we may think something looks cold, but when we touch it, it is hot, or we may believe a creaking floorboard or a branch blowing against a window is an intruder in our home. Descartes considered sensory deceptions such as these and reflected that they could be the work of a malignant being, an evil demon whose role is to fool us by sending us false sensory information (Fieser 2020). Such misconceptions are often used to good effect in literature, theatre and films.

When Descartes reasoned that all his knowledge may be false through being fooled by the 'demon', he came to doubt all that he previously held to be true and to exist. He even began to doubt his own existence. However, he realised that there was one thing that the demon could not falsify. He reasoned that when he thinks, he must exist or else he would not be able to think. Such reasoning led him to what he maintained was the one certain piece of *true* knowledge '*Cogito, ergo sum*' (I think, therefore I am). Following this, he held that through reason alone, knowledge and certain universal self-evident truths could be discovered, from which the sciences could then be deductively derived.

Mind–Body Split

Descartes was a devout Roman Catholic and he reasoned that God created two classes of substance that make up the whole of human reality. One class comprised thinking substances, or 'minds', and the other comprised extended substances, or 'bodies'. He rationalised that these were separate entities. This mind–matter split, called 'Cartesian dualism', assumes that we are rational individuals with rational minds and that our minds are separated from our bodies (Chinn et al. 2022).

Rationalism as a philosophy of science was very influential and Descartes's mind–body split underpins much of the biomedical model referred to in Chapter 1. Physicians were often trained to look for anatomical signs and physiological symptoms and come up with a diagnosis, irrespective of the patients' psycho-social-spiritual makeup. Similarly, when nurses assess a patient objectively from a physical and pathological perspective, while ignoring their thoughts, emotions and feelings, they are practising Cartesian dualism. We still hear experienced nurses referring to a 'head injury', a 'coronary' or a 'stroke' being admitted! This is reminiscent of the birthday cake analogy in Chapter 1 – by seeing only the slice, they miss the whole cake and its meaning (see Reflective Exercise 2.2).

Reflective Exercise 2.2

Theory – Cartesian Dualism in Practice

Next time you are in clinical practice, listen to the nursing handover. Do the nurses focus mainly on physical or psychological aspects of the patient, or do they consider both? Do they take any account of social factors? Do they mention that the patient has a very stressful job or a large family or is unemployed or do they focus mainly on the patients' presenting illness?

Empiricism

In contrast to rationalists, empiricists need data and evidence. They believe that knowledge is derived entirely from sensory experience (Reed & Crawford Sherer 2018). In other words, if something cannot be perceived through a person's senses, it does not exist. Those who favour empiricism criticise rationalism and deny the possibility of spontaneous ideas or *a priori* reasoning as a way of developing knowledge. Rather, they formulate concepts and propositions that attempt to explain the phenomena that they have experienced through their senses (Chinn et al. 2022: p. 11). These propositions may be turned into hypotheses (a form of proposition), which can be tested through experimental research. A simple example is the concept of dark clouds and rain. A proposition is that there is a positive relationship between dark clouds and rain. A testable hypothesis is that the presence of dark clouds always leads to rain. This is a result of observation and can be tested empirically. The end result is knowledge in the form of theory. As the opposite to rationalism, empiricism can be described as the 'research then theory' approach (McKenna et al. 2014), because the theory comes after the research that tests it. This type of knowledge development can also be called inductive or *a posteriori* reasoning (see Key Concepts 2.2).

Key Concepts 2.2

A priori **knowledge:** knowledge that arises before experience or, more accurately, without the need for experience seen in rationalism.

A posteriori **knowledge:** where knowledge emerges from experience. In this instance, it is termed *a posteriori* to denote that it is derived from empirical experience, which in all instances precedes it and is its source.

John Locke and Empiricism

The origin of empiricism can be traced to a number of English philosophers such as John Locke (1632–1704) and David Hume (1711–1776). Locke spent 20 years writing his *Essay Concerning Human Understanding*, postulating on how the mind collects, organises and makes judgements based on all the data that come to us through our senses, mainly seeing, hearing and touch, but also smell and taste. He had read Descartes but had rejected the rationalist philosophy as not being able to explain human understanding.

For Locke, there can be no instinctive knowledge: rather, everything we know must be gained from what we experience. He saw knowledge coming to us from the outside world impacting on our minds through our senses (Gordon-Roth & Weinberg 2021). Like the extract from the *Talmnd* outlined above, he viewed the mind at birth to be a blank slate, what he referred to as *tabula rasa* (Stokes 2015). As children develop, this slate is written on by their experiences.

Primary and Secondary Qualities

Hanck (2021) explored Locke's perceptions of primary and secondary qualities. Primary qualities are objective and include shape, solidity, number and motion. In contrast, secondary qualities are more subjective and include colour, smell and taste. The reason why they are termed secondary is that they are produced in our minds by the effect of primary qualities on our senses. To Locke, primary qualities really exist in the world and these influence the secondary qualities that exist in our minds. For example, the primary qualities of a cancerous tumour can be observed and its size, shape and position in the body measured. Less important for Locke would be the secondary qualities such as pain, fear and distress that the tumour produces in the patient's mind or that of the patient's family. Put very simplistically, from an empiricist perspective, cancer biologists may mainly be concerned with the size, position and type of cancerous growth, whereas nurses may mainly be concerned with the secondary qualities – the effect the growth was having on the patient and family. Neither may be right, but it could be suggested that biomedical scientists are educated to mainly prioritise the primary qualities, whereas nurses are educated to focus on the secondary qualities.

Auguste Comte and Positivism

Almost a century after Locke's death, the French philosopher Auguste Comte (1798–1857) gave empiricism a new twist. Comte is best remembered for being a student activist and an anti-Establishment figure, and he saw science as a means of changing and possibly overthrowing political institutions. One of his many claims to fame was that he founded the discipline of sociology as a means of applying the methods of science to the study of people and society.

In his six-volume publication, *Course of Positive Philosophy* (1830–1842), Comte criticised what he called negative philosophy, which he associated with woolly and abstract thinking. He favoured positive philosophy which used robust scientific methods to solve human problems and improve social conditions. From this, the word 'positivist' emerged. To Comte, scientists needed to classify or categorise confirmable observations in a rigorous manner, and this alone should be the basis for human knowledge and understanding (see Reflective Exercise 2.3).

In essence, positivism involves the following logic: our minds interpret the world through our senses, and because the world is subject to the laws of science, events outside the mind can be observed, described, explained and predicted. Therefore, to make sense of the outside world, all we have to do is to observe it and undertake experiments to test hypotheses that are formulated from such observations.

Reflective Exercise 2.3

Exploring Knowledge

To recap what we have covered so far in this chapter: knowledge is knowing that can be shared with others, and it comes from different sources such as rational thinking (reasoning) and sensory experiences (empirics).

In nursing practice, nurses develop knowledge by using reason or by what they experience while caring for patients. See if you can provide examples of each? Remember rationalist understanding comes without the help of experience and empiricist knowledge comes through what you encounter by seeing, hearing or touching.

Comte identified a hierarchy of six sciences which he argued were founded on systematic observation:

- astronomy
- biology
- chemistry
- mathematics
- physics
- sociology

These formed the 'gold standard' against which other disciplines could be judged. Readers will note that nursing is not included in this list. Comte would have perceived it as subjective and not worthy enough to be perceived as a meaningful approach to knowledge development. Therefore, reasoning, reflection and intuition as the sole basis for attaining knowledge were shunned and denigrated by positivists.

Throughout his life, Comte had been plagued by mental health problems and he had even attempted suicide on occasions. In his later years, his mental illness returned and with it a softening of his views regarding positivism. For instance, in some of his last writings, such as *The Catechism of Positive Religion*, he stated that the intellect should be the servant of the heart! Quite a turnaround, I think readers will agree.

However, it is for his earlier work on positivism that Comte will be best remembered (Lenzer 2017). Some scientists still argue that it was the only true source of knowledge. For positivists, objective truth exists, and the goal of science is to go out and discover it; to them, this forms our knowing and our knowledge base.

'The Vienna Circle'

At the turn of the 20th century in Austria, a group of scholars, mainly physicists, mathematicians and philosophers, including Moritz Schlick (1882–1936) and Ludwig Wittgenstein (1889–1951), formed an organisation called 'The Vienna Circle'. The members were very eccentric, and there were countless disagreements among them. Two of its members ended their lives through suicide and Schlick, the leader, was murdered (The Economist 2018). Nonetheless, during its existence, its fortnightly meetings were highly productive. It built on Comte's ideas and coined the term 'logical positivism', placing an even stronger emphasis on the importance of empirical research, induction and scientific verification.

For most of the first half of the 20th century, 'respected' scientists and scholars adopted the logical positivist view of science. For instance, Bertrand Russell was very supportive of the Vienna Circle's work. However, the philosophical force behind logical positivism weakened just prior to the Second World War when many of its members, who were Jewish, left Nazi Germany and Austria. Today, in the first third decade of the 21st century, it is seen as a spent force in scientific enquiry.

Popper: Principle of Falsification

One of the best-known members of the Vienna Circle was Sir Karl Popper, an Austrian, who was initially influenced by Descartes's rationalism. Popper argued that the way to true knowledge was by conjecture (developing theory through reason) and refutation (testing the theory through rigorous research to see if it could be proved as false). To him, the mark of a scientific theory is whether it makes predictions that can be falsified through testing (Popper 1989). Wisely, he also said that whenever a theory appears to you as the only possible one, take this as a sign that you have neither understood the theory nor the problem that it was intended to solve. This is an important lesson for nurses as they are often faced with a bewildering array of nursing theories.

Popper began to replace the Vienna Circle's emphasis on verification with his emphasis on falsification. In other words, theories should not be tested to see if they can be supported; rather, they should be tested to see if they can be proved wrong. If you test a theory nineteen times and it holds true, it may not hold true on the twentieth occasion. In Popper's view, we can learn much more from the twentieth test than from the previous nineteen. The example of the paper boat was used in Chapter 1. The same principle can be explained another way: let's say you were to construct a kite and test it to see if it will fly. It may fly perfectly the first 20 times you try it, but then on the next few attempts, it crashes to the ground. To Popper this falsification of the kite's reliability would be an important lesson and the creators would have to go back to the drawing board to come up with a better design of the kite (see Key Concepts 2.3).

Key Concepts 2.3

Popper's (1989) principle of falsification: theories should not be tested to see if they can be supported; rather, they should be tested to see if they can be falsified.

Like Comte, Popper also mellowed with age. He became critical of positivism and began to question the logical positivists' desire to reject subjectivity as a way of knowing (Reed & Crawford Sherer 2018). In what would seem to be a 'road to Damascus' change, Popper admitted that there was a place for intuition and imagination when scientific empiricism is being employed!

Post-positivist Empiricism

Today, thanks to philosophers like Karl Popper, logical positivism has been replaced in some quarters by post-positivist empiricism, a much milder form of positivism. Gortner (1993) was one of the few nurses to support the use of this form of empiricism in the development of nursing science. But she felt it was unfortunate that it is still being tarnished in the literature by being confused with logical positivism. In 1993, when referring to nursing theories, Gortner argued that Roy's (2003) Adaptation Theory 'in nursing reflects clearly the thinking of an empiricist scholar' (Gortner 1993: 481). The same can be said of the nursing theories of Henderson (1991), Neuman (1995) and Orem (1995).

Modern empiricists accept the shortcomings of verification and accept that the world is complex, and some behaviours and events can be reduced to their basics for study purposes and some cannot (Reed & Crawford Sherer 2018: 23). Nonetheless, in the 21st century, empiricism is still highly regarded as a research approach in the physical sciences of biology, physics and chemistry. In nursing too, we can agree that all of the thousands of experiments and quasi-experiments conducted by nurses are clearly based upon empiricism. We see the influence of empiricism again now in the evidence-based practice movement with its emphasis on the 'gold standard' of the randomised controlled trial (see Reflective Exercise 2.4).

Reflective Exercise 2.4

Nursing and Empiricism

Undertake a literature review for clinical nursing guidelines in your field of practice. See what research approaches were used to underpin the guideline. Was it a 'subjective qualitative' research design such as grounded theory or a phenomenological study? Alternatively, was it an 'objective quantitative' research design such as a randomised controlled trial?

Historicism

Each of us as human beings has our own experiences, memories and history, and they differ from those of other human beings. Therefore, we are unique and that means our knowing and knowledge are also unique. This is the basis for the philosophical position called historicism. Up until this point, we have dealt with knowledge that is objective and, for empiricists, can be perceived through the senses and can be measured.

The Italian astronomer Galileo Galilei (1564–1642) maintained that we should 'measure what is measurable, count what is countable, and what is not countable, make countable'. However, there are many phenomena of interest to nurses that cannot be measured. How would you calibrate compassion, measure empathy or quantify a presence? True rationalist or empirical principles could not be applied to these phenomena. For nursing, everything that can be counted does not necessarily count and everything that counts cannot necessarily be counted.

Historicism recognises that we are all influenced by our different history and different experiences, attitudes, values and beliefs. From these influences, we construct our own realities and we interpret events from this construction. Therefore, another term for this view is the interpretative-constructionist approach. In other words, we interpret what is real and construct this as our knowledge. Friedrich Nietzsche (1844–1900) famously stated that there are no facts – only interpretation.

According to Reed and Crawford Sherer (2018: 24), constructionists reject the view that there is objective truth and reality to be discovered. Rather, knowledge is constructed through social interactions among individuals and between people and their environment. Constructionists believe and assert that knowledge is a product of social interchanges and shared meaning. Therefore, cultural, social and historical factors are central to the development of knowledge. This knowledge is built through consensus with others, not through verification (see Reflective Exercise 2.5).

Reflective Exercise 2.5

Nursing and Historicism

Consider the following example. Two nurses observe an elderly patient getting out of bed, but they interpret it differently. One may believe that the patient is dependent and in danger of falling and should not be attempting to walk. The other may perceive the patient to be gaining independence and is therefore pleased that they are getting out of bed. They see the same thing but construct a different reality.

What would be your interpretation?

These nurses observe the same clinical phenomenon, yet past experience, reflection and intuition lead them to understand and interpret it differently. Furthermore, each may be attracted to a theory that describes and explains what they perceive. One might be attracted to Orem's self-care theory, whereas the other may be an advocate of the medical model, where the patient adopts a 'sick role'. Such theoretical influences affect how we make sense of the world around us. So, for different people, reality (and knowledge of that reality) is often a personal thing, the product of individual reflection, perception, perspective and purpose rather than being static and objective. Realising this, philosophers such as Toulmin (1972), Feyerabend (1977) and Kuhn (1977) challenged the positivist view and stressed the importance of history and perception in the development of knowledge. They rejected the idea of there being objective truths, arguing instead that the development of knowledge is a dynamic process and so there are no final and permanent truths.

Kuhn and Scientific Revolutions

Prior to Thomas Kuhn's seminal book, *The Structure of Scientific Revolutions* (1977), many scientists, particularly from the empiricist/positivist traditions, believed that different research studies built upon one another in a progression of the science, leading eventually to ultimate truth. For instance, Sir Isaac Newton said that 'If I have seen further, it is by standing on the shoulders of giants.' Here, Newton was stating that his work was built on the previous work of others.

In contrast, Kuhn (1922–1996) asserted that science progressed through a series of revolutionary steps. After each revolution, there is a period of 'normal science' where a particular paradigm (remember, we called this a 'world view' in Chapter 1) reigns supreme and scholars accept it as the agreed basis for knowledge and truth. Rejecting this paradigm during a period of normal science would be frowned upon by the scientific community. However, according to Kuhn, this paradigm is eventually questioned, leading to what he refers to as a 'scientific revolution'. This may be because that world view fails to deal adequately with some new phenomenon, or a new, more powerful paradigm has great explanatory power. As more evidence accumulates to show that the old way of thinking has outlived its usefulness, a 'paradigm shift' occurs. Contradicting Newton's giants analogy, Kuhn maintained that paradigm shifts are not built one upon another but are a completely new way of looking at or explaining reality. The new paradigm then becomes the focus for a new period of normal science, until the next revolution.

One example of this would be Ptolemy's (100–c. 170 CE) teaching that the Sun orbited the Earth. This paradigm held sway for centuries in what Kuhn would call 'normal science'. However, when Copernicus (1473–1543) challenged this with his theory that the Earth moved around the Sun, a paradigm shift took place. Galileo (1564–1642) proved this with his new invention (the telescope). Other examples include Newton's theory of gravity being replaced by Einstein's theory of relativity or the contemporary focus on community care as opposed to institutional care for those with mental health problems. Another paradigm shift was changing from a widely held view that the world was flat to accepting that it was round. Paradigm shifts occurred because the old paradigms were not able to explain new experiences or solve new problems. Kuhn's views did much to undermine the empirical/positivist view of science.

Such paradigm shifts are not always popular because they threaten the previous belief system, with which many people had invested. Galileo used his telescope to prove to leaders in the Roman Catholic church that the Earth went around the sun and not the previous 'normal science' that the sun went around the Earth. For this challenge to existing knowing and knowledge, he was imprisoned.

Laudan and Scientific Evolution

Laudan (1977) challenged Kuhn's view that knowledge development was a revolutionary process. Rather, like Newton, he believed that knowledge was developed in an evolutionary way with new knowing being influenced by and building upon previous knowing. This *evolutionary* approach of Laudan is an attractive one for nurses because it recognises a pluralistic view of knowledge development and application. After all, the problems facing nursing are forever changing and nurses must select the theory that is best suited to solving these problems.

Meleis and Scientific Convolution

Meleis (2017), the US-based Egyptian nurse metatheorist, famous for her development of the Transitions Theory of Nursing, had a different view. She argued that the revolutionary and evolutionary approaches to knowledge development are too simplistic on their own to explain nursing's experience of knowledge development. She coined the term 'convolution' to explain how nursing knowledge has developed. She maintained that nursing as a discipline has progressed not through evolution or revolution but through a convolution-ary series of peaks, troughs, detours, backward steps and crises. This gives the impression that knowledge development in nursing is confusing and uncoordinated. There may be some truth in this as nursing is still a young scientific discipline, one that Kuhn (1977) might place in a pre-paradigmatic stage of development.

The Influence of Phenomenology

A phenomenon is something, a fact, an event that is observed to occur or to exist. In their everyday work, clinical nurses observe numerous phenomena that they often have to make sense of. So, phenomenology is the study of the meaning of phenomena to a particular individual and a way of understanding people from the way things appear to them. Edmund Husserl (1859–1938) was a German philosopher and the founder of phenomenology. In contrast to the empiricists and positivists, he believed that science involved the exploration of perceptions, judgements, beliefs and other mental processes. He argued that, because of its refusal to accept anything other than observable facts and objective reality, positivism was not capable of dealing with human experience. He maintained that a better path to truth was to consider the 'essence' of things, and the best way of doing this was to interpret situations by exploring what meaning the mind has for those things (Husserl 1962 trans).

Therefore, the job of 'phenomenology' is to discover what 'lived experiences' are like for people (Neubauer et al. 2019). Understanding their 'lived experience' requires the use of reflection, which is the basis of phenomenology. While Descartes was sceptical about the external world (as discussed earlier), Husserl was sceptical about self-knowledge. Therefore, he recommended that phenomenologists should 'bracket existence'. This means that when they are exploring the essence of an occurrence or some phenomenon, they should suspend previous views and influences about it, as these would merely distort their true perception of it (see Key Concepts 2.4). In other words, when you come to investigate a phenomenon such as patient pain, you put to the back of your mind (bracket) everything you previously knew about patients' pain, as if you were noticing this for the first time. This is not unlike John Locke's 'tabula rasa' we described above. For a good example of nurses using Husserl's phenomenological approach, see Žiaková et al. (2020).

Key Concepts 2.4

Metatheorist: a person who studies and writes about theories. The best-known metatheorists in nursing are Afaf Meleis and Jacqueline Fawcett.

Metatheory: a theory of theories.

Heidegger and Hermeneutic Phenomenology

Another German philosopher, Martin Heidegger (1889–1976), maintained that as a way of generating knowledge, phenomenology should make evident what is hidden in everyday taken-for-granted experience. Hermeneutics, a branch of phenomenology much influenced by Heidegger, is based upon the idea that all texts and human activities are filled with meaning and can be subject to rigorous interpretations. This has its origins in the interpretation of religious texts, such as the Bible. Heidegger believed this approach could be applied to the interpretation of human behaviours. Therefore, within hermeneutics, to know is to understand through interpretation. In Heidegger's philosophical view, the understanding of phenomena is not about measuring, analysing, categorising or classifying. He famously defined phenomenology as letting 'that which shows itself be seen from itself in the very way in which it shows itself from itself' (Heidegger 1962: 58). So, to phenomenologists, science and knowledge generation is about taking account of meaning and perception rather than the detached objective measurement favoured by empiricists. However, it must have credibility and be no less rigorous or systematic. A good example of Heideggerian phenomenology is a study by Saletti-Cuesta et al. (2017).

Canadian philosopher van Manen (2017) took Heideggerian phenomenology a stage further, and his method has been used as a research approach by many nurses. An example of such a study can be found in the work of Errasti-Ibarrondo et al. (2018). We will return to van Manen's work later.

Phenomenology and Nursing

An example of phenomenology in nursing is Patricia Benner's (1984) work *From Novice to Expert: Excellence and Power in Clinical Nursing Practice*. In this landmark publication, Benner used a phenomenological approach to analyse experienced nurses' accounts of their practice; in other words, their lived experience. Benner then applied a 'model of skill acquisition', which proposed that in the acquisition and development of skills, students pass through five levels of competency: novice, advanced beginner, competent, proficient and expert. Novices and beginners need rules, but experts have a huge range of experience to draw on and no longer need rules. They have an 'intuitive grasp' of the situation and can immediately identify and concentrate on the important aspects (see Reflective Exercise 2.6). This could be one reason why novices like nursing models and theories whereas expert nurses have more difficulty accepting and adopting them, probably because they have their own personal models and theories based upon their experiences (McKenna et al. 2014).

Reflective Exercise 2.6

From Novice to Expert

Can Benner's ideas apply to you? Read Benner's five levels of competency and then assess yourself at the beginning of a clinical placement/practicum and at the end. Where do you think you start from? Are you a novice, advanced beginner, competent, proficient or expert? Did you think you progressed over the placement from one level to another? Do you recognise these levels in others. For instance, can you see that beginning student nurses are novices and advanced nurse practitioners are experts. What observations led to your judgement?

What would happen if you moved an expert nurse in the care of older people into an emergency department setting? Would they revert to being a novice again? Explain your answer.

Critical Theory

We referred earlier to the Vienna Circle, which was a group that believed staunchly in logical positivism. Contemporaneously, a rival group existed called the Frankfurt School, which was located at the University of Frankfurt am Main in Germany. It was established by Max Horkheimer, who became its director in 1930. The Frankfurt School gathered dissident Marxists and was very much anti-positivist in its teachings. They saw positivism as an inappropriate way of viewing knowledge development in the social sciences. Rather they favoured the critical theory approach (Chinn et al. 2022: 69).

Critical theory is a variant of phenomenology but goes further, stressing that meanings should not merely be elicited and interpreted but should be open to criticism (Habermas 1971). It is a very political philosophy.

There are three major concepts within critical theory:

- *Enlightenment:* knowledge of self in relation to the world and education of the oppressed in terms of their potential capacity to bring about change.

- *Empowerment:* social transformation through some form of educative process.
- *Emancipation:* a state of reflective clarity where people have a sense of themselves and can determine freely and collectively the directions they should take in life.

Therefore, its goal is to emancipate people from domination and oppression, and it goes further than just interpretation (Reed & Crawford Sherer 2018). Its focus on education, enlightenment, emancipation, empowerment, critique and change is an attractive perspective to many nurses who wish to leave behind subservience to the male-dominated medical model. Its popularity is reflected by the increase in the number of feminist and action research studies in nursing in recent years and, as such, may be perceived as a science of freedom. For an example of action research in nursing, see Okaisu et al. (2014).

Postmodernism

Postmodernism emerged in the later decades of the 20th century primarily as a reaction against the unrealistic assertions of positivism and the perceived empty promises of 'modernism' (Lyotard 1984). The central force within postmodernism was essentially scepticism – that is, the critical questioning of the knowledge presented by science, particularly the claims (where these existed) for discovering or establishing irrefutable absolute truth. A form of this was witnessed during the COVID-19 pandemic where scientific knowledge was challenged and questioned by society. This was not helped by some scientists recommending lockdown and isolating while others (e.g. in Sweden) were recommending 'herd immunity'. Confidence in objective scientific knowledge was shaken and challenged (McKenna 2021). This illustrated that knowledge is relative rather than absolute, to a greater or lesser extent context-bound or culture-specific, and often subject to multiple meanings (Chinn et al. 2022: 264). In relation to its central focus – the questioning of science's absolute and exclusive claim to 'truth' – the postmodern orientation served a useful purpose. But it also carried within its orientation some fatal shortcomings:

1. Its extreme and uncompromising rejection of all constructed knowledge. This, some might argue, was a totally preposterous position: to be sceptical of *all* knowledge to the extent of *rejecting* it would leave us in the extreme position of believing nothing and therefore (presumably) having no rational (knowledge) position upon which to base our actions. By querying all knowledge claims, even its own position on 'knowledge', and offering no constructive alternative way forward, postmodernism itself had nowhere to go, no way forward. It brought the world greater scepticism but no answers and no alternatives.

2. It is of course the case that even today critics of science speak of its excessive positivistic shortcomings. Indeed, this is not uncommon in nursing where the tendency to lean too much upon the natural or traditional sciences is criticised and labelled 'positivism'. As we discussed earlier, positivism as a movement had all but disappeared by the end of the 20th century, and the post-positivistic position was already taking a more balanced and reasonable position in respect of recognising the limits of science and the need to view knowledge claims in a sceptical and critical way. Indeed, it might be argued that, unlike postmodernism, post-positivism contained within it a balancing critique *and* a viable way forward (Reed & Crawford Sherer 2018).

In this section of the chapter, we have looked at three main philosophies of knowledge: rationalism, empiricism and historicism. All of these have influenced how knowledge is viewed by nurses and nursing. For example, early nurse theorists such as Neuman (1995), Orem (1995) and Roy (2003) were influenced by empiricism when they were developing their theories. Later nurse theorists, such as Watson (2005), were influenced by postmodernism. Rogers (1980) and Parse (1987) were heavily influenced by historicism. In the next section, we will look at types of knowledge and knowing with a specific focus on how nurses know.

How Do Nurses Know?

At the beginning of this chapter, we outlined the differences between knowledge and knowing. In this section, we will examine different types of knowing that are thought to be important in nursing; these are summarised in Table 2.2. We will look at two key authors – Carper (1978) and Kerlinger (1986) – both of whom discussed types of knowing; we will

TABLE 2.2   Types of knowledge.

1. **'Know that' – propositional knowledge; 'Know how' – practical knowledge;** 'Know why' – comprehendible knowledge	
2. Ways of knowing (Carper 1978)	Empirics Aesthetics Ethics Personal knowing
3. Categories of knowledge (Kerlinger 1986)	Empirical Tenacity Authority A priorism

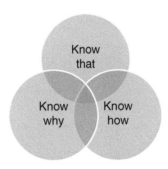

FIGURE 2.1   Venn diagram of interlapping 'Know that', 'know how' and 'know why' knowledge.

highlight how subsequent authors have contributed to their development. However, to set the scene, we will begin by differentiating between 'know that', 'know how' and 'know why' knowledge (Figure 2.1).

'Know That' or Propositional Knowledge

'Know that' knowledge is also called propositional knowledge as it is based upon reasoning and intentional thought processes. Above, we showed how a proposition is a relationship between two or more concepts. A *proposition* is an *idea* rather than a *thing* (an object that exists in the real world) or an *action* (some practical deed). More specifically, a proposition assumes the existence of the relationship between two or more concepts. But the assumption is still uncertain. That is, it is open to question until the relationship is adequately demonstrated. This is very different from 'know how' practical knowledge, which is not an idea being assumed but is demonstrated in action – we know how to *do* something by taking action or we do not.

'Know that' knowledge can be seen as emerging in two quite different ways, *a priori* and *a posteriori*, which we alluded to earlier in this chapter:

- *A priori* knowledge is knowledge that arises before experience or, more accurately, without the need for experience; think of Descartes's rationalism.
- *A posteriori* knowledge is where knowledge emerges *from* experience, and we make deductions arising from this. Knowledge in this form is what people usually mean when they speak of *scientific* knowledge – knowledge based on evidence that is derived through research. Think of Hume's empiricism (see above).

Therefore, when we think of 'know that' knowledge, we think of scientific knowledge that comes from empirical research.

'Know How' or Practical Knowledge

The process of attaining *practical* knowledge is perhaps more difficult to explain than *propositional* knowledge. Practical (unlike propositional) knowledge is largely to do with skills acquisition. It is, as we have noted, recognised as being fundamentally different from 'know that' knowledge. It is to do with manual skill and the associated psychomotor dexterity but also extends into something that is more cognitive and indicates skill and dexterity about what to do in particular circumstances, i.e. a form of practical wisdom. In nursing, it is often referred to as the craft or art of our profession (McKenna et al. 2014).

Such practical knowledge is not easily defined or *described* in rational language (language that is expressed in terms of logical reasoning, such as $2 + 2 = 4$). This is because it is *expressed* in the doing rather than the describing. Sometimes, such know how is termed *tacit knowledge* because it is more easily understood as something that resides in the individual, so that the term *personal knowing* is also used (Polanyi 1967). In essence, it is unspoken and indeed cannot be spoken of, except implicitly. It shows itself, quite literally, in the doing of an action.

In this form of knowledge, people can practise an activity until – no matter how complex – it becomes easier to do at increasingly higher levels of competence. We recognise a smoother and more refined performance of the skills. They become 'second nature', so that the person can perform them without having to think of what is being done in a rational fashion at all. Indeed, the person performing the skill *seems* to be doing it almost unconsciously and, to an extent, this is so. Benner (1984) described this level of skill expertise at the expert end of her continuum. However, it is important to recognise that what is happening here *is* a performance.

An example of this is seen with experienced airline pilots. They are skilled to fly the plane almost by touch and feel. They can be confronted by a wall of clocks and dials, yet they see the whole rather than individual instruments. This is sometimes referred to as the 'Gestalt'. To a trainee pilot, the complexity facing them in the cockpit is overwhelming, but for the experienced pilot, it forms a picture in which (almost without thinking) they can detect the most minor change that would need their attention.

It may seem that such acts are unconscious or habitual things, but that belies what is really going on. Complex patterns and subtle changes are being sensed, and refinements and adjustments are constantly being made without these being thought about in a logical step-by-step fashion. Indeed, to do this would immediately break the rhythm, interrupt the smooth performance and cause the expression of the 'skill' to deteriorate or even collapse. We might indeed argue that this is all habitual and that the person is doing it unconsciously.

There used to be a TV game show where members of the audience had to repeat against the clock a task undertaken by an expert. This could be spinning pizza dough above their head or dancing a tango or speed shuffling a deck of cards. Invariably, the unskilled audience members messed up. Like the expert airline pilots, the professionals were proficient through years of experience and could conduct the task with poise and style, almost without thinking.

Just because we realise that 'know that' knowledge is different from 'know how' knowledge, and that we cannot have propositions that directly guide know how, does not mean we cannot reflect upon its nature (see Reflective Exercise 2.7). We can indeed do this, and having a theory *about* know how is different from having a theory *of* know that (in the sense of a theory that actually guides it).

Reflective Exercise 2.7

'Know How' and 'Know That'

The notion of know how was introduced by the British philosopher Gilbert Ryle. His original publication (Ryle 1949) was the first modern statement to suggest that know how is different from know that and is a sophisticated form of knowing in its own right. The idea of know how is extremely important in nursing.

For this exercise, read further around the topic. You should not need to buy or read Ryle's original work as the internet is replete with descriptions of his original arguments. Spend some time exploring these and then proceed to write (up to a single A4 page maximum) a case for the importance of Ryle's concepts to nursing.

Knowing More Than We Can Tell

This knowing is also an awareness and indeed a highly honed and sensitive awareness within which the performers know the next step without knowing *how* they know this. The famous expression of Polanyi (1967) that 'we can know more than we can tell' is clearly at play here. It is also because the language of description is the language of 'know that' knowledge, theory and rational thinking; it is not suited to uncovering what is going on in a know how situation. Terms such as personal knowing, tacit awareness and intuitive responding are, in fact, almost alien to scientific language.

Practical Knowledge as Performance

Practical knowledge is a performance art or an expressive art form or skill, in that it exists exclusively within the act of doing. As may be clear from the preceding discussions, it is difficult to express in words and, when we try to do so, it is already in the past. In a sense, like a *Will o the Wisp*, it is already gone and beyond our grasp.

It is often the case that such *know how* knowledge is less valued than *know that* knowledge. Students often look with astonishment at experienced nurses who are performing a highly skilled task. The aesthetically pleasing art of what they are doing – almost without thinking – is perceived by the student to be *extraordinary* and they think they will never be as skilled. However, the expert nurse probably thinks it is *ordinary*, and one day, when qualified and experienced, the student too will perceive it as ordinary.

Similarly, an experienced nurse may be seen sitting and talking to a patient. To the untrained managerial eye, she is simply conversing, and should be working! However, the nurse may be assessing the patient, consoling them or preparing them for a procedure. The nurse is practising 'know how' knowledge, yet this may not be valued by their manager as much as 'know that' knowledge.

However, the suggestion that at least some aspects of practice are beyond our cognitive grasp (in terms of rational explanations) is rather amazing for nursing. We are accepting that a substantial amount of what nurses do is beyond our capacity to describe in rational or propositional terms. Furthermore, because it can only be expressed in the doing, it is also to some extent beyond the capacity of evidence-based healthcare. If the arguments presented here hold, there are important aspects of practice that are not amenable to evidence as they cannot be addressed in evidential (know that) terms at all. They may be referred to as 'practice-based evidence' rather than 'evidence-based practice'!

Practical Knowledge as Sophisticated Knowledge

While the examples used earlier are from fields such as aviation, the principles underlying such forms of knowing are similar in all practice knowing situations. This may seem a rather exotic claim to be making in respect of nursing. However, some of the skills involved in nursing require just as much in terms of dexterity and coordination of mind and body as does an activity such as juggling. And in nursing, we also find that our practice is every bit as creative and also involves the need to respond appropriately to often instantaneous and unplanned changes in patients' circumstances (see Reflective Exercise 2.8).

Reflective Exercise 2.8

Tacit Knowing

Picture the following scenario. During a clinical handover, a senior clinical nurse asks that you give particular attention to Mr Smith in Bay 3. When you ask why, she is unsure and cannot really explain why but asks you to do so nonetheless. He was admitted for observation because he was breathless, but the diagnostic tests did not show any abnormalities. The ward round is over, and one hour later, Mr Smith suffers a cardiac arrest. Thankfully, he survives. When you ask the staff nurse later how she knew there was something wrong, she is unable to tell you.

In your nursing career, you will see many examples of such tacit knowing, some that you yourself will undertake.

Join a small group of your fellow students or friends and try to explain what is going on here. You may wish to refer to Polanyi's (1967) work on tacit knowledge.

Gnostic and Pathic Touch

In an interesting paper, Max van Manen (2017), a phenomenologist and Dutch-born Canadian, differentiated between what he terms *gnostic* and *pathic* touch. In gnostic touch, the clinician is touching, feeling (palpating) to obtain knowledge. In this sense, they are not touching the other person in a personal or relational sense. The clinician is in an almost mechanical sense trying to feel through in order to gain knowledge (is there a swelling, a growth, and are the anatomical structures normally aligned?). They are feeling through the person's *body*. Therefore, we have the term 'diagnosis' (from the Greek terms *dia*, meaning distinguishing, looking through, to discern + *gnosis* meaning to know, knowledge). In contrast, *pathic* touch is a touching of or reaching out to the person. From its Greek origins of *pathos*, meaning suffering or hurt, we find that *pathic* touch reaches out to comfort or relieve pain. (See Reflective Exercise 2.9.)

There is a great deal of skill involved in both these touches. The diagnostic touch is only acquired through extensive anatomical and pathological study, experience and practice. There comes a time when the expert nurse's diagnostic powers (certainly in respect of the diagnostic touch or palpation) appear almost magical. They are every bit as astounding and awe-inspiring as a pilot landing a multimillion dollar jet in stormy weather.

This is also the case with pathic touch, which involves a reaching out, not to the physical body but to the person, in a healing way. This may involve highly developed skills of massage or manipulation, but sometimes, no less effective is the touch that conveys the way in which the nurse is simply present, being there *for* the person, reaching out to their loneliness and distress. We speak here of knowing when to reach out, whether to do so in silence or with voice as well as touch, the knowing how to listen, the knowing what to say or not, in each given moment. Furthermore, gnostic touch gathers clinical data in a one-way process.

Rogers (1980) was a well-known American nurse theorist. Her theory is not widely used, but it does stimulate nurses to think differently. Readers will know that we as human beings are three-dimensional – we have height, depth and width. Rogers (1980) believed that we had a fourth dimension, one that was like a sixth sense or an energy field. Therefore, according to Rogers, you can touch a person without actually touching them – their surrounding energy field means that you can move your hands over them without making contact and still pick up signs and symptoms of distress or lack of wellness. Aranha (2018) gave an example of Rogers's theory being applied in the nursing care of stroke patients.

Reflective Exercise 2.9

From Pathic to Sympathetic

Words commonly used in clinical practice (and indeed in other areas concerning human relations) are the terms *empathy* and *sympathy*. As you will see, these are derived from the Greek term *pathos*. You may recall that this term connotes feelings or emotions, often extended to include picking up hints that denote lack of well-being.

Conduct a Google search of sympathy and empathy. Consider how each may contribute to different nurse caring situations. Identify what you feel are examples of sympathy and empathy being acted out in your world. If you were a patient, how would you tell whether a nurse was being empathetic or sympathetic? To what extent are these examples accompanied by pathic touch?

In both the gnostic and pathic touch, there are tacit dimensions of knowing in the form discussed earlier. However, there is also a recognised need to integrate this with 'know that' knowledge. The diagnostic clinician is using a highly developed skill of palpation, but he or she must relate this to scientific knowledge of the anatomy, physiology and pathological processes of disease. Similarly, behind pathic touch, and the practical knowing of how and when to use this, there is a high level of knowledge derived from the psychological and social sciences and from the humanities (McCann & McKenna 1993).

'Know Why' or Comprehendible Knowledge

There is another dimension that is seldom explored and that is 'know why' knowledge, which could be called comprehendible knowledge. This goes a stage further than 'know how' and 'know that' knowledge. For example, a nurse may 'know how' to position a patient who has chronic obstructive airways disease so that they are more comfortable.

The nurse may also 'know that' research indicates that this is the best way to nurse such patients. But there is another dimension to this scenario; the nurse may 'know why' this is the case. They know that if such patients are nursed flat, their abdominal organs will press on their diaphragm and this will increase pressure on their lungs and cause greater difficulty with breathing. Globally, we are seeing more non-registered practitioners working in clinical settings. They are called support workers, nursing assistants or healthcare assistants. They often get a very practical training and so it is possible that when providing patient care, many have 'know how' knowledge, fewer have 'know that' knowledge and fewer still have 'know why' knowledge. The implications of this for patient safety are obvious (McKenna 2004) (See Reflective Exercise 2.10.).

Reflective Exercise 2.10

Different Ways of Knowing

- Practical knowledge is *know how*, contained in the doing, tacit, intuitive, personal, complex and performative.
- Propositional/theoretical knowledge is *know that*, descriptive, explanatory, predictive, prescriptive, contemplative, rational and justified.

These are some of the differences suggested between these two forms of knowing. Make a two-column table that differentiates the two types of knowing. Use these lists to construct your own brief (150-word) statement defining each type.

Identify examples where you used know that, know how and know why knowledge in your clinical practice.

While practical/know how and theoretical/know that knowledge forms are very different, they share one vitally important characteristic. They are both within the practice of nursing. They both contribute to safe and efficient treatment and care in respect of patients' health and well-being. In addition, they are not opposed or disruptive to each other but of necessity complementary. We need to know *what* to do (theoretical propositional knowledge), we need to know *how* to do it (practical know how) and we also need to know *why* we are doing it. In delivering optimum nursing care, all three are needed and are seen in Benner's (1984) expert nurse level.

Categories of Knowing

Carper's Ways of Knowing in Nursing

'Know how', 'know that' and 'know why' knowledge have been recognised as being very relevant to nursing practice. There has been a tendency to focus on 'know that' knowledge to neglect others, which is why the paper by Barbara Carper written in 1978 was so significant. In the first article in the first issue of a new US journal, *Advances in Nursing Science*, Barbara Carper identified four patterns of knowing in nursing. It proved to be a seminal paper and these four patterns of knowing were: *empirics*, the science of nursing; *aesthetics*, the art of nursing; *ethics*, moral knowing; and *personal knowing* (Figure 2.2).

Empirics
Considering our earlier description of empiricism, you can probably predict what type of knowing 'empirics' refers to. According to Carper, empirics represents the knowing that is obtained by rigorous observation or measurement. It provides knowledge that is verifiable, objective, factual and research-based. Empirics is organised systematically into scientific principles, theories and laws for the purpose of describing, explaining and predicting phenomena of special concern to nursing. The ability to quantify empirical data allows objective measurement that produces evidence that can be replicated by multiple observers or researchers (Carper 1992) and enables nurses to prescribe care. Empirics would correspond with 'know that' or propositional forms of knowledge.

37

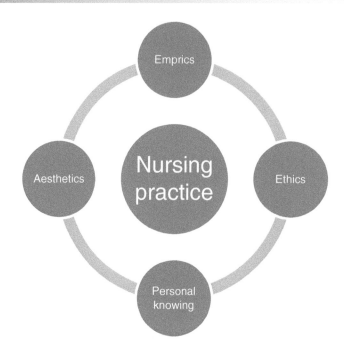

FIGURE 2.2 Patterns of knowing in nursing. Adapted from (Carper 1978).

Aesthetics

As you will have gathered from previous sections, empirics is perceived as having a narrow perspective. However, nursing practice may also be viewed as an art, and Carper acknowledged this in the pattern of knowing called 'aesthetics'. It gives us the knowledge that focuses on the craft of nursing that involves tacit knowledge, skill and intuition. It reflects Ryle's 'know how' knowledge and has its roots in the philosophy of historicism (see Reflective Exercise 2.7). Aesthetic knowledge is subjective, individual and unique. It enables us to go beyond that which is explained by existing laws and theories and accept that there are nursing phenomena that cannot be quantified, measured, categorised, classified or calibrated. Therefore, intuition, interpretation, understanding and valuing make up the central components of aesthetic knowing. For a systematic review of intuition in nursing, check out Holm and Severinsson (2016).

We would argue that, focusing on aesthetic knowing, nurses might place less emphasis on empirics. For instance, there are many research-based scales that are used to assess and predict the risk of suicide. But the nurse's clinical judgement based on experience and intuition may override what the scales tell us. Similarly, research evidence may provide guidance on the care of pressure sores or when patients can mobilise postoperatively, but the experience, intuitive expertise and knowledge of nurses may enable them to justifiably override the empirical guidance.

Ethics

Carper's third pattern of knowing is called 'ethics'. This type of knowing provides us with knowledge about what is right and wrong and what is good and bad, desirable and undesirable. It is expressed through moral codes and ethical decision-making. In everyday practice, nurses often have to make choices between competing interventions. These choices and judgements may have an ethical dimension, and to select the most appropriate position or action requires careful deliberation. For example, during the COVID-19 pandemic, nurses, as team members, had to decide on which patients were admitted to intensive care or who got access to a ventilator (McKenna 2020). For ethical reasons, some nurses made such judgements, even though the results of clinical trials or other studies (empirics) recommended other approaches. Similarly, we know of nurses who will not participate in electroconvulsive therapy for depression or therapeutic abortions, even though there is research evidence underpinning their effectiveness. Ethical evidence may also be used to

38

make decisions about the costs of treatment or whether terminally ill patients should be actively resuscitated after a heart attack. It may also be used by nurses when new effective drugs are available to help patients who have cancer or dementia but when they are too expensive for patients to access.

Personal Knowing

Like aesthetics, 'personal knowing' is subjective yet is about nurses being aware of themselves and how they relate to others. It represents knowledge that focuses on self-consciousness, personal awareness and empathy. If, as various nurse theorists argue, caring is an interpersonal process (Peplau 1992) where interactions and transactions between people are central (King 1981), then we must know ourselves, our own strengths and our weaknesses in order to be expert practitioners. Nurses do not possess exclusive ownership of an arsenal of surgical instruments or pharmaceutical products. What we have is ourselves and we can use this resource therapeutically to make a positive difference to patients. We can learn as much from a caring relationship as patients do and a good caring relationship will depend on our own self-regard, self-respect and self-perception. Therefore, personal knowing requires self-consciousness and self-awareness and active empathic participation on the part of the knower (Carper 1992). Here again, the influence of historicism is evident.

It is possible that nurses may sometimes reject empirical evidence because of their personal knowing. For example, consider the situation where a nurse is working with a patient or a family member who is going through a grief reaction. Despite research findings that suggest a linear movement through five stages – denial, anger, bargaining, depression and acceptance as if they happen in order, moving from one stage to the other – the nurse's personal experience of a family bereavement may provide them with an understanding that not everyone has to go through all these phases or in the order suggested by the research evidence.

As you reflect on these four patterns of knowing, you will note the complexity of nursing knowledge. The patterns are not mutually exclusive; there is overlap, interrelation and interdependence. By recognising that there are several legitimate ways of knowing, other than empirical knowing, Carper has made a valuable contribution to the examination of knowledge development in nursing.

Chinn et al. (2022) stated that:

- empirics removed from the context of the whole of knowing produces control and manipulation;
- removing ethics produces rigid doctrine and insensitivity to the rights of others;
- removing aesthetics produces prejudices, bigotry and lack of appreciation of meaning;
- removing personal knowing produces isolation and self-distortion.

Carper Reimagined

Carper's work has undergone careful analysis by many authors (Archibald 2012; Terry & Carr 2017; Willis & Leone-Sheehan 2019; Thorne 2020, Chinn et al. 2022; Lindell & Chinn 2022). Some have added extra patterns of knowing to Carper's original four. This is not surprising considering Carper's article was published 45 years ago. For example, Lindell and Chinn (2022) and Chinn et al. (2022) described 'Emancipatory Knowing' as the human capacity to be aware of and critically reflect on the social and cultural status quo and to figure out how and why it came to be that way. It centres on the knowing that is necessary to remove barriers that make health and well-being difficult or impossible for those from disadvantaged backgrounds and to ensure health and well-being.

They also highlight the importance of 'Sociopolitical Knowing' for nursing. It focuses on the policies and institutional practices that influence nursing practice. This makes sense, as healthcare is political, probably because most countries spend their greatest proportion of gross domestic product on their health services. In the United Kingdom, the National Health Service has always attracted political attention, while in the United States, 'Obamacare' had a major influence on the outcomes of political elections.

In 2019, Willis and Leone-Sheehan wrote a paper on 'spiritual knowing'. It will not surprise readers to learn that this type of knowing is linked closely to 'personal knowing'. The authors describe spiritual knowing as 'drawing upon wisdom deep within ourselves that reflects our experiences as healers and teachers oriented towards all that is good, wholesome, and healing in being human' (Willis and Leone-Sheehan 2019: 65). It is inclusive of, though not limited to, religious beliefs and practices. *Spiritual qualities* and experiences are consistent with notions of fostering well-being in nursing and are linked to compassion, care, kindness and empathy. These additions to Carper's patterns of knowing are not separate from them but integrated within them.

Experienced nurses use these patterns of knowing interchangeably. For instance, experienced palliative care nurses will be aware of the research and theoretical basis for providing analgesia (*empirics*) and have the skills and intuition to ensure the patient understands the treatment and is as comfortable as possible while receiving it (*aesthetics*). However, the issue of withholding analgesia because of the severe side effects and sometimes poor prognosis is a moral decision to be made with the patient and family (*ethics*). Knowing themselves and their inner resources is important in the construction of an interpersonal therapeutic relationship with the client (*personal knowing*). They will also respect the patient's ethnic, cultural and social background when planning and giving care (*emancipatory knowing*). This is also linked to the nurses taking account of the spiritual belief system of the patient *(spiritual knowing)*. Finally, the nurse will be aware of the political debates around issues such as the provision of the nursing workforce in palliative care and issues such as advanced care planning or assisted dying (*sociopolitical knowing*) (see Reflective Exercise 2.11).

Reflective Exercise 2.11

The Ways of Knowing

Construct a patient care situation where you would use all four of Carper's ways of knowing. If possible, also consider if there are aspects of the care that relate to sociopolitical, emancipatory and spiritual knowing.

This can be in any speciality or clinical setting. Try to see how the different patterns of knowing are linked and decide which is the most important for that particular scenario.

Identify another scenario where a nurse would ignore an intervention based on empirical evidence because of the primacy of some of the other ways of knowing. What are the legal and professional implications for her doing this?

Kerlinger's Ways of Knowing

Another way of thinking about knowing in nursing is through the work of Kerlinger (1986) (Figure 2.3). He also identified four ways of knowing.

- *Empirical* knowing is knowing something through rigorous research. Here 'hard evidence' is required in order to be certain that something is or is not true. Readers will note that this reflects an empiricist viewpoint.
- Knowing through *tenacity* is knowing something because it has always been believed to be true.

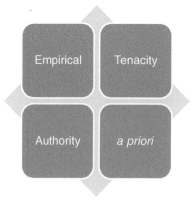

FIGURE 2.3   Ways of knowing. (Kerlinger 1986)/Houghton Mifflin Harcourt.

- Knowing through *authority* is knowing something because a respected or authoritative person or organisation said so.
- *A priori* knowing is knowing something because reason tells you it is true, an echo of Descartes's rationalist approach to knowledge creation.

(See Reflective Exercise 2.12.)

Reflective Exercise 2.12

Kerlinger's Ways of Knowing

From the experiences you have had on your nursing course so far, identify some examples of Kerlinger's four categories of knowing and where possible link them to Carper's patterns of knowing and to knowledge developed through: know that, know how and know why.

To illustrate Kerlinger's approach, consider the example of providing information to patients preoperatively to ensure better postoperative recovery. Nurses may believe this to be true 'it has always been done this way' (*tenacity*), because the clinical nurse manager told them so (*authority*) or because it is reasonable to assume that if a person gets information, they will be less anxious (*a priori*). You could also have identified Kerlinger's preferred *empirical* way of obtaining knowledge; nurses provide patients with information preoperatively because this practice was proven through the results of well-validated empirical research into preoperative preparation (see e.g. Boore 1978).

Like all physical scientists, Kerlinger felt comfortable building hierarchies of knowledge. In Kerlinger's scheme, the scientific empiricist method is supreme (see Figure 2.3) and intuitive knowledge occupies a more lowly position among the four. For a practice discipline like nursing, this is an inappropriate way of viewing the development of knowledge. Such hierarchies are seen in textbooks on evidence-based practice. For example, in 1997, Muir Gray identified what he called the hierarchy of evidence (Muir Gray 1997). This is illustrated in Figure 2.4.

In Muir Gray's hierarchy, you will notice that the top four levels are really about counting, and you will know from our previous discussion that this has its roots in empiricism. It is not unusual to hear the mantra that randomised controlled trials are the gold standard, the most highly prized source of knowledge. This is a false assumption as it depends on what knowledge you are seeking. If, for example, you want to know the possible causes of Alzheimer's disease, then yes the

41

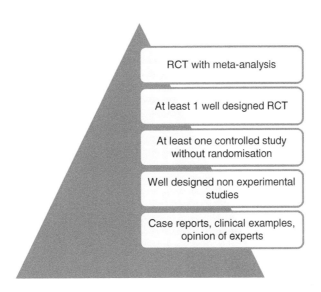

RCT with meta-analysis

At least 1 well designed RCT

At least one controlled study without randomisation

Well designed non experimental studies

Case reports, clinical examples, opinion of experts

FIGURE 2.4 Hierarchy of evidence (Muir Gray 1997)/with permission of ELSEVIER.

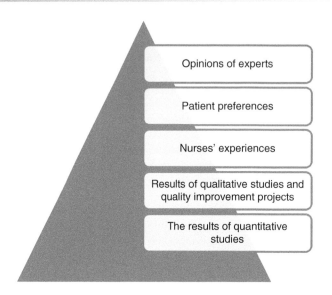

FIGURE 2.5   A proposed new hierarchy of evidence.

randomised controlled trial may well be the gold standard (empiricism). However, if you wanted to know the emotional effect a diagnosis of dementia has on patients and their families, then the gold standard may be a phenomenological study (historicism).

According to Muir Gray, word of mouth is not regarded as a good way of knowing. This is not the case in all professions. In the legal profession, such evidence is highly valued, and word of mouth is sufficient to put a person in jail for a long time, or, in some countries, be executed. But such sources are belittled in most textbooks and articles about evidence in nursing. It might be more useful to propose a new hierarchy, as in Figure 2.5 (McKenna 2010).

As with the previous hierarchy, this one also has inherent problems. How can you decide whether a patient's preference comes above or below the experience of nurses? It depends on the circumstances; hierarchies belong to the world of positivist quantification and categorising and the quality of knowledge required to nurse should not solely be tied to the quality of a research design (see Reflective Exercise 2.13).

Reflective Exercise 2.13

Frameworks for Knowing

We have described Carper's patterns of knowing and Kerlinger's categories of knowing.

Which one do you feel best represents your view, your own personal philosophy of knowing in nursing?

Consider how each might help inform your study and practice of nursing. Do you think there may be something in one scheme that is missing in the other? If so, how might the schemes be merged?

Does your nursing course teach interventions, based on hierarchies of knowing? Which one gets the most attention and deep down, which one do you prefer?

Developing Nursing Knowledge Through Reasoning

Inductive Reasoning

Every day, practising nurses experience a variety of patient phenomena. This could be pain, sleeping, mobilising, depression, etc. By taking note of patterns in those phenomena, it is possible to identify relationships that describe, explain or predict these phenomena and build up a body of theoretical knowledge. This is referred to as inductive reasoning and reflects moving from a specific situation to a general theory. The early empiricists championed this inductive method.

Qualitative research approaches from the historicist school of philosophy also use induction to generate theory ('know that' knowledge) from practice ('know how' knowledge).

For example, Sister Roy (1980) observed that patients adapted to their illness and surroundings. If they had pain in their right side, they lay on their left side or if they had a painful leg, they would limp by putting weight on the unaffected leg. Also, as individuals acclimatise to mountain living where the air is thinner, their body adapts by making more red blood cells to carry oxygen. In addition, when entering a darkened room, the rods and cones of a person's eye adapt. From similar observations, Roy developed her Adaptation Theory of Nursing. Here, induction from specific observations led to a general theory.

Deductive Reasoning

In contrast to inductive reasoning, deductive reasoning involves moving from the general to the specific situation. You will note elsewhere in this chapter that René Descartes favoured it as a key component of rationalism. Deductive reasoning traditionally involves the use of three propositions (two premises and one conclusion). In deductive reasoning, a conclusion follows from one or more statements that are taken as true. Aristotle (384–322 BCE) perfected this form of deductive argument, calling it a syllogism (Stokes 2015). The most famous example is shown in Key Concepts 2.5.

Key Concepts 2.5

Deductive reasoning is a method of reasoning where specific knowledge is made from general principles.

Example of a Deductive Argument – A Syllogism

All men are mortal	(first premise)	(axiom 1 or postulate 1)
Socrates is a man	(second premise)	(axiom 2 or postulate 2)
Therefore, Socrates is mortal	(conclusion)	(theorem)

Here, the reasoning goes from the general (all men) to the specific (Socrates). You can see that if the premises remained the same but we changed the conclusion to read 'Socrates is **not** mortal', then the deductive reasoning would be faulty. Similarly, if one of the premises was reversed, the unchanged conclusion would be wrong, and the reasoning would once again be faulty.

You could reverse the example and make it inductive reasoning. Here, the reasoning goes from a specific situation or example (Confucius, Socrates and Hannibal) to the general (all men). So, a series of discrete observations about phenomena are followed by a conclusion (see Key Concepts 2.6).

Key Concepts 2.6

Inductive reasoning is a method of reasoning where general knowledge is made from specific observations.

Example of an Inductive Argument

Confucius is a man and is mortal	(first premise)
Socrates is a man and is mortal	(second premise)
Hannibal is a man and is mortal	(third premise)
Therefore, all men are mortal	(conclusion)

Deductive reasoning in nursing normally starts with an established theory, and this (or a proposition from it) is tested in the real world of practice to see if it can be disproved – remember our earlier reference to Popper's (1989) work on refutation.

An example of deductive theory development in nursing is the work of Alligood (2021). She developed a mid-range theory by testing propositions from Rogers's (1980) nursing theory. This is a perfect example of deduction from the general (Rogers's theory) to the specific (Alligood's theory of creativity, actualisation and empathy). There are other examples where deductive research on the propositions of grand theories such as those of Henderson (1991), Peplau (1992) and Orem (1995) have led to the development of mid-range theories.

Retroductive Reasoning

Some nurse theorists will use a more deductive or a more inductive approach than others, but theory construction may include both; it is often not an either/or issue. This amalgamation of induction and deduction is referred to as retroduction. An example of this type of research would be that of Boore (1978), referred to earlier. Boore used an experimental design to test the theory that providing information to preoperative patients would reduce their stress levels postoperatively. Since a specific theory was being tested and applied, the method used was deduction. However, the results of this study led to new practices in how patients are prepared for surgery and a 'practice theory' of preoperative preparation was developed. Practice theories are often referred to as situation-specific theories. Here, Boore was also using induction where experiences within the research setting led to the development of a new, more clinically specific, theory.

Research as a Basis for Knowledge Development

Research is defined as 'the attempt to derive generalisable new knowledge including studies that aim to generate hypotheses as well as studies that aim to test them' (National Research Ethics Service [NRES] 2006: 2). With its emphasis on generalisation, it is possible with this terminology to see plainly the influence of empiricism. The contribution of the empiricist research approach to nursing knowledge cannot be denied and it should not be rejected completely. Internationally, there have been some very good research projects which, although having their basis in the experimental empiricist tradition, have contributed substantially to nursing knowledge.

New methods of research do not just happen; they are the products of much philosophical thought and discussion. One broad approach was based on what Wilhelm Dilthey (1833–1911) referred to as 'human science'. Readers will note from the following that it emanates from the *historicism* philosophy of science (discussed earlier). Human science recognises the effects that the researcher and the research participants/respondents have on what is being researched. Intuition, understanding, reflection, meanings and experiences are its central components. Within human science, the participants' 'lived experiences' are the core of explanations and meanings about things and are interpreted by them, not by outsiders. Humans are perceived as whole people, and breaking them down into components or parts, for example, Cartesian dualism, is dehumanising. Human science is often referred to as the *perceived view* as opposed to the *received view* of 'traditional' science. The differences can be seen in Table 2.3.

Chinn et al. (2022) accepted the importance of both views for the development of knowledge for nursing practice. In traditional science, an attempt is made to study the whole by looking at its parts, while in human science, an attempt is made to study the whole as it appears. In traditional science, knowledge is developed to describe, to explain and to predict; in human science, knowledge is developed to understand. In traditional science, theory is developed through defining, analysing and synthesising concepts and propositions; in human science, theory is developed through description and interpretation. Traditional science is directed towards uncovering cause-and-effect relationships and generalisations; human science is directed towards creating knowledge from common meanings, patterns and themes in descriptions.

Gadow (1990) did not think human science goes far enough in explaining how best to develop nursing knowledge. She believed the researcher should leave the personal and experience alone because there is no way to summarise (reduce) a life, a culture or any human situation. Also, qualitative research may be accused as no better than quantitative research, in that it treats experience as data. She appeared to argue that quantitative researchers may be more honest because they are 'up front' in calling the subject the object of their study (cited in Smith 1994). Nonetheless, it is heartening that nurses are beginning to accept and use methods of enquiry other than the empiricist approach to develop and test knowledge. This should have a powerful effect on identifying a body of knowledge that has particular relevance to patient care. In this way, 'know that' and 'know why' knowledge can enrich the 'know how' knowledge and vice versa.

TABLE 2.3 The received view versus the perceived view.

Received view	Perceived view
Objective	Subjective
Deduction	Induction
One truth	Multiple truths
Validation and replication	Trends and patterns
Justification	Discovery
Test theories	Evaluate theories
Prediction and control	Description/understanding
Particulars	Patterns
Reductionism	Holism
Generalisation	Individualism
Empirical positivism	Historicism

Reflective Exercise 2.14

Received View Versus the Perceived View

Form small groups in the class and discuss the received and perceived views of knowledge development. Take a show of hands as to group members' preferences. If everyone selected the perceived view, what does that say about the teaching received, or your fellow students – do you think this is unique to nursing?

If there is a mix of preferences, discuss the reasons for individuals' selections.

Also, discuss whether there are specific nursing problems that would lend themselves better to either a received or perceived view.

Mixed Methods

In the early decades of the 21st century, many nurse researchers realised that neither a quantitative nor a qualitative research approach can tell the whole story. One approach is to employ a quantitative method such as a closed-ended postal questionnaire to collect data from a large and dispersed sample. For example, a nurse researcher may survey patients on their attitudes to discharge from hospital. Once the data have been analysed, the findings will provide the researcher with statistical results on such attitudes. The researcher may then identify a small stratified or purposive sample and conduct interviews, the schedule of which will be informed by the results of the quantitative survey. This is a **quantitative then qualitative mixed-methods** approach. Obviously, the opposite strategy of a **qualitative then quantitative mixed-methods** approach could be used. For more information on mixed methods, see Shorten and Smith (2017).

Conclusion

This chapter has shown that there are many ways of knowing in nursing. It has highlighted the main philosophies of science underpinning how and why people develop knowledge. The armchair rationalist approach to knowledge development, popularised by Descartes, was influential in its day. However, by the mid-18th century, empiricists had set down the rules that were to influence subsequent healthcare research. Empiricism is still alive and well in nurses' use of randomised controlled trials, experiments and quasi-experiments. Roskoski (2019) pointed out that empiricism is a bridge linking nursing theory to nursing practice. Nonetheless, in the third decade of the 21st century, more nurse researchers have embraced phenomenology, an approach emanating from the tradition of historicism. In addition, we have seen an upsurge in nurses using a mixed-methods approach that combines the traditions of historicism with that of empiricism.

The importance of 'know how', 'know that' and 'know why' knowledge was discussed, and while the strengths of each have been highlighted, the need for nurses to embrace all three is crucial for a practice discipline. However, Carper's work reminds us that there are other ways of knowing and her views are reflected in the differences between the received view and the perceived view. There is a wealth of literature suggesting that nurses use several ways of knowing and that many of these do not fit neatly within empiricism. These include spiritual, sociopolitical and emancipatory knowing. These have built upon and enriched Carper's work and are being incorporated into contemporary nursing practice and research, leading in some cases to new theoretical perspectives.

In conclusion, all types of knowing and knowledge development are valuable. Placing one in a higher position than another is not helpful; it depends on what knowledge is being sought and what questions are being addressed.

Revision Points

- Knowing is defined as individual human processes of experiencing and comprehending the self and the world that can be brought to some level of conscious awareness. Knowledge is defined as the knowing that we can share and communicate to others.

- There are three key phases in the philosophy of knowledge development: rationalism, empiricism and historicism. All of these have influenced the evolution of nursing knowledge.

- Nurses use many different types of knowledge in their practice and three influences were identified:

- 'know how', 'know that' and 'know why' knowledge;

- Carper's ways of knowing, and more recent extensions of her work;

- Kerlinger's four categories of knowledge.

Useful Web Links

https://currentnursing.com/nursing_theory/nursing_theories_overview.html
https://currentnursing.com/nursing_theory/nursing_theorists.html
https://nursekey.com/outline-of-nursing-theories-and-frameworks-of-care/
https://nurseslabs.com/nursing-theories/
https://nursology.net/
https://uk.indeed.com/career-advice/career-development/nursing-theory
https://www.wgu.edu/blog/understanding-nursing-theories2109.html

References

Alligood M.R. (2021) *Nursing Theorists and Their Work*, 10th edition. New York: Mosby.

Aranha P.R. (2018) Application of Rogers' system model in nursing care of a client with cerebrovascular accident. *Manipal Journal of Nursing and Health Sciences*, **4**(1), 50–56.

Archibald M.M. (2012) The holism of aesthetic knowing in nursing. *Nursing Philosophy*, **13**(3), 179–188. DOI: 10.1111/j.1466-769X.2012.00542.x

Barnhart C.L. & Barnhart R.K. (1976) *The Worldbook Dictionary Field*. Chicago, IL: Enterprises Educational Corporation.

Benner P. (1984) *From Novice to Expert: Excellence and Power in Clinical Nursing Practice*. Menlo Park, CA: Addison-Wesley.

Boore J.R.P. (1978) *A Prescription for Recovery*. London: Royal College of Nursing.

Carper B.A. (1978) Fundamental patterns of knowing in nursing. *Advances in Nursing Science*, **1**(1), 13–23.

Carper B.A. (1992) Philosophical inquiry in nursing: an application. In Kikuchi J.F. & Simmons H. (eds) *Philosophic Inquiry in Nursing*. Newbury Park, CA: Sage.

Chinn P.L., Kramer M.K. & Sitzman K. (2022) *Knowledge Development in Nursing: Theory and Process*, 11th edition. St Louis: Elsevier.

Errasti-Ibarrondo B., Jordán J.A., Díez-Del-Corral M.P. & Arantzamendi M. (2018) van Manen's phenomenology of practice: how can it contribute to nursing? *Nursing Inquiry*, **26**, 1. DOI: 10.1111/nin.12259

Feyerabend P. (1977) Consolidation for the specialist. In Lakatos I. & Musgrave A. (eds) *Criticism and the Growth of Knowledge*, pp. 32–47. Cambridge: Cambridge University Press.

Fieser J. (2020). *Continental Rationalism. In The History of Philosophy*. https://www.coursehero.com/file/132302889/Epistemological-Theories1doc/

Freud S. (1949) *An Outline of Psychoanalysis*. New York: W.W. Norton.

Gadow S. (1990) Response to 'personal knowing: evolving research and practice'. *Scholarly Inquiry in Nursing Practice*, **4**(2), 167–170.

Gordon-Roth J. & Weinberg S. (eds) (2021) *The Lockean Mind*. Abingdon: Oxon Routledge.

Gortner S.R. (1993) Nursing's syntax revisited: a critique of philosophies said to influence nursing theories. In Nicoll L.H. (ed.) *Perspectives on Nursing Theory*, 3rd edition, pp. 236–254. Philadelphia, PA: J.B. Lippincott.

Habermas J. (1971) *Knowledge and Human Interests*. Boston, MA: Beacon Press.

Hanck T. (2021) Locke on primary and secondary qualities. In Gordon-Roth J. & Weinberg S. (eds) *The Lockean Mind*, pp. 275–292. London: Routledge.

Heidegger M. (1962) *Being and Time*. New York: Harper & Row.

Henderson V.A. (1991) *The Nature of Nursing. Reflections after 25 Years*. New York: National League for Nursing.

Holm A.L. & Severinsson E. (2016) A systematic review of intuition—a way of knowing in clinical nursing? *Open Journal of Nursing*, **6**, 412–425. DOI: 10.4236/ojn.2016.65043

Husserl E. (1962) *Ideas: General Introduction to Pure Phenomenology*. New York: Collier.

Kerlinger F.N.B. (1986) *Foundations of Behavioural Research*, 3rd edition. New York: Holt, Rinehart & Winston.

King I. (1981) *A Theory of Nursing: Systems, Concepts, Process*. New York: John Wiley & Sons Inc.

Kuhn T.S. (1977) *The Structure of Scientific Revolutions*, 3rd edition. Chicago, IL: Chicago University Press.

Laudan L. (1977) *Progress and its Problems: Towards a Theory of Scientific Growth*. Berkeley, CA: University of California Press.

Lenzer G. (2017) *Auguste Comte and Positivism: The Essential Writings*, 3rd edition. New York: Taylor & Francis.

Lindell, D. Chinn, P. (2022). *Aesthetic Knowing* Blog. Nursology. https://nursology.net/category/aesthetic-knowing/

Lyotard J.-F. (1984) *The Postmodern Condition: A Report on Knowledge*. Minneapolis, MN: Minnesota University Press.

McCann K. & McKenna H.P. (1993) An exploration of touch between nurses and elderly patients in a continuing care setting in Northern Ireland. *Journal of Advanced Nursing*, **18**, 838–846.

McKenna H.P. (2004) 'Role drift' to unlicensed assistants: risks to quality and safety. *Quality and Safety in Health Care*, **13**(6), 410–411.

McKenna H.P. (2010) Critical care: does profusion of evidence lead to confusion in practice? *Nursing in Critical Care*, **15**(6), 285–290.

McKenna H.P. (2020) Covid-19: ethical issues for nurses. *International Journal of Nursing Studies*, **57**(110), 103673. DOI: 10.1016/j.ijnurstu.2020.103673

McKenna H.P. (2021) *Research Impact: Guidance on Advancement, Achievement and Assessment*. New York: Springer Nature.

McKenna H.P., Pajnkihar M. & Murphy F.A. (2014) *Fundamentals of Nursing Models Theories and Practice*. London: Wiley Blackwell.

Meleis A.I. (2017) *Theoretical Nursing: Development and Progress*. Philadelphia, PA: Walters Kluwer Publishers.

Muir Gray J.A. (1997) *Evidence-Based Health Care*. Edinburgh: Churchill Livingstone.

National Research Ethics Service [NRES] (2006) *Differentiating Audit, Service Evaluation and Research, Version 1.1*. London: NHS Health Research Authority.

Neubauer B., Witkop C.T. & Varpio L. (2019) How phenomenology can help us learn from the experiences of others. *Perspectives on Medical Education*, **8**(2), 90–97.

Neuman B. (1995) *The Neuman Systems Model*, 3rd edition. Norwalk, CT: Appleton and Lange.

Okaisu E.M., Kalikwani F. & Wanyana G. (2014) Improving the quality of nursing documentation: an action research project: original research. *Curationis*, **37**(2). https://hdl.handle.net/10520/EJC163017

Orem D.E. (1995) *Nursing Concepts of Practice*, 5th edition. St. Louis, MO: Mosby, Inc.

Parse R.R. (1987) *Nursing Science: Major Paradigms, Theories, and Critiques*. Philadelphia, PA: Saunders.

Peplau H.E. (1992) Interpersonal relations: a theoretical framework for application in nursing practice. *Nursing Science Quarterly*, **5**, 13–18.

Polanyi M. (1967) *The Tacit Dimension*. London: Routledge and Kegan Paul.

Popper K. (1989) *Conjectures and Refutations: The Growth of Scientific Knowledge*, revised edition. London: Routledge.

Reed P.G. & Crawford Sherer N.B. (2018) *Nursing Knowledge and Theory Innovation, Advancing the Science of Practice*, 2nd edition. New York: Springer.

Rogers M.E. (1980) *An Introduction to a Theoretical Basis of Nursing*, 2nd edition. Philadelphia, PA: F.A. Davis & Co.

Roskoski J. (2019). *What is empiricism in Nursing Theory*? https://careertrend.com/list-7429101-barriers-applying-nursing-theory.html

Roy C. (1980) The roy adaptation model. In Riehl J.P. & Roy C. (eds) *Conceptual Models for Nursing Practice*. Norwalk, CT: Appleton-Century-Crofts.

Roy C. (2003) Reflections on nursing research and the Roy adaptation model. *Igaju-syoin Japanese Journal*, **36**(1), 7–11.

Ryle G. (1949) *The Concept of Mind*. Chicago, IL: Chicago University Press.

Saletti-Cuesta L., Tutton E., Langstaff D. & Willett K. (2017) Understanding patient and relative/carer experience of hip fracture in acute care: a qualitative study protocol. *International Journal of Orthopaedic and Trauma Nursing*, **25**. DOI: 10.1016/j.ijotn.2016.09.002

Shorten A. & Smith J. (2017) Research made simple: mixed methods research: expanding the evidence base. *Evidence Based Nursing*, **20**(3). DOI: 10.1136/eb-2017-102699

Smith M.C. (1994) Arriving at a philosophy of nursing: discovering? constructing? evolving? In Kikuchi J.F. & Simmons H. (eds) *Developing a Philosophy of Nursing*. Newbury Park, CA: Sage.

Stokes P. (2015) *Philosophy: 100 Essential Thinkers*. London: Arcturus Publishing Ltd.

Terry L. & Carr G. (2017) Expert nurses' perceptions of the relevance of Carper's patterns of knowing to junior nurses. *Advances in Nursing Science*, **40**(1), 85–102.

The Economist (2018) *The vienna circle – their significance and impact for today*. https://cla.umn.edu/austrian/news/vienna-circle-their-significance-and-impact-today

Thorne S. (2020) Rethinking Carper's personal knowing for 21st century nursing. *Nursing Philosophy*, **21**(4). DOI: 10.1111/nup.12307

Toulmin S. (1972) *Human Understanding*. Princeton, NJ: Princeton University Press.

Van Manen M. (2017) But is it phenomenology? *Qualitative Health Research*, **27**, 6. DOI: 10.1177/1049732317699570

Watson J. (2005) *Caring Science as Sacred Science*. Philadelphia, PA: F.A. Davis.

Willis D.G. & Leone-Sheehan D.M. (2019) Spiritual knowing: another pattern of knowing in the discipline. *Advances in Nursing Science*, **42**(1), 58–68. DOI: 10.1097/ANS.0000000000000236

Žiaková K., Čáp J., Miertová M., Gurková E. & Kurucová R. (2020) An interpretative phenomenological analysis of dignity in people with multiple sclerosis. *Nursing Ethics*, **27**(3), 686–700.

CHAPTER 3

Theory from Practice and Practice from Theory

Outline of Content

In this chapter, the relationship between theory and practice is explored in depth. The idea that practice is based upon or guided by theory and the extent to which practice influences theory development are considered. Building upon theory definitions in the first chapter, different forms of theory are considered. As theory is linked to science, the discussion is extended into the relationship between science and practice.

Learning Outcomes

At the end of this chapter, you should be able to:

1. Outline how theories may be classified in terms of both their sophistication and their abstraction

2. Describe Dickoff and James's (1968) four levels of theory and provide an example of each

3. Explain the differences between situation-specific theory, mid-range theory, grand theory and meta-theory, giving some examples

4. Discuss closing the theory–practice gap

5. Discuss the contribution of science to nursing and society

Introduction

In Chapter 1, we defined theory as a statement used to describe, explain or predict phenomena that increases knowledge, and in Chapter 2, we explored different categories and types of knowledge that nurses might use in their practice. In this chapter, we refocus on nursing theory, looking at the relationship between theory and practice. We will explore:

Fundamentals of Nursing Models, Theories and Practice, Third Edition. Hugh P. McKenna, Majda Pajnkihar and Dominika Vrbnjak.
© 2025 John Wiley & Sons Ltd. Published 2025 by John Wiley & Sons Ltd.
Companion website: www.wiley.com/go/nursingmodels3e

- the early developments of theory in nursing;
- what levels of theory might be appropriate for nursing;
- the relationship between theory and practice;
- closing the theory–practice gap and consider some of the strengths and limitations of science for nursing and the wider society.

First Steps – Reflecting on Theory

In Chapter 1, we aimed to highlight the importance of theory for nursing. We presented a logical argument to support the need for theory in nursing, hoping to engage you further in this discussion. Now, we shift our focus and encourage you to think deeply and reflect on theoretical and practical issues.

Drawing from the sociologist Thomas Merton's insights in his 1969 book, we are reminded that assumptions can often prevent us from achieving a deep understanding, leading us to superficially engage with concepts rather than fully comprehend them. This insight invites us to revisit and examine critically our foundational beliefs, especially regarding theory in nursing.

In Chapter 1, we defined theory as 'statements that link (by propositions) ideas – phenomena (concepts, when a name is given to a phenomenon) about the world as experienced through our senses, thus creating knowledge'. However, within this notion are assumptions about the composite terms: ideas, concepts, propositions and knowledge. Therefore, when we say that theory is concerned with concepts and the propositions that link them, in extending knowledge about the world, we are making assumptions about several things. We make suppositions about what concepts and propositions are. We make assertions about knowledge, but what we mean by knowledge and knowing may be problematic, as we have discovered in Chapter 2.

This is relevant to you personally. As Merton suggested, we invite you to revisit or reflect on key issues to deepen your understanding of theory and its practical application. Your success depends on taking essential notes, either written or mental, to support further exploration of these issues.

We claim that the relationship between theory and practice is vitally important in nursing. But within this apparently straightforward statement, there exists a few potential pitfalls. Not only about what theory is and what we mean when we say 'practice' but also about the terms that lie hidden within theory and practice: knowledge, knowing, concepts, propositions, skill, praxis, wisdom and so on. This is why we are identifying the essentially reflective nature of this chapter at its beginning. It is a call to reflect on previous positions in respect of theory, knowledge and practice, not only as presented in Chapters 1 and 2 but also what you may have learned about theory previously. It is also a call to reflect inwards about your own assumptions and understandings. However, it may be useful to undertake the activity in Reflective Exercise 3.1 first.

Reflective Exercise 3.1

Retrospective

Before you proceed, review what has been discussed about theory and its relevance to nursing, access the Wikipedia website to search for 'theory' and 'nursing theory'. (Remember that Wikipedia is an open-source Internet encyclopaedia that readers can contribute to themselves, so the quality is only as good as the contributors, whose expertise may vary widely.)

Review the descriptions of theory from Chapter 1 and compare them with the definitions and discussions of theory (and nursing theory) found on Wikipedia. Write out your reflections (in no more than 400 words) and, if possible, discuss them with your peers/fellow students and/or teacher.

The Questions Begged

Our chapter 'Theory from practice or practice from theory?' raises some fundamental questions:

- Does theory go beyond describing, explaining or predicting our practice?
- If so, does it inform, advise, guide or even direct or prescribe our practice?
- Does practice itself provide the most appropriate source of theory for nursing?
- If theory *does* emerge from practice, what do we do with it after it is mined from the practice situation?
- Can we assume a reflexive and cyclical relationship between theory and practice, wherein practice is the source of theory, and theory, in turn, informs practice?
- If practice is in some way faulty, what does this mean for the theory derived *from* it? And, in any case, might it be argued that theory derived from practice in one set of circumstances may not apply well to practice under different circumstances?
- Apart from theory derived from nursing practice, does theory from other sources (including non-practice sources of theory), or sources that are not theoretical at all, inform nursing practice?

We could continue asking such questions, leading to detailed discussions. Typically, these questions generate even more questions. Reflecting on Thomas Merton's work (1969), when we attend to something, we find progress hindered because of a lack of clarity with respect to things we had taken for granted. The answers to all the above questions depend on how we define 'practice' and 'theory' (see Reflective Exercise 3.2).

Reflective Exercise 3.2

Defining 'Practice'

In this and previous chapters, we have started to define theory. In this chapter, we are looking at the relationship between theory and practice. As you will have several practice placements on your course, make a note of your understanding of what 'practice' means.

Developing Nursing Theory

It is important to understand how the historical and cultural contexts shaped the development of nursing theory. As you saw in Chapter 1, much of the significant early theorising in nursing arose in the United States in the 1950s, 1960s and 1970s. Nurses in the United States wanted to clearly identify what the differences were, if any, between nursing and medicine, and to do this, they had to try to begin to define nursing. Thus, some important and influential definitions of nursing were published at that time (see Reflective Exercise 3.3).

Reflective Exercise 3.3

Look up Nightingale's (*1859*/1980) theory and her definition of nursing. Do you think this definition still has relevance for nursing today? Consider the relevance of the physical environment on patient health and recovery.

Additionally, nurses at that time wished to try and develop nursing as a profession. The major professions, such as law and medicine, commanded a great deal of respect, authority and autonomy with a characteristic of a profession being that it had a unique body of knowledge. Johnson (1959) emphasised that for any profession to thrive, it must explicitly establish its theoretical foundations; and nursing is no exception. However, it was clear that nursing did not appear to have that but used knowledge from other disciplines, in particular medicine. To achieve professional status and to clearly demarcate nursing from medicine, nursing needed to try to develop itself as a discipline and to do so it had to develop a knowledge base unique to nursing. However, nurses had to agree on several key things, such as what might constitute the unique focus of the discipline of nursing. Should nursing develop its own theories of nursing or should it just 'borrow' theories from other disciplines and apply them to nursing? From Chapter 1, you will recall that what emerged from this period in the US was what were referred to as 'nursing models', sometimes called 'grand' theories, and the authors of these became very well known (see Reflective Exercise 3.4).

Reflective Exercise 3.4

Examples of Nursing Models/Theories

The works by Roy (1980), Orem (1995) and Roper et al. (2000) are examples of what might be called nursing models or grand theories (see Key concepts 3.1). If any of these are not familiar to you, do an Internet search (e.g. nursology.com) to find out about the theory and how the theorist defined nursing.

Key Concepts 3.1

Differences Between Models and Theories

Remember, there is ongoing debate about the distinction between models and theories in nursing. Some make a distinction between models and theories (e.g. Jacquline Fawcett), and some argue that all models are essentially theories (e.g. Afaf Meleis), but there are just different types of theory. This will be discussed further in this and later chapters.

Theories – The Building Blocks of Models and 'Grand' Theories

These early nurse theorists tended to use theories from other disciplines. So, for example, Peplau (1992) used Harry Stack Sullivan's theory of interpersonal relations as a starting point for her theory. Orem (1995) drew on Abraham Maslow's (1954) hierarchy of needs – originating from psychology in thinking about individuals having self-care deficits. Roy (1980) used systems theory (von Bertalanffy) in thinking of individuals as systems that need to adapt. In doing so, she studied the work of Harry Helson on how the retina of the eye adapts to different levels of light. Nurse theorists integrated these theories with their own ideas and nursing experiences to develop unique nursing theories.

As we shall see, there are issues about using theories (we might term them *imported or borrowed* theories) that do not emanate from nursing practice, and indeed may have little support among practising nurses in their day-to-day work. There is always some risk that where attempts are made to adopt such imported unmodified theory in its totality, it will be less amenable to the problems and issues of nursing practice and consequently less accepted by practising nurses. This is understandable; such theories were initially constructed for other purposes. Indeed, even attempts not simply to *adopt* the theory but merely to *adapt* it to nursing are not always successful. There is the added danger that by using borrowed theories, nurses will contribute more to the discipline it was borrowed from than to nursing itself. Read more about the dangers and benefits of borrowing theory from other disciplines for application in nursing in Chapter 7.

The development of nursing models and theories were attempts to try and define nursing and thus, by implication, identify the skills, attributes and knowledge nurses might need. These models and theories were intended to provide a framework for delivering nursing care, and you may still see examples of them being used in practice today. Crucially, for the purposes of this chapter, it was hoped that from these early 'nursing models' *nursing* theories would develop that could be tested by *nursing* research to develop *nursing* knowledge and *nursing* science (see Reflective Exercise 3.5).

Reflective Exercise 3.5

Models and Theories

Search for 'Orem theory generation and testing' on Google Scholar. Explore the results to determine if any theories derived from Orem's self-care model have been empirically tested in clinical practice. This exercise will help you understand the practical application and validation of theories in nursing.

Levels of Theory

Along with recognising the need to formally identify types of knowledge used by nurses, there was also much debate about what kinds of theories might be useful for nurses and nursing. However, as we will outline in Chapter 5, the naming and categorisation of theories is a complex area in the literature. In this chapter, we will look at the categorisation of theory in two main ways (Figure 3.1):

- levels of *sophistication* of the theory;
- levels of *abstraction* of the theory.

Levels of Theory: Sophistication

To illustrate theory in terms of levels of sophistication, we will draw on a landmark paper, written in 1968 by two non-nurse philosophers, James Dickoff and Patricia James. As we discussed earlier, a key issue in the 1960s was whether nursing could develop 'nursing' knowledge and what kind of theory was best suited to and most appropriate for a practice discipline such as nursing. The influential paper by Dickoff and James (they also wrote another paper in the same year with Ernestine Wiedenbach, who was a nurse) argued that nursing was a practice discipline and therefore needed particular types of theory. Consequently, they identified four levels of theory for nursing, designed to describe, explain, predict or prescribe phenomena:

53

- Factor-isolating theory, which *describes* and names concepts.
- Factor-relating theory, which relates concepts to one another and *explains*.
- Situation-relating theory, which is the interrelationship among concepts or propositions and can *predict*.
- Situation-producing theory, which *prescribes* actions to reach certain outcomes.

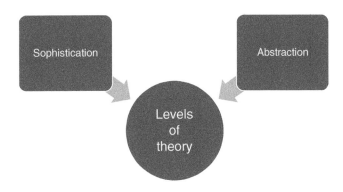

FIGURE 3.1 Categorisation of theory.

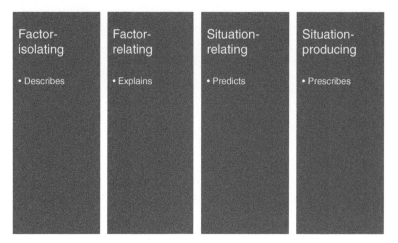

FIGURE 3.2   Levels of theory (Dickoff & James 1968).

They also proposed two crucial arguments:

1. In ascending order each of these levels builds on previous levels, so factor-isolating theory is a precursor of factor-relating theory and so on (Figure 3.2).
2. As a practice discipline, nursing requires situation-producing theory so that nurses can, with a degree of certainty, prescribe interventions that lead to desired outcomes for patients.

They asserted that we must adequately *describe* the concepts within a situation before we can *explain* how these are linked by propositions. Only then can we suggest cause–effect or *predictive* relationships when we have such explanations available. Finally, we cannot take the risk of advocating or *prescribing* actions or interventions until we have firm grounds for claiming predictive relationships. Prescriptive theory is the most sophisticated level of theory that emerges from the development of the three preceding levels. For a practical discipline like nursing, prescriptive theory is the best that can be had. However, compared with established disciplines such as medicine or law, this kind of theory in nursing is relatively new. This means that we do not have many prescriptive theories. However, we have an increasing number of descriptive and explanatory theories which, in time and with rigorous research, are expected to evolve into predictive and prescriptive theories (Figure 3.3).

In Figure 3.3, it can be seen that at the two lower levels, theory simply demonstrates that something is so, and *why* it is so in terms of propositions that link the defining concepts. At the two higher levels, one particular way in which concepts are linked (the cause–effect form of linkage or relationship) is the essential factor.

Predictive and Prescriptive Theory

Sometimes, the difference between predictive and prescriptive theory can be unclear. Indeed, occasionally authors suggest that strong predictions will inform practice and, in this context, are prescriptive theories. In such an argument, prescriptive theory is no different from predictive theory (other than that we are stating that only well-tested or 'strong' predictive theory should inform our actions). In one sense, this is exactly what prescriptive theory is. Rather than saying (as does predictive theory) the following:

if such an action is taken in these circumstances, *then this will be the outcome…*

the prescriptive theory says something like:

in order for this outcome to be achieved, you must *do the following…*

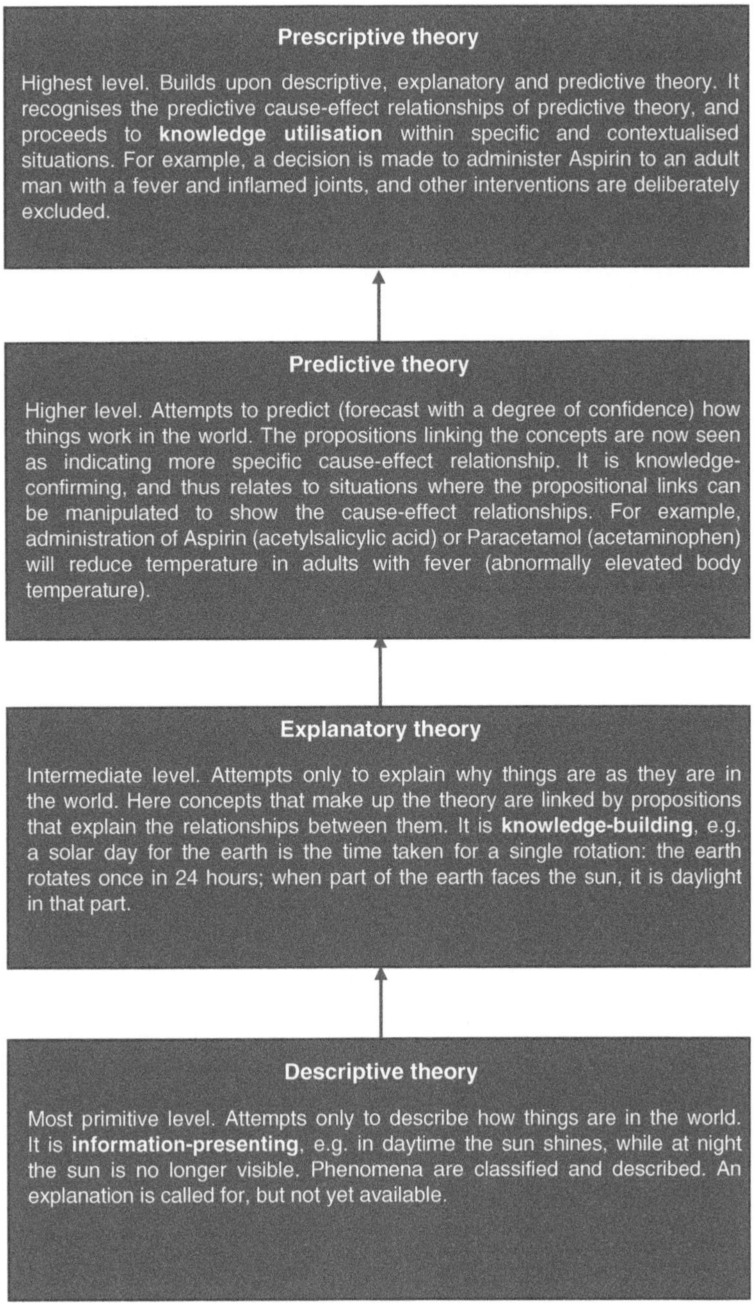

Prescriptive theory

Highest level. Builds upon descriptive, explanatory and predictive theory. It recognises the predictive cause-effect relationships of predictive theory, and proceeds to **knowledge utilisation** within specific and contextualised situations. For example, a decision is made to administer Aspirin to an adult man with a fever and inflamed joints, and other interventions are deliberately excluded.

Predictive theory

Higher level. Attempts to predict (forecast with a degree of confidence) how things work in the world. The propositions linking the concepts are now seen as indicating more specific cause-effect relationship. It is knowledge-confirming, and thus relates to situations where the propositional links can be manipulated to show the cause-effect relationships. For example, administration of Aspirin (acetylsalicylic acid) or Paracetamol (acetaminophen) will reduce temperature in adults with fever (abnormally elevated body temperature).

Explanatory theory

Intermediate level. Attempts only to explain why things are as they are in the world. Here concepts that make up the theory are linked by propositions that explain the relationships between them. It is **knowledge-building**, e.g. a solar day for the earth is the time taken for a single rotation: the earth rotates once in 24 hours; when part of the earth faces the sun, it is daylight in that part.

Descriptive theory

Most primitive level. Attempts only to describe how things are in the world. It is **information-presenting**, e.g. in daytime the sun shines, while at night the sun is no longer visible. Phenomena are classified and described. An explanation is called for, but not yet available.

FIGURE 3.3 The utility of theory in nursing.

However, to be accepted as having such prescriptive power, prescriptive theory must have gone beyond merely establishing the cause–effect relationship. We must have considered the evidence for the cause–effect relationship. We must have considered the 'expected utility' of one or some actions as opposed to others, and we will have taken account of the context. In the example within the 'prescriptive theory' box in Figure 3.3, only the decision (give the patient aspirin) is presented. But behind this, there are a few other things that have taken place, e.g.:

- The strong evidence that aspirin *does* reduce temperature is confirmed.
- There is recognition that paracetamol would also reduce temperature but may be more toxic under certain conditions.

- The fact that while aspirin and paracetamol will relieve pain equally well (as strong empirical evidence indicates no significant difference), aspirin also has anti-inflammatory properties and this person has joint inflammation.
- Although aspirin may be contraindicated in some cases (e.g. young children and people with bleeding disorders), there is no evidence to exclude its use with this particular person – the theory takes account of context and the individual case.
- The evidence clearly shows that immersion in chilled water will also reduce temperature (but in this case, it would be distressing and uncomfortable for the person).
- There is clear evidence that other methods to reduce temperature, such as tepid sponging or electric fans, are ineffective.

Behind a prescriptive theory, as indicated earlier, there is a large body of supporting evidence (obtained through research and a systematic review of research findings), and a strong foundation of decision-making that has taken account of *context* and *expected utility*. Importantly, the theory is stated in *prescriptive terms*. In real-world situations, it is presented within treatment protocols or care guidelines, and this is the link to evidence-based practice and the hierarchy of evidence that we discussed in Chapter 2. To be so placed, it must, by definition, be tested theory, and very well tested indeed. Theory testing is an issue we address in Chapter 8. For now, we note that a cause–effect theory that is still not well tested can still be termed a predictive theory. However, where there is a prescriptive theory, there is an assumption that one of the essential attributes is that it has already been well tested. Therefore, such theories are not just predicting, they also aim to operate on the world and do things in it; they are thus termed 'situation-producing theories' (Dickoff & James 1968; Slevin 2003; McKenna et al. 2014). Situation-producing theories prescribe specific activities to achieve defined goals and address nursing therapeutics and the consequences of interventions. These theories advocate for change, predict intervention outcomes and outline the interventions, expected results, client types and conditions under which they apply (Meleis 2018; McEwen & Wills 2019, 2023).

Application to Practice

Clinical nurses analyse practice situations to improve the effectiveness of their practice. They do try to think about (or *describe*) the nature of nursing situations; they further attempt to make sense of (or explain) what is happening in these situations and, on this basis, try to forecast (or *predict*) what would be the outcome of actions they undertake. Based on such predictions they may even stipulate (or *prescribe*) nursing actions. This process mirrors the theoretical construction of nurse scientists and theorists, although the spontaneous, day-to-day theorising by clinical nurses, especially in the absence of other theoretical guidance, differs from formal theory construction. This does not mean it is unimportant or insignificant. When we think of theory as being of the different types outlined earlier, we see that – whether on a smaller scale during clinicians' practice or in more formal theory-construction situations – they are, in fact, of increasing degrees of sophistication, as indicated in Figure 3.3 (see Reflective Exercise 3.6).

For example, one of the most well-known nursing theories, Peplau's Theory of Interpersonal Relationships, can be recognised as a descriptive theory (Peterson & Bredow 2020). Another, lesser-known example of descriptive theory is by Sacks and Volker (2015), which describes the process by which hospice nurses identify and respond to their patients' suffering (McEwen & Wills 2023). Watson's Theory of Human Caring is a prominent example of an explanatory theory (Peterson & Bredow 2020; Butts & Rich 2022). The Theory of Health-Related Outcomes of Resilience in Middle Adolescents (Scoloveno 2015, in McEwen & Wills 2023) and the Theory of the Well-Being Supportive Physical Environment of Home-Dwelling Elderly (Elo et al. 2013) are other examples of explanatory theories. Orlando's Theory of the Deliberative Nursing Process stands as an example of a predictive theory (Peterson & Bredow 2020). A mid-range theory of diabetes self-management mastery (Fearon-Lynch & Stover 2015) and the Caregiving Effectiveness Model (Smith et al. 2002) are other examples of predictive theories (McEwen & Wills 2023). Prescriptive theories are relatively rare in the nursing literature (Peterson & Bredow 2020; McEwen & Wills 2023). The Neuman System Model is one of only a few considered prescriptive in nature. Walling's (2006) Theory of Medical Acupuncture for nurse practitioners and Auvil-Novak's (1997) Theory of Chronotherapeutic Intervention for Postsurgical Pain can be considered as prescriptive theories as well (McEwen & Wills 2023).

Reflective Exercise 3.6

Does the Theory Have a Use?

We have referred to how, in theorising, nurses are describing, explaining, predicting and perhaps even prescribing. In an important seminal paper, the authors Dickoff and James (1968) described these different theoretical positions (we might see them as theory types) as follows:

- factor-isolating theory, which *describes*;
- factor-relating theory, which *explains*;
- situation-relating theory, which *predicts*;
- situation-producing theory, which *prescribes*.

Furthermore, they see these as progressively more sophisticated theoretical positions. It is not possible to prescribe unless you can predict. It is not possible to predict unless you can explain. Before you explain, you must first describe. Taking it from the opposite direction, unless the basic ideas or building blocks of a theory (remember, in Chapter 1, we called them concepts) are sound, it will be difficult to explain relationships between them and proceed from this to the prediction of causal relationships and prescribing actions.

Undertake a brief literature review on the idea of a situation-producing theory and the influence of Dickoff and James's seminal work. Write a brief report of your review. You may find sharing and discussing this with your peers/fellow students useful.

Levels of Theory: Abstraction

The paper by Dickoff and James was very important in suggesting what level of theory nurses might need to develop based on the assumption that nursing is a practice discipline. They outlined these levels in terms of their sophistication, with each level building upon the previous one. We have seen before that theories consist of concepts that are linked together as propositions or statements, which are then connected to form a theory. Some of these statements might be very focused with a clear identification of the ideas within them. However, some theory statements might be quite unclear, abstract and have a very wide focus rather than a narrow one. The understanding of this led to different ways of classifying theories within nursing based on how *abstract* the theory is (Figure 3.4).

The classification of nursing theories by levels of abstraction shows slight variations among authors. Walker and Avant (2019) classified theories into four levels – metatheories, grand theories, mid-range theories and practice theories. Im and Meleis (2021a, 2021b) classified theories into grand theories, mid-range theories and situation-specific theories.

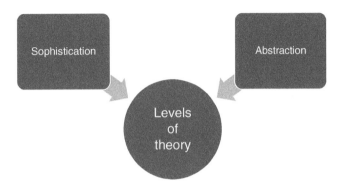

FIGURE 3.4 Levels of theory.

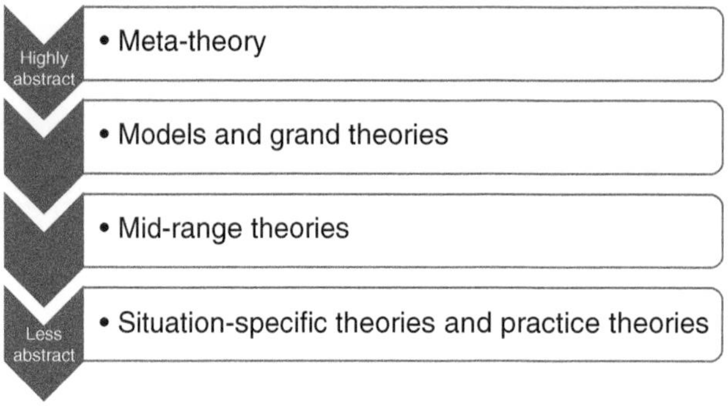

FIGURE 3.5 Levels of theory-abstraction.

Fawcett (2021) also delineated four levels: conceptual models, grand theories, mid-range theories and situation-specific theories. Peterson and Bredow (2020) outlined theories as grand theories, mid-range theories and practice theories. McEwen and Wills (2019) classified theories into metatheories, grand theories, mid-range theories and practice theories, which are sometimes referred to as micro theories or situation-specific theories (McEwen & Wills 2019, 2023; Peterson & Bredow 2020).

We will discuss four main categories (Figure 3.5).

Meta-theory

This is *about* theory, rather than being itself a *form* of theory and is at the most abstract level (above grand theory) (McEwen & Wills 2023). Meta-theory is not a theory in itself, but concerns the nature and assumptions of nursing theory (Walker & Avant 2019). Nurses may also think about theory and its importance to nursing and nursing practice, which might be seen as *theories of or about theories*. A theory of theories suggests that we take some position on the nature of theories, their purpose and how we might make practical use of them. It could be stated that the authors of this book are meta-theorists.

Therefore, 'meta-theory' usually means a critical appraisal or evaluation of theory and the outcome of such a critique would be some understanding (as previously suggested, we might call this a theory) about theory itself. This is a highly complex critical activity (McKenna 1997; McEwen & Wills 2007, 2023). Clearly, if we are to promote theory, and if it is to be used to inform our practice, it must be evaluated. We will return to this topic in detail later in the book. In Chapters 1 and 2, you learned that two of the best-known nursing meta-theorists were Afaf Meleis (2012, 2018) and Jacqueline Fawcett (2005). They have written some very important texts in which they provided an overview of the development of nursing theory and also conducted detailed critical analysis and evaluation of some of the best-known models and theories. However, it's important to note that Fawcett did not use meta-theory in her classification of theories according to her level of abstraction (Fawcett 2022).

Grand Theories

Grand theories are abstract, providing a broad perspective on the goals and structure of nursing practice (Walker & Avant 2019). These are also referred to by some authors as conceptual models, however, not Fawcett, who distinguishes grand theories from conceptual models (Fawcett 2021); and you will learn more about this theory–model controversy in Chapter 5. Early in the development of the discipline, grand theories were developed to address questions regarding the nature, mission and goals of nursing (Im & Meleis 2021a, 2021b). They aimed to explain broad areas within the discipline (McEwen & Wills 2019, 2023) and often addressed issues at a level of abstraction that is not easily amenable to research testing, and they are not intended to be reducible to testable hypotheses. They are intended to provide world views, help us map out our discipline's areas of activity, give general future direction and so on. Such theory is too abstract to be restated and/or tested in empirical terms.

However, while a grand theory as a whole may be untestable, one or more of its concepts or propositions could be tested. For example, Roper, Tierney and Logan's (grand) theory is very broad and abstract (Roper et al. 2000). However,

2 of the 12 activities of daily living are 'maintaining a safe environment' and 'mobilising'. You could imagine a situation where researchers tested the relationship between these two concepts to uncover new knowledge of use in clinical nursing. In this scenario, the researcher is not testing the grand theory in its entirety, but rather specific concepts and propositions derived from it. This principle is applicable to other grand theories as well.

When we think of nursing theory, we tend to think of 'models of nursing' and, as you can see, these are referred to as 'grand theories'. Meleis (2012, 2018) saw these early nursing grand theories as reflecting four schools of thought:

- needs theorists (Orem 1958; Abdellah et al. 1960; Henderson 1966; Roper et al. 1983);
- interaction theorists (Peplau 1952; Orlando 1961; Wiedenbach 1964; Travelbee 1966; King 1968; Paterson & Zderad 1976);
- outcome theorists (Johnson 1959; Levine 1966; Rogers 1970; Roy 1970);
- caring/becoming theorists (Watson 1979; Parse 1981).

Such grand theories offer a broad framework to guide nursing practice, research and education. Because they were so broad, they did not always fit well into every aspect of nursing practice and were sometimes considered too complicated and jargonistic to be useful for practising nurses. This perception may have been influenced by their American origin, reflecting a healthcare system and nursing education system distinct from those in Europe. Also, their high level of abstraction posed challenges for empirical testing, complicating the process of deriving more applicable nursing theories from them through research.

Mid-Range Theories

The scope of mid-range theories is narrower than that of broad-range or grand theories (McEwen & Wills 2019, 2023). These are theories that are still expressed in terms that are sufficiently linked to the specific setting so as to at least allow for testable hypotheses or research goals to be stated. Such theories are broad enough to retain a view of the discipline and its general progression, yet specific enough to identify the empirical work that could provide evidence for practice.

During the 1990s and early 21st century, there was a shift from grand theories toward mid-range theories (Figure 3.6). As suggested earlier, grand theories are broad and abstract and do not easily lend themselves to application or testing. In contrast, mid-range theories are moderately abstract and inclusive but are composed of concepts that are measurable and propositions that can be tested. At their best, mid-range theories balance the need for precision with the need to be sufficiently abstract (Merton 1968). They have fewer concepts and propositions within their structure, are presented in a more testable form, have a more limited scope and have a stronger relationship with research and practice.

Mid-range theory tends to focus on concepts of interest to nurses, such as pain, empathy, grief, self-esteem, hope, comfort, dignity and quality of life. They bridge the theory–practice and research–practice gaps, offering knowledge that can be directly applied in patient-care settings.

As was seen from the Roper, Logan and Tierney example in the section on 'Grand Theories', some mid-range theories might have their basis in grand theories. For example, the mid-range theory of 'self-care deficit' grew out of Orem's (1980) grand theory of 'self-care'. Orem's theory served also as a foundation for a mid-range Theory of Self-Care of Chronic Illness developed by Riegel, Jaarsma and Strömberg (2012) and a mid-range Theory of Weight Management by Pickett, Peters and Jarosz (2014) (McEwen & Wills 2019). This supports the assertion that a major function of grand theories is to act as a source for mid-range theory (Smith 1994; Peterson & Bredow 2020). However, mid-range theories can also emerge directly from practice or research. For example, Swanson's (1991) mid-range theory of 'caring in perinatal nursing' was inductively developed from studies in three perinatal settings and Burkhart and Hogan's (2008, 2020) mid-range theory of Spiritual Care in Nursing Practice was developed using grounded theory research. The Theory of Unpleasant Symptoms by Lenz and Pugh (2018) is an example of derivation from practice. Similarly, Mishel (1990) developed a mid-range Uncertainty in Illness theory. Meleis and colleagues developed a mid-range theory of transitions in nursing, starting from concept analysis (Schumacher & Meleis 1994) to the formulation of a model and subsequently a mid-range theory (Meleis et al. 2000).

Some mid-range theories originate from a combination of both nursing and non-nursing theories. For example, the mid-range theory Facilitated Sensemaking by Davidson (2010) is derived from Roy's adaptation model and Weick's business model of sensemaking. There are also examples of mid-range theories derived from non-nursing disciplines. Theory

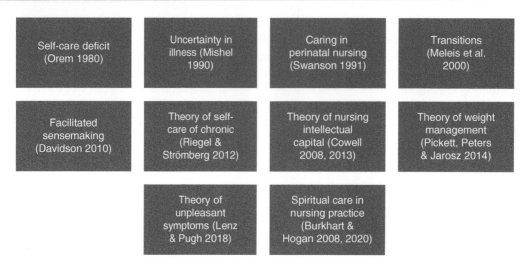

FIGURE 3.6 Examples of mid-range theories.

of Nursing Intellectual Capital by Covell (2008; Covell & Sidani 2013) is such an example where theory was derived from intellectual capital theory using Walker and Avant's strategy of theory derivation. Another example is the Health Promotion Model by Pender, Murdaugh and Parsons (2015), which was derived from the expectancy-value theory and social-cognitive theory (Peterson & Bredow 2020).

Despite their origin, mid-range nursing theories are characterised by their balance between breadth and focus, permitting generalisations across settings, a limited number of clearly articulated concepts and the ability to generate testable hypotheses (McEwen & Wills 2019). The list of mid-range theories has expanded significantly over the past two decades (Alligood 2018c; McEwen & Wills 2019, 2023), with the examples provided above representing just a selection.

Practice Theory

The literature presents a range of terms for theories that are less abstract, more specific and narrower in scope than mid-range theories (Peterson & Bredow 2020). The designation 'practice theory' is commonly used, but the term microtheory is also employed and refers to theory that is expressed in concrete and researchable terms and is very specific to a knowledge issue. The most recent addition to this terminology is 'situation-specific theory', introduced by Im (2005) and Im and Meleis (1999, 2021a, 2021b).

Practice theories have the most limited scope and level of abstraction. They are developed for a particular nursing context. Theories at this level impact nursing practice more directly than broader, abstract theories. These practice theories offer frameworks for nursing interventions and activities, proposing potential outcomes or the impact of nursing practises (Smith & Parker 2015). So, practice theories are very specific in their clinical focus, narrower in scope than mid-range theory and more concrete in their level of abstraction. Jacox (1974: 10) defined 'practice theory' as 'a theory that says – given this nursing goal (producing some desired change or effect in the patient's condition), these are the actions the nurse must take to meet the goal (produce the change)'.

In terms of sophistication, practice theories relate to Dickoff and James's (1968) highest level of theory – situation-producing theory. The essence of practice theory is a defined goal and the recommended actions to attain that goal (Walker & Avant 2019). Recently, there has been a growing interest in examining the practices of nurses to recognise that they not only use various types of knowledge in their work but also engage in theorising and using different types of theory (Peterson & Bredow 2020). You will recall from Chapter 1 that nurses in their practice constantly theorise and draw on their knowledge of practice to make clinical decisions as to the best course of action to help the patient. As well as 'formal' theories, it is important to recognise the informal theories nurses use daily. Some examples of 'formal' practice theories are The Praxis Theory of Suffering (Morse 2005), The Theory of Breastfeeding (Nelson 2006) and The Theory of Health Promotion for Preterm Infants (Mefford 2004) (in Butts & Rich 2022).

Im and Meleis (1999) introduced the concept of situation-specific theory and called it a variant of mid-range theory that highlights the importance of context in theory application. But some, as Peterson and Bredow (2020) referring to Jacox, claimed that all situation-specific theories are practice theories. Situation-specific theory underscores the necessity of considering the unique contexts where the theory will be applied. This specificity is crucial due to the variability among different populations, practice areas and clinical approaches. Situation-specific theory is tailored to meet the specific needs of a particular group within a distinct context (Im & Meleis 2021a, 2021b; Chinn, Kramer & Sitzman 2022). A distinctive aspect of situation-specific theories is their focus on sociopolitical, cultural and historical contexts, which uniquely influence their application and development (Peterson & Bredow 2020) (see Reflective Exercise 3.7).

Reflective Exercise 3.7

Levels of Theories

Navigate to the Nursology website, which serves as a comprehensive resource for nursing. Access the directory of theories and models and explore different types of nursing theories. Spend some time exploring the directory to familiarise yourself with the different types of theories available. Take note of how they vary in scope, focus and application. Within the directory, you can also find a section specifically dedicated to situation-specific theories. Look up the Situation-Specific Theory of Heart Failure Self-Care by Riegel and Vaughan Dickson. Review the details and context of this theory. Consider the impacts of sociopolitical, cultural and individual factors as discussed in the theory.

Using Theories in Practice: An Example

Let us consider an example from practice to illustrate these levels of theory. A nurse working in a gynaecological ward cares for women who suffer early miscarriages (loss of the foetus in the early stages of pregnancy). On the ward, the nursing care is framed by the work of Orem (1995) and her grand theory of self-care. Orem's ideas have been described as a 'model' or a grand theory because they are abstract and not directly testable by research. Orem, an early nursing theorist writing at the end of 1950s, believed that individuals have varying capacities for self-care. Sometimes, illness can impair this capacity, at which point the nurse's role is to compensate for the person's self-care deficits until they can independently care for themselves again. The nurse working on the gynaecological ward focuses on helping the woman safely through the surgical procedure until she is capable of self-care and then assists in planning a safe discharge home.

However, a grand theory like Orem's may not provide enough specific guidance for nurses caring for women after a miscarriage. Therefore, in addition to the grand theory, the nurse might also use a mid-range theory, such as that of Swanson (1991). This theory is more focused on the psychological needs of women experiencing miscarriages, particularly emphasising their emotions. It specifically guides the nurse to concentrate on the emotional needs of the woman by listening to and attending to the woman and offering interventions such as counselling. Swanson's mid-range theory has a narrower focus than Orem's grand theory and can therefore be tested by research.

It might be argued that Swanson's theory, although it places a much welcome emphasis on the need for emotional care, makes an assumption that all women need that kind of emotional care. This assumption may not be suitable, as individual women are likely to react very differently to their experience of miscarriage. Furthermore, the emphasis on emotional care might overlook other crucial aspects, such as the physical pre- and postoperative care needed. Consequently, experienced gynaecological nurses might also rely on their own practice theory, which is developed through years of experience in caring for women after miscarriages. This includes the 'tacit knowledge' discussed in Chapter 2. Through experience, a nurse might recognise that women's feelings post-miscarriage vary significantly, leading to a careful individual assessment to determine the most appropriate care approach. So, in addition to using Orem's grand theory and Swanson's mid-range theory, the nurse will also draw on practice theory similar to 'theories in use' (Argyris & Schön 1974) to care for the woman. This approach enables the nurse to identify and respond to the specific emotional needs of the woman and her partner, decide on the most suitable intervention and ensure that the woman is guided safely and efficiently through the surgical process.

The grand theory of self-care of Orem and the mid-range theory of Swanson are presented above to support the treatment of the patient. For comparison, we also searched for a situation-specific self-care theory (SST) for the treatment of the patient. Some SSTs have been presented, but due to the characteristics of SSTs, such as the specificity of their focus on sociopolitical, cultural and historical contexts, unique environments and clients and limited generalisation and abstraction, we cannot offer an example for use. It might be a limitation of SSTs, that they are too narrow and too specific. The nurse is theorising and drawing on theories. Some of these theories would be at different levels of abstraction and sophistication, as we have discussed earlier. However, the aim was to produce nursing knowledge and nursing theory that informed practice. So, for the scenario described, the aim would be the development of prescriptive theory, which would identify the optimum nursing intervention for women experiencing miscarriages.

Summary – Categorising Theory

So far in this chapter we have looked at levels of theory and have identified two broad ways of thinking about such levels: sophistication and abstraction (see Key Concepts 3.2).

Key Concepts 3.2

Categorising Theory

In this chapter, we have categorised theories:

1. In terms of their *sophistication*, where we drew on the work of Dickoff and James (1968) and identified four levels: factor-isolating, factor-producing, situation-relating and situation-producing.
2. In terms of their *level of abstraction*, where again we identified four types: meta-theory, grand theory, mid-range theory and practice theory.

62

However, others speak of just two theory types – grand theory and mid-range theory (Fawcett 2005). According to Fawcett (2005), mid-range theories are specific enough to allow empirical indicators to be drawn from them. These empirical indicators (later renamed empirical research methods) are, by definition, concrete and specific, which allow data to be collected and tested to validate the mid-range theory. Fawcett does not see these indicators as theories, but they fill that space containing what others define as practice theory or micro-theory.

You may find all this a little confusing: after all, we speak of theory as being of different levels of sophistication (descriptive, explanatory, predictive and prescriptive) and also of different levels of abstraction (practice, mid-range theory, grand theory and meta-theory). But Fawcett (2005), as illustrated in Figure 3.7, perhaps presented an easier way of thinking about theory:

- Grand theory provides broad direction to the discipline.
- Mid-range theory provides testable hypotheses for operational practice.

For another alternative, see Reflective Exercise 3.8.

We summarise the main differences between grand theories, mid-range theories and situation-specific theories according to the authors presented above.

Grand and mid-range theories rarely take into account sociopolitical, cultural and/or historical contexts and are limited in describing the diversity of phenomena in patient experiences and responses, health, systems and nurses' interpretations of phenomena that characterise each patient–nurse encounter (Im & Meleis 2021a, 2021b). Situation-specific theories are situated in a social and historical context and are not developed to transcend time, socially constraining structure or politically constraining situations. They are theories that are more clinically specific, reflecting a particular context, and may include plans for action.

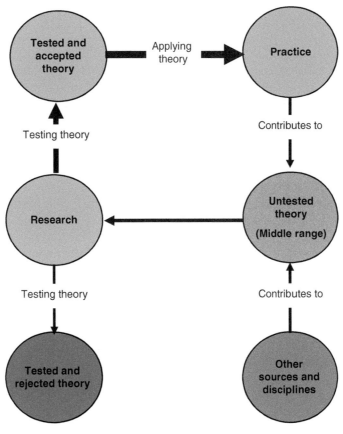

FIGURE 3.7 Propositional theory: from conception to application.

Reflective Exercise 3.8

Nursing Cannot Have Theories!

In an interesting editorial, Edwards and Liaschenko (2003) presented the following argument (not as their own position, but as one advanced by others):

(a) Nursing requires practical knowledge.
(b) Practical knowledge is distinct from propositional knowledge.
(c) Theories are set out in propositions.
(d) Therefore, there cannot be a theory of nursing.

We found in previous chapters that theory is indeed about propositional knowledge: theory was defined as concepts linked by propositions. But is the argument outlined above convincing? Are practical and propositional types of knowledge different, and if so, is propositional (theoretical) knowledge to be excluded from nursing? Using literature on nursing theory, seek out three points in favour of and three against the latter position.

The Relationship Between Theory and Practice

In Chapter 1, we made a case for the indispensable role of theory in nursing. So far in this chapter, we have defined what theory is and outlined different levels of theory. Moving this discussion forward, it is valuable to reflect on the relationship between theory and practice, the concept of a theory–practice gap and the interconnected issue of the relationship between science and practice. Theory and practice can be related in various ways. Figure 3.8 illustrates some possible configurations, and in the remainder of this chapter, the relationship is explored further.

We can note that the idea is as follows: the theory that will be most useful and appropriate is that which emerges from the situation being studied (as opposed to theory imported from other situations). In effect, data are not being collected from the situation to test a previously posited theory – the usual approach in research. Instead, by analysing the data, it is claimed that theory will emerge from it.

However, in Figure 3.8, practice is shown to be informed by theory that is practice grounded or by theory from other sources. Importantly, it is also illustrated that practice may be informed from other non-theory sources. It would be easy to assume from Figure 3.8 that such other 'non-theory' sources play a minor role in this matter. We speak here of knowledge derived from sources such as the arts – literature, painting and poetry – or ethics, all of which differ from the propositional knowledge characteristic of theory.

Closing the Theory–Practice Gap

Nursing is a professional discipline, and nursing theories, however complex or abstract, are practical in nature and reflect the phenomena nurses use to shape how they think, act and be in the world (Smith & Parker 2015). The idea of *praxis*, discussed in Chapter 1, allows for no separation and indeed no distinction between theory and practice. The argument was that practice is by definition informed by some theory, that indeed *praxis* is a form of practice we might term 'living theory': good practice is good theory in action. However, some do see practice and theory as separate and discrete entities and some view the two concepts as not only separate but also discordant ideas. Even in those instances where it

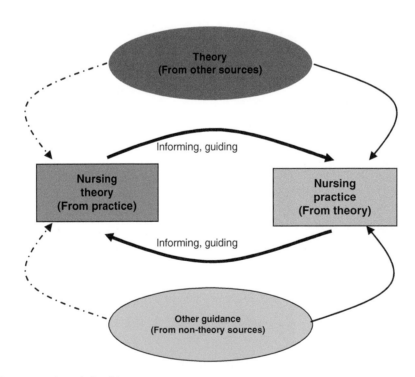

FIGURE 3.8   The theory–practice relationship.

is argued that theory and practice are, in fact, complementary, it is recognised that there is a challenge to be faced in bringing theory and practice together. Smith and Parker (2015) emphasised that nursing students should be willing to accept new ways of thinking, knowing and being within the field of nursing. Investigating structures of nursing knowledge and understanding the nature of nursing as a professional discipline provide a framework to clarify nursing theory.

Over the decades, there have been fewer and fewer publications about the separation of theory and practice or the so-called theory–practice gap. So much so that the term theory–practice gap has become almost shorthand for referring to the whole debate surrounding theory and the difficulties people have experienced in bringing theory into practice. For some, this is not a matter of concern: the two terms are not only separate but desirably so. This, it may be recalled, is a view sometimes expressed by those who see nursing as practical and not involving theory. It is also a view held by those who see theory as largely conjecture and not a valid aspect of science, arguing instead that practice must be based upon the best scientific empirical evidence. However, for others, theory is viewed as essential. It is the basis of science, and theory tested through research is seen to be the basis of best practice. Here, any separation of practice from theory is seen as problematic.

There is a growing body of literature and evidence that theories have become linked to and underpin practice. Evidence clearly shows that as the science and discipline of nursing have developed, theories are being applied and underpin practice. Smith and Parker (2015) highlighted how nursing is defined beyond mere functions, emphasising the role of nursing theories in shaping educational curricula and practice frameworks. They discussed the impact of applying these theories in healthcare settings, specifically in hospitals pursuing magnet status, and how this is aligned with enhancing theoretical applications in nursing. They highlighted the potential benefits of nursing theories in advancing scientific knowledge and improving practice in various healthcare environments.

The increasingly strong link between theory and practice is represented by the increasing development of theories according to different levels of abstraction, the increasing level of knowledge of nurses in practice and the development of reasoning to develop theories for the needs of practice.

Closing the Gap Between Theory and Practice

In Chapter 1, we described the relationship between theory and practice in nursing, offering various definitions of theory and its functions. We also explored why there might be a perception that theory is not used in practice.

We now argue for closing the theory–practice gap:

- In the discipline of nursing, nurses are scientists in all domains, guided by common values, knowledge and processes that guide their professional thinking and actions (Smith & Parker 2015).
- Development of nursing knowledge is the result of theory-based research (theoretical framework) of theoretical nursing research for application in practice, while practice knowledge enriches nursing theory (Smith & Parker 2015).
- Theories represent the real world as seen by the theoretician. Chinn stated, *theories create mental models of 'the way the world is'* (Chinn 2021: 29).
- Understanding the importance of nursing theory has become increasingly clear to both the discipline and the nursing profession as nursing has evolved (Alligood 2018a).

Educators play an essential role in demonstrating the value of theory to practising nurses and preparing them comprehensively for its application. As Meleis (2021) highlighted, academic programmes are crucial in advancing nursing theory. Courses in philosophy, theory development and knowledge advancement in graduate programmes are important as they facilitate theoretical dialogues and contribute to the evolution of the third-, fourth- and fifth-generation theorists. These academic programmes are vital for promoting the dissemination and enhancement of theoretical work in nursing (Meleis 2021). Yancey (2015) also stressed the necessity for nursing education programmes to have a solid theoretical foundation to educate nurses and advance nursing science and highlighted the significance of incorporating nursing theories into curricula to ensure the discipline's development. Many nursing schools, particularly in the United States, have applied nursing theories to guide curriculum development in their BSc, MSc, ANP, PhD and DNP programmes (Smith & Parker 2015; Chism & McLain 2022).

On the other hand, healthcare organisations have also been more active in promoting attention to theoretical applications in nursing practice. Numerous hospitals, aiming for recognition of Magnet® status, have implemented nursing theoretical perspectives into their professional practice models to guide nursing practice within their facilities (Smith 2018; Duffy, 2022). For example, many US acute care hospitals have adopted Watson's theory as a component of

65

their professional practice models (Duffy 2022). Watson's theory provides a philosophical framework that aligns with the Magnet model's emphasis on creating a supportive environment for nurses to thrive. The quality of the practice environment significantly impacts care quality and nurse retention, and theory-guided practice contributes to greater nurse job satisfaction (Smith 2018).

Significant contributions to theory-based education and practice have been made by Jean Watson through her Watson Caring Science Institute (n.d.). The Institute supports institutions in their sustainable commitment to integrating caring science within practices and policies, aiming to transform and broaden the notion of health and healing for its staff as well as the patients, families and communities it serves. Another example is the Anne Boykin Institute for the Advancement of Caring in Nursing (n.d.), which promotes the universal visibility and significance of caring in nursing. We need to emphasise that there are more examples of other theories that are serving as conceptual frameworks for nursing education programmes or as frameworks for practice models in health systems, not only in the United States (Butts & Rich 2022).

With the intensive development of nursing research and theories in the last decades, the core of knowledge/science applied and used in practice has been intensively published. This has also been supported by the raising of educational levels for nurses. Furthermore, it has become clear (as it has been for several decades in the United States and to a lesser extent in the United Kingdom) that practice nurses need postgraduate education. This represents a major shift, emphasising the understanding of the theoretical core of knowledge, research methods and supporting practice – theory and evidence-based informed practice for optimal patient care.

The important issue in all of this is as follows: theory does enhance practice and the practice situation is a testing field for theory, wherein it can be both tried and refined. In addressing closing the theory–practice gap, there may be issues in respect of how science is linked to the practical world, particularly where theory is seen as a part of science. Closing the gap between science and practice will be considered now.

Closing the Science–Practice Gaps

The theory–practice gap in nursing may be influenced by the perception that scientific knowledge, or propositional knowledge, does not necessarily connect with the real world. Theories, as part of this scientific endeavour, are often viewed as detached from reality. However, if you recall from Chapter 1, we have argued that theory plus research equals science and in Chapter 2, it was suggested that we need to know *what* to do, *why* we do it and *how* to do it, and one without the other will not suffice.

Alligood (2018c) explained that as research and knowledge development expanded, it became clear that research without conceptual and theoretical frameworks produced isolated information rather than the core of nursing knowledge. Fawcett (2021) claimed that nurse scientists engage in research to develop and test new mid-range and situation-specific theories as well as test existing ones derived from nursing conceptual models and grand theories. The theories produced through this research provide the necessary basis for evidence-based practice. The primary objective of this research is to create practice guidelines, including assessment formats and intervention protocols. Fawcett (2020) also argued that as theories themselves constitute evidence, no gap exists between theory and practice. She further supported the integration of theory and practice by asserting that while there might be no existing theory that fits a particular practical action, this suggests that any action not founded on theory indicates a need for developing new theories. Thus, evidence-based practice is equivalent to theory-based practice (Fawcett 2022).

Nursing theories play a crucial role by providing a conceptual framework that guides the integration of research findings into clinical decision-making and patient care. Nurses can design and implement interventions that are more targeted and personalised, addressing the unique needs and experiences of patients and aligning with the core principles and values of the nursing profession (Karnick 2016; Baptiste 2023). As nursing continues to evolve, maintaining this synergy between theory and science is crucial for advancing the profession and, most importantly, ensuring the quality of care and well-being of the patient (Baptiste 2023).

Closing the gap between science and practice can also be supported by the expansion of the philosophy of nursing science, growth and use of mid-range and situation-specific theories and nurses embracing different methodologies, quantitative, qualitative and mixed methods to explore unanswered nursing questions (Alligood 2018b). Im and Meleis (2021a, 2021b) stressed the importance of diverse methodological approaches, especially in the development of situation-specific theories in nursing. They emphasised the belief that limiting these approaches is not advisable for the growth of nursing knowledge and explained how this diversity can enrich the discipline through varied research projects, practice situations and conceptualisations, ultimately advancing nursing knowledge.

You will learn more about the relationships between research and theory in Chapter 8. In this chapter, we have aimed to make arguments about closing the theory–practice gap by also addressing the closing science–practice gap.

Closing the Gap: The Role of Technology, Digitalisation and Artificial Intelligence

Advancements in technology, including digitalisation and artificial intelligence (AI), are helping to bridge the gap between theory and practice. These technologies enhance knowledge dissemination, facilitate collaboration and promote evidence-based practice through data-driven decision-making. By providing practitioners with access to *how-to* knowledge, technology addresses key barriers to integrating research findings into clinical settings. Tools such as electronic order sets and decision support systems are pivotal in incorporating research into daily clinical decisions (Harrington 2017), and the integration of AI aims to deliver more personalised and high-quality patient care (Pailaha 2023).

Despite the benefits, the rapid incorporation of technology in nursing poses risks of placing too much focus on technology at the expense of patient care (Krel et al. 2022). It is crucial for nurses to understand how technological changes influence their relationships with patients (Pepito et al. 2023) and to ensure that these technologies complement rather than replace the uniquely human elements of nursing care, maintaining ethical standards (Stokes & Palmer 2020).

Before we continue, since we have touched on the emerging issue of integrating technology and AI in nursing, we must consider how this integration can enhance clinical practice while preserving the essential human touch. This discussion leads us into Reflective Exercise 3.9, where we will explore the impact of AI on evidence-based practices, decision-making in clinical settings and the indispensable human elements of nursing care.

Reflective Exercise 3.9

Exploring Impact of AI in Nursing

Discuss with your peers how AI can support the implementation of evidence-based practices in nursing. Can AI help close any gaps between current research and clinical applications? Can AI replace the decision-making of nurses in clinical settings? Why or why not? What elements of nursing care should always be maintained by human professionals?

Sitzman and Watson (2017) highlighted the ongoing journey of adapting to these technological advances while addressing the accompanying human-technological challenges. They emphasised the importance of integrating human caring and compassion to maintain our humanity amidst these changes. They also illustrate how Watson's theory can guide nurses in navigating the digital landscape. Similarly, Locsin's theory of Technological Competency as Caring in Nursing offers a framework that empowers nurses to leverage technology in a way that enhances their ability to know and care for patients as whole persons, rather than allowing technology to detract from the core nursing value of caring (Locsin & Purnell 2015).

Science (and Theory) Failing – or Saving – the World

Science has progressed from a time when ethical implications were often overlooked, as illustrated by the Manhattan Project at Los Alamos, where the intense distress and guilt experienced by scientists over the devastation caused by the atomic bombs highlight the deep moral conflicts involved. Today, scientists recognise their responsibility to be mindful of the consequences of their work. In nursing, this moral consciousness is manifested especially in a commitment to social justice, addressing structural inequities in healthcare and developing policies that are inclusive and adaptive to global crises such as climate change, migration and conflict.

As Fields et al. (2021) stressed, the COVID-19 pandemic showed the essential role of global alliances and partnerships in safeguarding the health and well-being of all individuals. While the COVID-19 pandemic significantly disrupted the work of nurse scientists, they have played a crucial role not only in minimising the spread of COVID-19 but also in leading research in care delivery science and implementation science, which translates knowledge into practice. Furthermore, nurse scientists can participate in studies aimed at preventing future outbreaks of other infectious diseases. The COVID-19 pandemic reminded us of the importance of conducting robust science. It emphasized the need for reproducibility in scientific research. This situation underscored the importance of reproducibility in scientific inquiry (Pickler et al. 2020; McKenna & Thompson 2023).

In 2015, every United Nations member state unanimously agreed to pursue the sustainable development goals (SDGs) within the 2030 Agenda for Sustainable Development, a comprehensive set of objectives aimed at improving global economic, social and environmental conditions. The nursing profession plays a crucial role in realising these goals, starting with enhancing awareness through education and a commitment to research, as well as active participation in both local and global decision-making processes (Fields et al. 2021; Sensor et al. 2021).

Disrupting structural inequities, particularly in contexts of poverty, has profound implications for healthcare globally. Wars and conflicts, such as those in Ukraine and Gaza, along with widespread unrest, exacerbate these inequities, severely disrupting nursing services and increasing health risks among civilian populations. Concurrently, climate change contributes to health emergencies by affecting living conditions and food security, intensifying the challenges faced by millions of migrants. These migrants, often fleeing environmental disasters or conflict, encounter additional barriers in accessing healthcare, further highlighting the urgent need for inclusive health policies that address these multifaceted challenges. Kalogirou et al. (2020) emphasise that nurses have been slow to respond to climate change, often not seeing it as a professional issue. Adopting a planetary health perspective is recommended as a theoretical foundation for nursing education, research and practice. Embracing this perspective could advance the nursing profession and guide healthcare systems toward a climate-resilient future.

This intersection of crises underscores the critical need for international cooperation and robust healthcare systems that can withstand and adapt to complex global changes. According to Chinn (2021) and her concept of emancipatory nursing, this approach integrates into various aspects of the nursing field, including practice, theory, research, policy and education, emphasising its fundamental goal of promoting social justice within these areas.

To some extent, the modern scientific community is still polarised into two camps. On the one side, a largely green and populist grouping is concerned with ensuring that science does not harm our environment and that its 'discoveries' are geared towards ecological protection and the benefit of society in general. On the other side, a largely opportunist and capitalist grouping is concerned with acquiring profit for the few (sometimes even to the extent that others are harmed). Thus, some science is seen as supporting for-profit industry and technology that increases hothouse gases and deliberately facilitates technology that underpins unethical practices such as the sale of high-tar tobacco products in the developing world. Conversely, other science is seen as supporting such beneficial technologies as the development of largely harmless wind turbine energy and facilitating the development of safe technology, including the development of pharmaceuticals by ethically acceptable research.

One danger in the emergence of a moral conscience and the establishment of ethical positions is that one might end up taking 'the moral high ground', not only claiming but also believing that one knows best. If the belief that 'science' knows best in a moral sense comes together with an equally strong belief that science is the only real source of knowledge and, furthermore, that it is capable of uncovering knowledge to solve most, if not all, of our problems, the claims being made are not only extreme but dangerous. This is because, allied to the belief that science knows best – indeed, that only science really *knows* at all – is an almost blind faith in its capabilities and an equally blind rejection of alternatives (as presented in religion, law or other forms of non-scientific thought) (see Reflective Exercise 3.10). This may be viewed as a naïve and misguided position at best or as an arrogant and deceptive position at worst.

Reflective Exercise 3.10

From Science to Utopia

There is a view that science can solve all the problems of humankind – that, as we advance our sciences and our technologies, we will eradicate disease and need, construct ideal living environments and create a perfect and harmonious world for living.

However, such faith in science may be naïve. The term *scientism* is used to describe this. Scientism is the view that the natural sciences are the only valid sources of factual knowledge about the world (Williams 1983). There is an almost blind faith in what is viewed as hard science, believing that science will solve all our problems, leading us into a new and better world.

For now, draw upon your own experience to date in clinical settings. Do you feel that there is too much faith being placed in the technologies of science? Is this more characteristic of some groups than others? In particular, compare medical and nursing staff – do they differ in their alignment to the scientific orientation, and if so, why?

It is important to emphasise that during the COVID-19 pandemic, science scepticism emerged, also within the nursing profession. Ideologies and worldviews significantly influenced this scepticism. During COVID-19, one group of scientists recommended herd immunity (e.g. in Sweden) as a means of building up immunity. Alternatively, others recommended strict lockdown. Which scientists were right and did this confuse the community and undermine faith in science? The origins of scepticism about COVID-19 often closely align with those of climate change scepticism (Rutjens et al. 2021).

Science (and Theory) Disappointing the World

It is important to remember that, especially from the mid to late 20th century, scepticism about science extended beyond moral concerns. The movement known as positivism, which was discussed in Chapter 2, had exerted an influence well beyond the bounds of the laboratory and the academy. The fundamental 'positivist' position saw science as a quest for real or genuine true knowledge. This could only be achieved by observing – that is, through sensing and experiencing – how things were and how things worked in the world. In effect, the only genuine knowledge was that procured through empirical (experiential) means, by the objective identification and measurement of phenomena.

The positivists' claims for absolute truth were persuasive. They fit well with significant scientific discoveries that *did* greatly benefit humanity. Furthermore, the devaluing of other forms of knowledge in comparison to this persuasive position was also in turn compelling. Society, having previously placed its faith in religion and law, now saw science as the route to a new Utopia. Science would eradicate poverty and disease; it would allow us to develop new technologies that would make life a veritable heaven upon earth. Consider the labour-saving devices that we have in our homes or that we carry on our person.

Unfortunately, while science led to the invention of life-saving technologies like penicillin and electricity, it also resulted in harmful developments like thalidomide – a highly toxic medicine for unborn infants – asbestos that fireproofed buildings yet caused cancer and nuclear weapons. It became clear that science could not guarantee absolute truth or fully harness nature to our advantage, and its products might sometimes be harmful. This acknowledgement does not diminish the significant benefits that science and technology have provided, which are crucial to the well-being of people, all living things and the environment. The impacts of past inventions such as antibiotics and electricity are at least matched by modern technologies like the Internet, which supports initiatives like distance education and telemedicine. However, what has changed is the growing realisation that the products of science and technology can also be harmful and potentially destructive on a global scale.

It might be suggested on the basis of the latter arguments that the relationship between science and practice is a complex one. Science, we have seen, does lead to technological advances that have a direct impact on practice. Intercontinental air travel, modern antibiotics, high-technology food processing, laser technology and automobile travel have all had profound practical implications for how we live today. But the relationship is complicated and not without its negative aspects. In a sense, we are deceived into the false security of a brave and bright new world. But this is an illusion. The costs of modern super-antibiotics are the ravages of superbugs and methicillin-resistant *Staphylococcus aureus* (MRSA) infections. The costs of increasingly available air travel are massive increases in hothouse gases and global warming. And the cost of such technology that relieves us of burdens of activity (such as physical toil) includes the consequences of sedentary living: obesity, hypertension, cardiac disease and cancers.

The COVID-19 pandemic serves as another potent example of both the power and the limits of modern science. On the one hand, scientific research facilitated the rapid development of vaccines, showcasing technology's potential to effectively address global health crises. On the other hand, the pandemic exposed vulnerabilities in global public health systems, led to disruptions in healthcare that delayed treatment for other diseases and caused a rise in mental health issues, such as anxiety and depression, exacerbated by social isolation and economic uncertainties. Additionally, it highlighted economic disruptions and the societal costs associated with managing such a crisis, including the potential long-term consequences of COVID-19.

It is important to recognise that by the latter half of the 20th century, a more reasoned and realistic outlook on the limits of science had emerged. As discussed in Chapter 2, this still broadly positivistic perspective, known as *post-positivism*, adopted the more balanced view that scientific evidence can only be viewed as the best available knowledge until and if or when it is refuted. This perspective in a sense reinforced the link between theory (making conjectures) and practice (seeking refutations through actions based on testing those theories – i.e. research). Such outlooks are definitive of the post-positivistic orientation.

We can see that by exploring ontological and epistemological questions, nursing scholars have investigated the foundational aspects of nursing and articulated the meaning of nursing science from diverse philosophical perspectives. Today, we observe nurse scholars and practitioners, instead of practising under some specific paradigms, use multiple paradigms, methodologies and approaches to develop nursing knowledge. It might be that nurse scholars should focus on developing mid-range theories and situation-specific theories, which are developed to help nurses determine their actions in particular clinical situations, thereby advancing nursing knowledge and guiding nursing practice (Younas & Parsons 2019). This is also supported by Im and Meleis (2021a, 2021b) who advocated philosophical diversity in nursing theory. They stressed the necessity of philosophical, theoretical and methodological plurality in nursing and explained how pluralism aligns with the goals of nursing and the development of SST. They detail three major philosophical roots – postempiricism, critical social theory and feminism, and hermeneutics – as foundational to SST.

To conclude, contemporary nursing benefits from a multi-paradigmatic approach and diverse methodologies, enhancing effective nursing praxis. Nurse scholars and practitioners are encouraged to continue using various paradigms, methodologies and approaches, rather than limiting themselves to specific ones, to further develop nursing knowledge (Deeb et al. 2024).

Science and Nursing Theory

Early nursing theorists in the 1950s through the 1970s, heavily influenced by the prevailing scientific perspectives of their time, aimed to develop nursing theories that could be empirically tested or refuted. However, this goal was not entirely successful, leading to a shift towards mid-range and situation-specific theories that are more applicable to current practical issues but lack broad generalisability. Additionally, criticisms from scholars like Donald Schön in *The Reflective Practitioner* showed the limitations of propositional (technical-rational) knowledge in professional practice, advocating for a more reflexive approach to adapt to the dynamic and ever-changing nature of real-world problems (Schön 1983). This reflects a broader trend in nursing theory to move from static reflection on established knowledge to a more dynamic and adaptive reflexive approach in practice.

Reflection in and on action also has limitations. What may be required is a movement from a position of *reflection* on what is (or was in the past) knowable, to a more *reflexive* orientation to dynamic changing processes. As the argument runs here, such is the dynamic and changing nature of the world that our past knowledge and previous experiences are of limited value in addressing new and previously unencountered phenomena and the problems they present. We must therefore develop reflexive approaches – wherein the nature of what we encounter challenges us to respond appropriately.

The future of nursing knowledge development is difficult to predict precisely. However, it is reasonable to expect certain changes based on current trends and priorities within the nursing field and broader society worldwide. The advancement of nursing knowledge will increasingly rely on nurses who possess robust analytical skills to identify areas needing research, like nurses with advanced nursing practice and doctor of nursing practice degrees (Rodgers 2022). You will learn more about new roles in nursing in Chapter 4. All activities – whether administrative, clinical or research oriented – should be conducted with an understanding of the essential connections between the discipline of nursing, its knowledge base, including the organisation of knowledge into theories and nursing practice (Rodgers 2022).

The Questions Begged – Some Answers

We have concerned ourselves in this chapter with how practice and theory are related and posed a number of questions at the outset. The fundamental questions (by definition binary in nature), which are even contained within our chapter title, are as follows:

- Does our practice derive from theory?
- Does our theory derive from our practice?

The questions are not simple to answer, and we can return to our opening quotation from Merton (1969). As we delve into these issues, we uncover inconsistencies and ambiguities. This chapter has shown that seemingly simple questions are, in fact, complex and multifaceted. If this exploration has made you more sceptical and critical of superficial statements about the relationship between theory and practice, you have accomplished a great deal.

Fortunately, from this chapter, we can add some comments about the relationship between theory and practice, as follows:

1. We must recognise the close complementary relationship between theory and practice, including the knowledge of practical doing that we term 'know-how'. We must know *what* the best thing is to do in practice situations (through knowledge derived from tested theory), and we must know *how* to do it (through the development of practical know-how).

2. We recognise different levels of theory in terms of sophistication and abstraction.

3. There are different sources of theoretical knowledge, and these can be seen as emerging from other disciplines through being adopted or adapted to the nursing purpose; or emerging from the nursing field itself as theory derived from practice; or indeed from all these sources (e.g. where the practice context helps us to adapt non-nursing theory to the nursing context).

4. Knowledge used in practice must be thoroughly tested and presented as the best information or evidence available, as in evidence-based practice. Theory, even where it is constructed from reliable evidence, should be tested for its fitness for purpose.

5. We recognise the distinction between theory and theorising and also the case for recognising that we all theorise (attempt to make sense of our environment), as a fundamental characteristic of being human.

6. Given that nurses themselves theorise about their practice, we recognise that there is no such thing as practice without theory. We therefore recognise the need to ensure that this valuable, context-bound theory is also nurtured and, where possible, explicated and tested.

7. Insofar as nurses do themselves theorise and are also presented with theory that may inform their practice, there is a need to develop within nursing practice a sceptical and critical approach to theory, particularly where it has not or cannot be adequately tested.

8. We have demonstrated that theory is derived from science and in turn contributes to science. To the extent that theory is indeed sometimes recognised as part of science (the conjectural, creative part that relates to and indeed guides the doing or research part), there is a need to view critically what has been and what can be achieved by science and theory.

9. There is a particular need to recognise the risks that have emerged from science, some of a global nature and the ways in which these risks impact on our practice.

10. There is a need to look to the future that is unfurling, and how we might respond indicates the importance of embracing nursing theories, especially mid-range and SST theories.

Conclusion

The relationship between theory and practice has been explored in detail. The definitional statements of the theory were extended into classifying theory in terms of increasing sophistication (as in descriptive, explanatory, predictive and prescriptive theory) and increasingly abstract properties (as in meta-theory, grand theory, mid-range theory and situation-specific theory). The relationship was further explored in terms of how theory may inform practice and how, in turn, practice may inform theory and contribute to theory construction. This discussion was carried forward into the issue of the relationship between science and practice, given that theory is most often recognised as a part of science.

In the link between science, theory and practice, we have cited the philosophical diversity in nursing theory and the need for philosophical, theoretical and methodological pluralism in nursing. Grand theories and conceptual models represent an important philosophical and historical aspect of the theoretical underpinning of nursing. However, with the development of mid-range and situation-specific theories, we are slowly closing the gap between theory and practice and theory and science.

Revision Points

- Theory was defined as statements that link (by propositions) ideas (concepts) about the world, thus creating knowledge.

- It was argued that theory development and use are vital for nursing practice. However, there is an argument that as nursing requires practical knowledge it cannot develop theories, which, by their nature, rely on propositions.

- Two possible ways of categorising theory were identified: on the basis of the sophistication or abstraction of the theory.

- In terms of sophistication, Dickoff and James's (1968) four levels of theory were provided as an example: factor-isolating, factor-relating, situation-relating and situation-producing theories.

- In terms of abstraction, different levels of theory were identified: situation-specific, mid-range, grand and meta-theory.

- Despite the importance of theory for nursing, there is a theory–practice gap and there are many possible causes for this gap and various ways of closing the gap.

- As theory is linked to science, the positive and negative contributions of science to nursing and society were explored.

Additional Reading

Deeb A.M., Vaughan C., Puddester R. & Curnew D. (2024) Embracing paradigmatic diversity in nursing: the stadium model in nursing. *Advances in Nursing Science*, **47**(3), 274–228.

Fawcett J. (2020) Thoughts about nursing science and nursing sciencing revisited. *Nursing Science Quarterly*, **33**(1), 97–99.

Younas A. & Parsons K. (2019) Implications for paradigm shift in nursing: a critical analysis of Thomas Kuhn's revolutionary science and its relevance to nursing. *Advances in Nursing Science*, **42**(3), 243–254.

References

Abdellah F.G., Beland I.L., Martin A. & Matheney R.V. (1960) *Patient Centred Approaches to Nursing*. New York: Macmillan.

Alligood M.R. (2018a) Introduction to nursing theory: its history and significance. In Alligood M.R. (ed.) *Nursing Theorists and Their Work*, 9th edition, pp. 2–10. St. Louis, MO: Elsevier.

Alligood M.R. (2018b) State of the art and science of nursing theory. In Alligood M.R. (ed.) *Nursing Theorists and Their Work*, 9th edition, pp. 573–578. St. Louis, MO: Elsevier.

Alligood M.R. (2018c) *Nursing Theorists and Their Work*, 9th edition. St. Louis, MO: Elsevier.

Anne Boykin Institute for the Advancement of Caring in Nursing (n.d.) https://nursing.fau.edu/outreach/anne-boykin-institute/index.php – accessed 15 June 2024.

Argyris C. & Schön D.A. (1974) *Theory in Practice: Increasing Professional Effectiveness*. London: Jossey-Bass.

Auvil-Novak S.E. (1997) A middle-range theory of chronotherapeutic intervention for postsurgical pain. *Nursing Research*, **46**(2), 66–71.

Baptiste D. (2023) Integrating nursing theory into evidence-based practice: bridging the gap between research and patient-centered care. *Journal of Nursing & Health Sciences*, **9**(4), 1–2.

Burkhart L. & Hogan N. (2008) An experiential theory of spiritual care in nursing practice. *Qualitative Health Research*, **18**(7), 928–938.

Burkhart L. & Hogan N. (2020) Spiritual care in nursing practice (SCiNP). In Peterson S.J. & Bredow T.S. (eds) *Middle Range Theories: Application to Nursing Research and Practice*, 5th edition, pp. 116–125. Philadelphia, PA: Wolters Kluwer.

Butts J.M. & Rich K.L. (eds) (2022) *Philosophies and Theories for Advanced Nursing Practice*, 4th edition. Burlington: Jones & Bartlett Learning.

Chinn P.L. (2021) Equity and social justice in developing theories. In Im E.O. & Meleis A.I. (eds) *Situation Specific Theories: Development, Utilization, and Evaluation in Nursing*, pp. 29–37. Cham: Springer.

Chinn P.L., Kramer M.K. & Sitzman K. (2022) *Knowledge Development in Nursing: Theory and Process*, 10th edition. St. Louis, MO: Elsevier.

Chism L.A. & McLain N. (2022) The essentials of the doctor of nursing practice: a philosophical perspective. In Butts J.M. & Rich K.L. (eds) *Philosophies and Theories for Advanced Nursing Practice*, 3rd edition, pp. 47–66. Burlington: Jones & Bartlett Learning.

Covell C.L. (2008) The middle-range theory of nursing intellectual capital. *Journal of Advanced Nursing*, **63**(1), 94–103.

Covell C.L. & Sidani S. (2013) Nursing intellectual capital theory: testing selected propositions. *Journal of Advanced Nursing*, **69**(11), 2432–2445.

Davidson J.E. (2010) Facilitated sensemaking: a strategy and new middle-range theory to support families of intensive care unit patients. *Critical Care Nurse*, **30**(6), 28–39.

Deeb A.M., Vaughan C., Puddester R. & Curnew D. (2024) Embracing paradigmatic diversity in nursing: the stadium model in nursing. *Advances in Nursing Science*. (ahead of print)

Dickoff J. & James P. (1968) A theory of theories: a position paper. *Nursing Research*, **17**(3), 197–203.

Duffy J.R. (2022) Theories focused on caring. In Butts J.M. & Rich K.L. (eds) *Philosophies and Theories for Advanced Nursing Practice*, 4th edition, pp. 447–464. Burlington: Jones & Bartlett Learning.

Edwards S. & Liaschenko J. (2003) On the quest for a theory of nursing. *Nursing Philosophy*, **4**, 1–3.

Elo S., Kääriäinen M., Isola A. & Kyngäs H. (2013) Developing and testing a middle-range theory of the well-being supportive physical environment of home-dwelling elderly. *Scientific World Journal*, **13**, 945635.

Fawcett J. (2005) *Contemporary Nursing Knowledge: Analysis and Evaluation of Nursing Models and Theories*, 3rd edition. Philadelphia, PA: F.A. Davis.

Fawcett J. (2020) Thoughts about nursing science and nursing sciencing revisited. *Nursing Science Quarterly*, **33**(1), 97–99.

Fawcett J. (2021) Middle-range theories and situation-specific theories: similarities and differences. In Im E.O. & Meleis A.I. (eds) *Situation Specific Theories: Development, Utilization, and Evaluation in Nursing*, pp. 39–48. Cham: Springer.

Fawcett J. (2022) Using theory in evidence based advanced nursology practice. In Butts J.M. & Rich K.L. (eds) *Philosophies and Theories for Advanced Nursing Practice*, 3rd edition. Burlington, Cham, Switzerland: Jones & Bartlett Learning.

Fearon-Lynch J.A. & Stover C.M. (2015) A middle-range theory for diabetes self-management mastery. *Advances in Nursing Science*, **38**(4), 330–346.

Fields L., Perkiss S., Dean B.A. & Moroney T. (2021) Nursing and the sustainable development goals: a scoping review. *Journal of Nursing Scholarship*, **53**(5), 568–577.

Harrington L. (2017) Closing the science-practice gap with technology: from evidence-based practice to practice-based evidence. *AACN Advanced Critical Care*, **28**(1), 12–15.

73

Henderson V. (1966) *The Nature of Nursing: A Definition and its Implications for Practice, Education and Research*. London: Collier Macmillan.

Im E.O. (2005) Development of situation-specific theories: an integrative approach. *Advances in Nursing Science*, **28**(2), 137–151.

Im E.O. & Meleis A.I. (1999) Situation – specific theories: philosophical roots, properties, and approach. *Advances in Nursing Science*, **22**(2), 11–24.

Im E.O. & Meleis A.I. (2021a) *Situation Specific Theories: Development, Utilization, and Evaluation in Nursing*. Cham: Springer.

Im E.O. & Meleis A.I. (2021b) Situation-specific theories: philosophical roots, properties, and approach. In Im E.O. & Meleis A.I. (eds) *Situation Specific Theories: Development, Utilization, and Evaluation in Nursing*, pp. 13–27. Cham: Springer.

Jacox A.K. (1974) Theory construction in nursing: an overview. *Nursing Research*, **23**(1), 4–13.

Johnson D.E. (1959) The nature of a science of nursing. *Nursing Outlook*, **7**, 291–294.

Kalogirou M.R., Dahlke S., Davidson S. & Yamamoto S. (2020) Nurses' perspectives on climate change, health and nursing practice. *Journal of Clinical Nursing*, **29**(23–24), 4759–4768.

Karnick P.M. (2016) Evidence-based practice and nursing theory. *Nursing Science Quarterly*, **29**(4), 283–284.

King I. (1968) A conceptual frame of reference for nursing. *Nursing Research*, **17**(1), 27–31.

Krel C., Vrbnjak D., Bevc S., Štiglic G. & Pajnkihar M. (2022) Technological competency as caring in nursing: a description, analysis and evaluation of the theory. *Zdravstveno Varstvo*, **61**(2), 115–123.

Lenz R.R. & Pugh L.C. (2018) Theory of unpleasant symptoms. In Smith M.J. & Liehr P.R. (eds) *Middle Range Theory for Nursing*, 4th edition, pp. 179–214. New York: Springer Publications.

Levine M.E. (1966) Adaptation and assessment: a rationale for nursing intervention. *American Journal of Nursing*, **66**(11), 2450–2453.

Locsin R.C. & Purnell M. (2015) Advancing the theory of technological competency as caring in nursing: the universal technological domain. *International Journal for Human Caring*, **19**, 51–54.

Maslow A.H. (1954) *Motivation and Personality*. New York: Harper & Row.

McEwen M. & Wills E.M. (2007) *Theoretical Basis for Nursing*, 2nd edition. Philadelphia, PA: Lippincott Williams & Wilkins.

McEwen M. & Wills E.M. (2019) *Theoretical Basis for Nursing*, 5th edition. Philadelphia, PA: Wolters Kluwer.

McEwen M. & Wills E.M. (2023) *Theoretical Basis for Nursing*, 6th edition. Philadelphia, PA: Wolters Kluwer.

McKenna H. (1997) *Nursing Theories and Models*. London: Routledge.

McKenna H.P., Pajnkihar M. & Murphy F.A. (2014) *Fundamentals of Nursing Models Theories and Practice*. London: Wiley Blackwell.

McKenna H.P. & Thompson D.R. (2023) Fake news, the research reproducibility crisis. *International Journal of Nursing Studies*, **138**. DOI: 10.1016/j.ijnurstu.2022.104396

Mefford L.C. (2004) A theory of health promotion for preterm infants based on Levine's conservation model of nursing. *Nursing Science Quarterly*, **17**, 260–266.

Meleis A.I. (ed.) (2012) *Theoretical Nursing: Development and Progress*, 5th edition. Philadelphia, PA: Wolters Kluwer/Lippincott Williams & Wilkins.

Meleis A.I. (ed.) (2018) *Theoretical Nursing: Development and Progress*, 6th edition. Philadelphia, PA: Wolters Kluwer/Lippincott Williams & Wilkins.

Meleis A.I. (2021) Development of situation-specific theories: an integrative approach. In Im E.O. & Meleis A.I. (eds) *Situation Specific Theories: Development, Utilization, and Evaluation in Nursing*, pp. 49–65. Cham: Springer.

Meleis A.I., Sawyer L.M., Eun O.I., Hilfinger-Messias D.K. & Schumacher K. (2000) Experiencing transitions: an emerging middle-range theory. *Advances in Nursing Science*, **23**(1), 12–28.

Merton R.K. (1968) *Social Theory and Social Structure*. New York: Free Press.

Merton T. (1969) *My Argument with the Gestapo: A Macaronic Journal*. New York: Doubleday & The Abbey of Gethsemane.

Mishel M.H. (1990) Reconceptualisation of the uncertainty in illness theory. *The Journal of Nurse Scholarship*, **22**, 256–261.

Morse J.M. (2005) Creating a qualitatively-derived theory of suffering. In Zeitler U. (ed.) *Clinical practice and development in nursing*, pp. 83–91. Aarhus, Denmark: Center for Innovation in Nurse Training, Center for Innovation in Nurse Training.

Nelson A.M. (2006) Toward a situation-specific theory of breastfeeding. *Research and Theory for Nursing Practice*, **20**(1), 9–27.

Nightingale F. (1859/1980) *Notes on Nursing: What It Is and What It Is Not*. Edinburgh: Churchill Livingstone.

Orem D.E. (1958) *Nursing: Concepts of Practice*. New York: McGraw Hill.

Orem D.E. (1980) *Nursing Concepts of Practice*, 2nd edition. New York: McGraw Hill.

Orem D.E. (1995) *Nursing Concepts of Practice*, 5th edition. St. Louis, MO: Mosby, Inc.

Orlando I. (1961) *The Dynamic Nurse Patient Relationship. Function, Process, and Principles*. New York: G.P. Putnam & Sons.

Pailaha A.D. (2023) The Impact and Issues of Artificial Intelligence in Nursing Science and Healthcare Settings. *Open Nursing*, **9**, 23779608231196847.

Parse R.R. (1981) *Man-Living-Health: A Theory of Nursing*. New York: John Wiley & Sons.

Paterson J.G. & Zderad L.T. (1976) *Humanistic Nursing*. New York: John Wiley & Sons.

Pender N., Murdaugh C. & Parsons N.A. (2015) *Health Promotion in Nursing Practice*, 7th edition. New York: Prentice Hall.

Pepito J.A.T., Babate F.J.G. & Dator W.L.T. (2023) The nurses' touch: an irreplaceable component of caring. *Nursing Open*, **10**(9), 5838–5842.

Peplau E.H. (1952) *Interpersonal Relations in Nursing: A Conceptual Frame of Reference for Psychodynamic Nursing*. New York: G.P. Putnam & Sons.

Peplau H.E. (1992) Interpersonal relations: a theoretical framework for application in nursing practice. *Nursing Science Quarterly*, **5**, 13–18.

Peterson S.J. & Bredow T.S. (2020) *Middle range theories: application to nursing research and practice*, 5th edition. Philadelphia, PA: Wolters Kluwer.

Pickett S., Peters R.M. & Jarosz P.A. (2014) Toward a middle-range theory of weight management. *Nursing Science Quarterly*, **27**(3), 242–247.

Pickler R.H., Abshire D.A., Chao A.M., Chlan L.L., Stanfill A.G., Hacker E.D. et al. (2020) Nursing science and COVID-19. *Nursing Outlook*, **68**(5), 685–688.

Riegel B., Jaarsma T. & Strömberg A. (2012) A middle-range theory of self-care of chronic illness. *Advances in Nursing Science*, **35**(3), 194–204.

Rodgers B.L. (2022) The evolution of nursing science. In Butts J.M. & Rich K.L. (eds) *Philosophies and Theories for Advanced Nursing Practice*, 4th edition, pp. 17–46. Burlington: Jones & Bartlett Learning.

Rogers M.E. (1970) *An Introduction to a Theoretical Basis of Nursing*, 1st edition. Philadelphia, PA: F.A. Davis.

Roper N., Logan N. & Tierney A. (1983) *Using a Model for Nursing*. Edinburgh: Churchill Livingstone.

Roper N., Logan W. & Tierney A.J. (2000) *The Roper-Logan-Tierney Model of Nursing Based on Activities of Living*. Edinburgh: Churchill Livingstone.

Roy C. (1970) Adaptation: a conceptual framework for nursing. *Nursing Outlook*, **18**(3), 42–45.

Roy C. (1980) The Roy adaptation model. In Riehl J.P. & Roy C. (eds) *Conceptual Models for Nursing Practice*. New York: Appleton-Century-Crofts.

Rutjens B.T., van der Linden S. & van der Lee R. (2021) Science skepticism in times of COVID-19. *Group Processes & Intergroup Relations*, **24**(2), 276–283.

Sacks J.L. & Volker D.L. (2015) For their patients: a study of hospice nurses' responses to patient suffering. *Journal of Hospice & Palliative Nursing*, **17**(6), 490–500.

Schön D.A. (1983) *The Reflective Practitioner: How Professionals Think in Action*. New York: Basic Books.

Schumacher K.L. & Meleis A.I. (1994) Transitions: a central concept in nursing. *Journal of Nursing Scholarship*, **26**(2), 119–127.

Scoloveno R. (2015) A theoretical model of health-related outcomes of resilience in middle adolescents. *Western Journal of Nursing Research*, **37**(3), 342–359.

Sensor C.S., Branden P.S., Clary-Muronda V., Hawkins J.E., Fitzgerald D., Shimek A.M. et al. (2021) Nurses achieving the sustainable development goals: the united nations and sigma. *American Journal of Nursing*, **121**(4), 65–68.

Sitzman K. & Watson J. (2017) *Watson's Caring in the Digital World: A Guide for Caring When Interacting, Teaching, and Learning in Cyberspace*. New York: Springer.

Slevin O. (2003) Nursing as a profession. In Basford L. & Slevin O. (eds) *Theory and Practice of Nursing: An Integrated Approach to Caring Practice*, 2nd edition. Cheltenham: Nelson Thornes.

Smith M.C. (1994) Arriving at a philosophy of nursing: discovering? constructing? evolving? In Kikuchi J.F. & Simmons H. (eds) *Developing a Philosophy of Nursing*. Newbury Park, CA: Sage.

Smith M.C. (2018) Disciplinary perspectives linked to middle range theory. In Smith M.J. & Liehr P.R. (eds) *Middle Range Theory for Nursing*, 4th edition. New York: Springer Publications.

Smith C.E., Pace K., Kochinda C., Kleinbeck S.V., Koehler J. & Popkess-Vawter S. (2002) Caregiving effectiveness model evolution to a midrange theory of home care: a process for critique and replication. *Advances in Nursing Science*, **25**(1), 50–64.

Smith M.C. & Parker M.E. (2015) *Nursing Theories and Nursing Practice*, 4th edition. Philadelphia, PA: FA Davis.

Stokes F. & Palmer A. (2020) Artificial intelligence and robotics in nursing: ethics of caring as a guide to dividing tasks between AI and humans. *Nursing Philosophy*, **21**(4), e12306.

Swanson K.M. (1991) Empirical development of a middle range theory of caring. *Nursing Research*, **40**(3), 161–166.

Travelbee J. (1966) *Interpersonal Aspects of Nursing*. Philadelphia, PA: F.A. Davis.

Walker L.O. & Avant K.C. (2019) *Strategies for Theory Construction in Nursing*, 6th edition. Boston, MA: Pearson.

Walling A. (2006) Therapeutic modulation of the psychoneuroimmune system by medical acupuncture creates enhanced feelings of well-being. *Journal of the American Academy of Nurse Practitioners*, **18**(4), 135–143.

Watson J. (1979) *Nursing: The Philosophy and Science of Caring*. Boston, MA: Little, Brown.

Watson Caring Science Institute (n.d.) https://www.watsoncaringscience.org/ – accessed 15 June 2024.

Wiedenbach E. (1964) *Clinical Nursing: a Helping Art*. New York: Springer Publication Company.

Williams R. (1983) *Keywords*, 2nd edition. London: Fontana.

Yancey N.R. (2015) Why teach nursing theory? *Nursing Science Quarterly*, **28**(4), 274–278.

Younas A. & Parsons K. (2019) Implications for paradigm shift in nursing: a critical analysis of Thomas Kuhn's revolutionary science and its relevance to nursing. *Advances in Nursing Science*, **42**(3), 243–254.

CHAPTER 4

Nursing Theories and New Nursing Roles

Outline of Content

The impact of worldwide advances in healthcare systems on the roles of healthcare professionals has been dramatic. In particular, the introduction of new and innovative advanced nursing practice roles to meet these new challenges is described. Particular attention is paid to the use of theory to inform nursing practice in circumstances where methods of care delivery are changing, and new advanced nursing practice roles are developing.

Learning Outcomes

At the end of this chapter, you should be able to:

1. Define what is meant by 'role'
2. Outline the background to the development of new advanced practice roles in nursing
3. Identify implications for nursing associated with the development of these new roles
4. Discuss the contribution of role theory in analysing new nursing roles
5. Discuss the influence of the biomedical model on new nursing roles and outline alternative models
6. Argue the importance of nursing theories for new roles in nursing

Introduction

Advancements in health technology, professional knowledge, skills, patient needs and expectations have transformed healthcare into a dynamic field. These changes, evident in healthcare systems worldwide, are influencing the type of care provided and the format of its provision. The rapid and complex changes occurring in health systems globally provide

Fundamentals of Nursing Models, Theories and Practice, Third Edition. Hugh P. McKenna, Majda Pajnkihar and Dominika Vrbnjak.
© 2025 John Wiley & Sons Ltd. Published 2025 by John Wiley & Sons Ltd.
Companion website: www.wiley.com/go/nursingmodels3e

opportunities for nurses to expand and advance their roles, better meeting and responding to the needs of the populations and systems they serve (Oulton & Caldwell 2017; Lusk et al. 2019).

Many countries worldwide have implemented reforms to introduce advanced nursing roles, aiming to enhance access to care, improve quality and reduce healthcare costs (Maier, Aiken & Busse 2017; ICN 2020). While countries are at different stages of developing these roles, with different educational preparation, role definition, scope of practice, regulatory requirements and terminology, these roles continue to expand and evolve to meet the changing demands of healthcare systems worldwide (ICN 2020). There is a well-established and growing body of research evidence indicating that nurses in new roles provide quality, safe and effective care (Maier, Aiken & Busse 2017; Oulton & Caldwell 2017).

The scope of advanced nursing practice (ANP) extends beyond traditional nursing and overlaps with medicine due to its autonomous nature, encompassing direct and indirect care, as well as illness prevention and treatment (ICN 2020). Therefore, it is not surprising that advanced practice nurses (APNs) often struggle with identity issues and feel lost when trying to find nursing theories to guide their work (Zhang 2024).

While advanced nursing practice is at various stages of development and implementation worldwide, the literature suggests that this trend will continue into the future, especially as more countries embrace this role (Oulton & Caldwell 2017; Brownwood & Lafortune 2024). As the role of advanced practice nurses becomes established globally (Wheeler et al. 2022), it is crucial to explore how nursing theories can support and guide their practice.

In this chapter, we will:

- briefly overview the background to the development of these advanced practice roles in nursing with a consideration of some implications of these new roles;
- consider role theory and the biomedical model to discuss whether these might have some relevance to new nursing roles;
- examine how nursing theories can support and guide practice within these new roles.

Defining Role

The concept of role is difficult to define and analyse due to its multidimensional nature. Perhaps the most common definition is that a role refers to the set of prescriptions defining what the behaviour should be in a specific job, such as nursing, or in a particular social position, such as being a mother (see Key concepts 4.1). Along with a role comes *expectations* of how the person should behave, and this is an important component of defining the role.

🔍 Key Concepts 4.1

Defining a Role

Role: a set of prescriptions defining what the behaviour should be in a specific job (e.g. nursing) or in a particular social position (e.g. being a mother).

Background to the Development of New Roles in Nursing

As already stated, it is recognised that the identification and context of advanced nursing practice varies in different parts of the world (ICN 2020). In 2002, ICN provided an official position on advanced practice nursing and continues to promote a common vision that fosters a greater understanding among international nursing and healthcare communities regarding the development of new roles (ICN 2020). The International Council of Nurses Nurse Practitioner/Advanced Practice Nurse Network (ICN NP/APNN) periodically analyses advanced practice nursing roles (Wheeler et al. 2022).

Regardless of work setting or practice focus, APNs are practitioners who provide safe and competent patient care and have achieved education, typically requiring at least a master's degree. They have roles or levels of practice with increased levels of competency and capability that are measurable beyond those of generalist nurses. These nurses have acquired the ability to explain and apply the theoretical, empirical, ethical, legal, care giving and professional development required for advanced practice nursing. They have defined APN competencies and standards that are periodically reviewed to ensure they remain current. Furthermore, their practice is influenced by global, social, political, economic and technological factors (ICN 2020: 9).

APNs provide care across the entire health continuum, from health promotion and illness prevention to curative, rehabilitative and supportive services. They serve individuals, families, groups and communities throughout all stages of life. They work in various sectors, including both public and private, and in diverse geographic locations, ranging from urban to rural settings (Oulton & Caldwell 2017).

The Clinical Nurse Specialist (CNS) and Nurse Practitioner (NP) are two types of APNs that are most frequently identified internationally (Maier, Aiken & Busse 2017; ICN 2020) (see Reflective Exercise 4.1).

Reflective Exercise 4.1

New Nursing Roles

Find the latest ICN guidelines on advanced practice nursing and search for the glossary section. Identify and note the terms related to advanced nursing practice (ANP) and advanced practice nursing (APN), as well as advanced practice nurses (APNs), focusing specifically on the roles of Clinical Nurse Specialist (CNS) and Nurse Practitioner (NP).

79

Some Implications of the New Nursing Roles

The development of these advanced practice roles in nursing has not been unproblematic and was characterised by inconsistency in role development, titles and how individuals might be prepared for these roles. Hamric and Tracy (2019) highlighted several implications for education, regulation and credentialing, research and practice of advanced practice nursing.

Implications for Advance Practice Education

All APNs are required to have at least a master's degree in advanced nursing practice. However, professional organisations in the United States are advocating for the doctoral preparation of advanced practice nurses through the Doctor of Nursing Practice (DNP) degree (Hamric & Tracy 2019). It is important to note that the DNP is not a role, but a degree focused on practice, in contrast to the PhD, which is research focused (Chism & McLain 2022).

To progress as a discipline, advanced practice nurses must be educated to think theoretically and develop and utilise a unique knowledge base. They must also understand the importance of integrating perspectives from other disciplines into their practice. One of the core competencies of advanced practice nursing is also evidence-based practice. If you recall from Chapter 3, the theories constitute evidence, and evidence-based practice is equivalent to theory-based practice (Fawcett 2022a). Nursing theories therefore should be placed as a formative foundation in advanced nursing practice curricula (Wood 2020). It is the responsibility of nurse educators to prepare APNs as experts in applying knowledge and excelling in evaluating, applying and supporting theory-based interventions to ensure person-centred care (Chism & McLain 2022). Excluding theories from the curriculum risks losing the central unifying focus of the discipline and discipline-specific knowledge, which forms the core identity and relevance of advanced nursing practice. APNs should know, understand and use nursing theories (Wood 2020).

Implications for Regulation and Credentialing

Regulatory mechanisms specific to each country provide the foundation for APNs through professional regulations and policies. These mechanisms grant APNs the authority to diagnose, prescribe medications, order diagnostic tests and therapeutic treatments and refer clients or patients to other services or professionals. They also allow APNs to admit and discharge clients or patients from hospitals and other facilities. Officially recognised titles for nurses working as APNs must be protected and conferred through legislation. Additionally, legislation and policies from authoritative entities should include forms of regulatory mechanisms like certification, credentialing or authorisation that are specific to the country's context (ICN 2020). APNs must practise and should be certified in the specific population focus and role for which they have been educated (Hamric & Tracy 2019).

Implications for Research

There is substantial evidence that APNs deliver safe, high-quality and efficient care (Maier, Aiken & Busse 2017; Oulton & Caldwell 2017). Despite this, establishing clear links between advanced practice nursing and specific patient outcomes continues to be a significant research priority (Hamric & Tracy 2019). In countries with established DNP programmes, further exploration is needed to compare the outcomes of different educational pathways, such as master's versus DNP programmes, particularly in relation to the experiences of graduates and patient outcomes (Hamric & Tracy 2019). Translation evidence-based practice change (Hamric & Tracy 2019) and quality improvement projects, which are similar to predictive theories, tested by experimental research are most relevant research focus of APNs (Fawcett 2022b). There is also a need for more research on the applicability of traditional nursing theories to contemporary advanced practice (Oulton & Caldwell 2017).

Implications for Practice Environments

APNs retain their direct patient care activities. These roles require considerable autonomy and authority and must demonstrate a higher level of responsibility and accountability. Their roles should be structured in practice environments to allow them to enact advanced nursing skills rather than be simply substitutes for physicians (Hamric & Tracy 2019).

Using Theory to Understand New Roles in Nursing

In Chapter 3, we focused on the importance of theory and the different levels of theory in terms of both sophistication and abstraction that may be appropriate for nursing. In this section, we look again at the contribution of theory to understanding the development and impact of these new roles in nursing (see Reflective Exercise 4.2).

Reflective Exercise 4.2

Reviewing Levels and Types of Theory

If you need to, refer back to Chapter 3 to review the different levels and types of theory that were identified.

Any discussion on the development of APN has to consider, for example, the boundaries between medical and nursing practice and the roles of both doctors and nurses, especially when nurses expand their remit into what might be deemed traditional medical territory. Therefore, to understand the contribution of theory to APN, we will consider role theory, the impact and influence of the biomedical model and, finally, how nursing theories have a contribution to make to these new nursing roles.

Role Theory

It is important to understand role theory in the context of new role developments in nursing. Two key terms describe this phenomenon: role expansion and role extension. Role expansion means that nurses retain their occupational focus but work within an expanded scope. For example, if a nursing role focused on health promotion, then widening their role in health promotion signifies role expansion. In contrast, role extension occurs when nurses extend their remit into the baili-wick of another discipline, almost 'amoeba like'. Hence, nurses taking on tasks such as prescribing or minor surgery would be considered role extension (see Reflective Exercise 4.3). This can lead to role confusion, role overlap and role conflict. These issues arise at the boundary where doctors are shedding duties that were once entirely within their scope, and nurses are taking on these duties. If both parties do not simultaneously realise and agree on these changes, role conflict and confusion can occur. During such transitions, the quality of care and patient safety can be compromised (McKenna 2004).

Reflective Exercise 4.3

Extended and Expanded Nursing Roles

Look up the differences between extended and expanded nursing roles. From your own experience of practice, give some examples of each. Consider whether this is a good thing or a bad thing for the nursing profession.

Using a Sociological Perspective on Role

Theories regarding roles can be found in the social sciences, particularly in sociology and psychology. Drawing on theories within sociology, it is possible to see different ways of thinking about role and these are framed within two broad categories of thinking about society. The first is structural functionalism, where the successful fulfilment of roles is viewed as crucial for the stability of the social system. A key theorist, Talcott Parsons, proposed the idea of the 'sick role' (Parsons 1952). Unlike the biomedical model, which views illness as a 'biomedical, mechanical breakdown', Parsons saw illness as a 'deviation' from social norms, needing authorisation. In an illness situation, both the doctor and the patient are assigned roles, each with associated duties, rights and obligations. These roles help structure expectations for how both the patient and the doctor should perform.

Another broad perspective is that of 'agency', where individuals are social actors and have the autonomy and capacity to shape the world around them. Within this perspective, individuals play a role in presenting themselves within the social world (Goffman 1959). Goffman used the metaphor of a theatre in which individuals play their roles according to the situation or context in which they find themselves. For example, when caring for patients, a nurse will adopt a specific role and behave in ways that meet the expectations others have of a nurse. Goffman referred to this as 'front-stage' behaviour – the behaviour that aligns with others' expectations within a particular context. However, Goffman also described 'back-stage' behaviour. Here, out of the sight of patients, nurses may act in ways that differ from their front-stage behaviours, which may or may not align with the expectations of their professional role.

For the purposes of this chapter, there are theories that can be used to explain the concept of role. These are not nursing theories but can be applied to nursing to try and understand important issues regarding roles and how they may impact nursing. The development of APN meant that there was a change in the roles of both the individuals involved and the nursing role in general. By changing their roles, pioneering APNs acquired new knowledge and skills, expanding their practice into medical territory. Using sociological perspectives, these theories help us understand the role's part in complex social systems like healthcare. With each role comes specific expectations of behaviour and practices. Therefore, it is very disturbing when individuals or occupational groups such as nursing do not conform to these expectations. Role theory represents a collection of concepts and a variety of propositions in the form of hypothetical predictions of how people will perform in a given job, or under what circumstances certain types of behaviour can be expected. Key to this are the expectations of how people should behave when they are in a particular social position (Hindin 2007). Concepts within role theory include:

- role norms
- role set
- role stress
- role confusion
- role overlap
- role conflict

Role Norms and Role Set

A structural functionalist perspective remains influential in thinking about roles. 'Role norms' are the ideas within a group that specify what members ought to do and what they are expected to do in given circumstances (Biddle & Thomas 1966). Additionally, there are role expectations held by members of the 'role set' that surround an individual, exerting pressures on them and their performance in a given situation (Biddle & Thomas 1966). The 'role set' refers to the role relationships associated with occupying a particular social status (Merton 1966). For instance, a 'role set' for a nurse would typically comprise nursing colleagues, other health professional colleagues, patients and representatives from their employing organisation.

The consideration of role is of particular relevance to those involved in creating new roles in nursing. After all, the context in which they work is changing, and therefore the perceptions and expectations of their role (from themselves, other professionals and patients) are also changing.

Role Stress and Strain

82

Role stress is a situation of increased role performance demand, while role strain is a subjective feeling of frustration, tension or anxiety in response to role stress (Bryczynski & Mackavey 2019: 84). There is some evidence that the introduction of new roles into nursing has resulted in examples of role stress and strain for the nurses involved.

Inter- and intra-professional challenges, along with confusion surrounding role development and professional isolation, contribute to potential role stress among those in new nursing roles. New roles can lead to feelings of isolation, burnout and role dissonance (see Reflective Exercise 4.4), especially when there is minimal support from the organisation and managers (Choi & De Gagne 2016). Additionally, keeping up with new technologies can also be an issue (Bryczynski & Mackavey 2019: 84).

Reflective Exercise 4.4

Burnout and Nursing

Look up the term 'burnout' as applied to nursing. In particular, investigate what are the factors that might cause burnout, what are the signs and what might be the possible effects on nurses themselves.

The innovative nature of some roles can also mean that accessibility to colleagues in similar roles is difficult. Lack of collegial interaction, lack or absence of preceptorship and reduced peer support are challenges of APNs (Torrens et al. 2020; Pajnkihar et al. 2021).

McKenna et al. (2005) found that linking with colleagues who shared similar jobs and theoretical perspectives was important for personal and professional identity, as well as providing a resource for support and debriefing. Additionally, if different advanced practitioners use different theories to inform their practice, this could encourage isolation and mean that best practices are not shared.

Role Conflict

Role conflict occurs when role expectations are perceived to be mutually exclusive or contradictory (Bryczynski & Mackavey 2019: 84). APNs may experience conflicts due not only to the varying demands of their role but also to intraprofessional and interprofessional conflicts.

Intraprofessional conflicts often arise from poor relationships among peers and differing perceptions of roles and responsibilities. Dynamics in interdisciplinary teams can be particularly challenging due to role overlap when two or more autonomous health professionals develop similar roles at the practice level. This is the case with APNs who perform medical activities, such as requesting diagnostic exams and prescribing treatments (Rodríguez et al. 2024). If not agreed, planned and supported, the introduction of these new activities can lead to role conflict, role overlap and role confusion (McKenna et al. 2003). Furthermore, nurses in new roles often face challenges fitting into the traditional hierarchical structure of hospitals, which can lead to role ambiguity and lack of autonomy (Bridges et al. 2003; McKenna et al. 2004; Noyes 2022).

One possible reason for role conflict, especially where advanced nursing practice and new roles are evolving, is a lack of clarity in expectations, blurred responsibilities and uncertainty regarding role implementation, known also as role ambiguity (Bryczynski & Mackavey 2019). In some healthcare services, a lack of awareness exists about the differences between nurse specialists and APNs (Gutiérrez-Rodríguez et al. 2019). This can lead to ambiguity regarding the development, scope of practice and impact of these roles. Where regulation and governance are in place, the role of the advanced practice nurses is clearly defined and structured. However, many countries lack such governance and regulation (Cooper et al. 2019).

Summary

A sociological perspective, particularly a structural-functionalist approach, emphasises that new roles bring new behaviours which can often challenge people's expectations of how an individual should behave. This can result in role conflict and role stress. An agency approach emphasises the autonomy of the individual to shape and create new roles and, hence, new expectations of their behaviour. Both approaches can be helpful in increasing understanding of the impact these new roles might have on nursing practice (see Reflective Exercise 4.5). They can also help prepare nurses for their new roles, especially if they are aware of these possible consequences.

Reflective Exercise 4.5

The Use of Non-Nursing Theories to Shed Light

Thus far, we have considered what is meant by the term 'role'. We have also recognised that it has certain dynamic attributes. You have been introduced to role theory, which, like all theories, is composed of a number of concepts linked by statements called propositions. Some of these concepts include role expansion, role extension, role norms, role set, role stress, role confusion, role overlap and role conflict.

You can see that a theory from the social sciences (role theory) can help to describe, explain and possibly predict behaviour that is of importance in understanding nursing. We suggest that you consult the literature and identify another non-nursing theory that impacts how nurses work. For example, you might focus on learning theory, the theory of planned action or communication theory. Write a page about it, including its main concepts and how these relate to each other. You could usefully discuss this with your fellow students.

The Influence of the Biomedical Model on Nursing Roles

Previously, we have looked at some sociological role theories to help us to understand how theories from another discipline such as sociology can lead to increased understanding of the nursing role within healthcare systems. In this section, we explore the biomedical model, which has had a significant influence on new advanced practice roles. The development of advanced nursing roles has significant implications for the education and training of nurses. These roles often require nurses to learn advanced assessment, diagnostic and prescribing skills, traditionally found within the realm of medical practice. As a result, nursing education programmes have had to evolve to incorporate the necessary knowledge and skills for these functions. This integration ensures that nurses in advanced practice roles are well-prepared to meet the demands of their expanded responsibilities.

A Brief History of the Biomedical Model

The biomedical model has a long history, and it is no surprise that it has influenced the development of some nursing theories and nursing roles while impeding others. The scientific basis for the biomedical model can be traced back to Hippocrates, Aristotle and Galen. You will recall from Chapter 2 that in the early 17th century, Descartes fostered the notion of the body as a machine. Disease was viewed as the consequence of breakdown and the physician's task was to repair the machine. Most physicians based their treatment philosophy on this fundamental tenet of reductionism. This implied that all behavioural phenomena must be conceptualised in terms of physiochemical principles (Engel 1977). Over the years, this basic precept was accepted not only by many healthcare professionals but also by the public.

Criticism and Limitations of the Biomedical Model and Shift to Alternative Models

The limitations of the biomedical model have been highlighted for several decades, primarily for treating illness as a condition of isolated bodily parts rather than addressing the whole person (Rocca & Anjum 2020) and neglecting the social, psychological and behavioural aspects of individuals and illness (Farre & Rapley 2017). While the biomedical model has some significant benefits in treating illness, such as advances in medical cures that alleviate symptoms and facilitate early patient discharge, it is not holistic. Proposed alternative views, such as the bio-psychosocial model by Engel in 1977, recovery-oriented approach (Davidson 2008 in State of Victoria, Department of Health 2011) and trauma-informed healthcare model (Harris & Fallot 2001) emerged from dissatisfaction with the biomedical model. The recovery-oriented approach emphasised holistic well-being and individual strengths (State of Victoria, Department of Health 2011). Trauma-informed care models can help nurses to understand and respond to the impact of vulnerable patients' previous healthcare experiences, as these are likely to influence the responses and adherence to treatment plans.

There are also other models of advanced practice blending nursing and medical orientations, such as Schuler's Model of Nurse Practitioner Practice and Dunphy and Winland-Brown's Circle of Caring: A Transformative, Collaborative Model. Other models proposed either by professionals or by individual authors are also described in the literature (Tracey 2019).

Today, it is generally accepted that illness and health are the result of an interaction between biological, psychological and social factors (Wade & Halligan 2017). Solely relying on medical models for caring practices can overlook the significant nursing component in patient care. While the medical model focuses on disease management, it may neglect the crucial human caring aspect that nursing provides. Nurses in new roles should acknowledge the benefits and the contributions of the biomedical model. However, APNs must provide holistic care, which recognises psychological, social, emotional, cognitive and spiritual dimensions and their relationships (Tracey 2019).

The Relevance of Existing Nursing Theory to New Nursing Roles

Theory can guide advanced nursing practice and education, as well as practice and outcomes-based research. This research focuses on implementing evidence-based findings to achieve the safest, most beneficial and most satisfying healthcare outcomes (McFarland & Eipperle 2008).

You will recall from Chapter 3 that in terms of abstraction, there are different levels of theory: situation specific theory, mid-range, grand and meta-theory (see Reflective Exercise 4.6). We will focus on the first three levels. Remember, situation-specific theories are often called practice theories and sometimes micro-theories.

Reflective Exercise 4.6

Grand, Mid-Range and Situation-Specific Theories

Go back to Chapter 3 and refresh your memory as to the differences in these types of theories.

It will be argued that grand theory may have limited value for those nurses who have taken on new roles. In contrast, the less abstract and more easily operationalised mid-range, situation-specific theories have become crucially important for such nurses.

Relevance of Existing 'Grand' Nursing Theories

The majority of grand theories were formulated many decades ago. The obvious point to consider is whether these old theories formulated in the 1950s and 1960s are still relevant to the new roles that nurses are undertaking in the 21st century. We did identify some examples of grand theories in Chapter 3.

Historical Overview of the Development of Nursing Theories

As we saw from Chapter 1, Hildegard Peplau (1952) has been given credit for formulating the first contemporary theory in nursing in her development of the 'theory of interpersonal relations'. After leaving Columbia University, she developed her theory retroductively – inductively by reflecting on a long career in psychiatric nursing and deductively through the influence of the psychiatrist Harry Stack Sullivan's (1953) interpersonal relations theory. Peplau's work influenced later theorists who used interaction and 'interpersonal relationships' as a basis for their work, such as Johnson (1959) and Hall (1959). More will be uncovered about these theories in Chapter 6.

The 1960s saw the publication of theories by Abdellah et al. (1960), Orlando (1961), Wiedenbach (1964), Levine (1966), Travelbee (1966) and King (1968). Among these theorists, Abdellah, Orlando and Travelbee were undoubtedly influenced by Peplau. We would argue that many of the new roles undertaken by nurses require expertise in interpersonal relationships. It underscores the centrality of the nurse–patient relationship and the importance of skilled communication and interprofessional skills, which are essential for APNs to engage patients, assess their needs and provide personalised evidence-based care.

De Leon-Demare (2015) researched interactions between APNs and patients in primary care settings and suggested using King's theory of goal attainment as a framework for describing and guiding APNs–patient interactions. The findings encourage APNs to be more reflective in their practice. By recognising disturbances in clinical encounters and viewing them as opportunities for mutual goal setting, APNs can become more person centred. The application of King's theory by APNs in clinical encounters reinforces the nursing foundations underlying APN.

In the mid-1960s, Henderson, Wiedenbach and Orlando, previously students at Columbia University in New York, worked as lecturers in the Yale School of Nursing. Here theorists began to study how nurses practised and the effect this had on patients. Myra Levine, while also working at Yale, put forward her Conservation Model (Levine 1966). It was also at Yale that the philosophers Dickoff and James (1968) wrote their seminal work on a 'theory of theories', referred to in Chapter 3. Their work led nurses to realise that they, as practising nurses, could make a major contribution to the formulation and use of theory.

The rapid growth in the number of nursing theories witnessed in the 1960s continued into the 1970s, with the work of Roy (1970), Rogers (1970), Orem (1971), Neuman and Young (1972), Riehl (1974), Adam (1975), Paterson and Zderad (1976), Leininger (1978), Watson (1979) and Newman (1979).

While the 1980s witnessed an acceptance of the significance of theories for nursing in Europe, in North America at least there seems to be a slowing down of the number of theories being developed. There, only three new grand nursing theories were published in the 1980s, by Parse (1981), Fitzpatrick (1982) and Erickson et al. (1983). Interestingly, Parse and Fitzpatrick constructed their theories not from first principles but from Martha Rogers's earlier theory (1970). This 'borrowing' of theory from other nurse theorists represented a new and interesting departure for nursing theory development.

While there was a slowing down in the development of new theories in the United States, there was a surge in theory development in the United Kingdom. Although Nightingale's teachings are held up to be the first attempts at nurse theorising (Nightingale 1859/1980), the United Kingdom did not boast a pedigree of theory development. It was not until the 1980s and 1990s that some British nurses followed their American counterparts and began to formulate grand theories, including work by McFarlane (1982), Roper et al. (1983), Stockwell (1985), Wright (1986), Clark (1986), Minshull et al. (1986), Green (1988), Bogdanovic (1989), Friend (1990), Yoo (1991) and Slevin (1995).

'Grand' Theories and APN

Despite being criticised for their practical application, as will be discussed further in Chapter 5, there are examples in the literature of grand theories being used to guide the work of APNs (Zhang 2024). These examples highlight the relevance of grand theories in providing a philosophical foundation and guiding principles for APN. Presented below are just some examples.

Abumaria et al. (2015) discussed adapting Levine's theory as a framework for adult-gerontology primary care nurse practitioners to provide care for older adults. As their role is to deliver quality care to adult and older adult populations, focusing not only on healthcare management but also on advocacy, leadership in collaborative care, advanced planning and navigating healthcare delivery systems, Levine's theory could foster effective interventions, particularly in long-term care settings.

Orem's theory has also been suggested for implementation in the practice of APNs. Geden, Isaramalai and Taylor (2001) discussed the implementation of Orem's theory into the primary care practice of APNs to help maintain a nursing perspective by emphasising the individual as a unified whole, not divisible into parts. This theory views individuals as capable agents with the potential to develop, mature and engage in self-care. It offers a language to describe nursing actions and patient outcomes, allowing APNs to study the effects of their practice through nurse-sensitive outcomes. For example, a patient's acceptance of having asthma is an outcome sensitive to nursing intervention, which benefits the patient, the APN and the healthcare system. Findings were supported by Yip (2021) in a case study illustrating how an APN used Orem's theory-led practice in a primary healthcare setting, demonstrating the theory's application to case management.

McFarland and Eipperle (2008) suggested Leininger's theory to serve as a foundational basis for the educational preparation, primary-care contextual practice and outcomes-focused research endeavours of APNs. Her theory can guide APNs by framing cultural knowledge, predicting similarities and differences among cultures and gathering essential cultural care information for holistic assessments. It can help to discover caring and healing values, beliefs and practices within various groups and establish a caring and healing system essential for integrated and appropriate care.

Bernick (2004) discussed Watson's theory as a guide for APNs in caring for older adults. Guided by this theory, a nurse focuses on the human responses of individuals, families and groups to their health and illness situations, aiming to facilitate caring and healing. The advanced practice role also demands specialised knowledge and skills grounded in ethical and moral values to understand the needs and challenges faced by older persons and their families. This knowledge informs practice but does not solely determine the priority of care and concern.

Watson's theory could also positively influence APNs' job satisfaction. Horner (2020), in a mixed methods study, investigated whether mentoring based on this theory positively influences APNs' job satisfaction. It was found that through Watson's theory, a reciprocal relationship between mentors and mentees can provide new APNs with a sense of community and direct availability. This mentoring relationship can also enhance job satisfaction, which is crucial for retaining APNs.

Relevance of Existing 'Mid-Range'

Mid-range theories discussed in Chapter 3 are essential for practice disciplines. These theories are particularly relevant for developing new nursing roles, as APNs need research-based theories that can be operationalised to enhance patient care.

As we saw in Chapter 3, there are many mid-range theories with the potential to be readily applied to practice. Some emerged from the 'grand' theories, such as Orem's mid-range theory of self-care deficit, and some emerged inductively from practice. The example we gave was Swanson's (1991) mid-range theory to be used in perinatal nursing and readers will recall that we presented miscarriage as an example.

There are other mid-range theories on menstrual care, family care-giving, relapse among ex-smokers, uncertainty in illness, peri-menopausal process, self-transcendence, personal risk-taking and illness trajectory, quality caring, symptom management theory, etc. The advantage of mid-range theories is that they can be applied readily to practice. From the previous discussion, it has been stressed that nurses in new roles are often professionally isolated (McKenna et al. 2005). Mid-range theories can provide them with the theoretical and professional security that autonomy and accountability in new roles require. Nonetheless, it is important to be aware of the threat they pose to communication and collaboration between generalist and specialist nurses and across different specialties.

Some examples of using mid-range theories in APN practice can be found in the literature (Zhang 2024). For instance, Newcomb (2010) used Symptom Management theory to explain how APNs care for children with asthma. Sangster-Gormley et al. (2013) discussed how Kolcaba's Comfort Theory and Antonovsky's Sense of Coherence theory can be used to illuminate the holistic nature of APN and result in person-centred outcomes. Hansen and Dysvik (2022) discussed the importance of the integration of nursing theories in APNs, selecting and discussing several mid-range theories to guide future theory development within APNs' education. These include Coordination and Organisation theory by Allen (2014), Critical Caring theory by Falk-Rafael and Betker (2012), Transition theory by Meleis (2010), Bureaucratic Caring theory by Ray (2018) and Technological Competency as Caring theory by Locsin (2015). They concluded that these theories could extend holistic approaches to caring within complex healthcare environments (Hansen & Dysvik 2022).

Lewis et al. (2019) suggested that a pragmatic mid-range theory New BITTEN (Betrayal history by health-related institutions, Indicator for healthcare engagement, Traumas related to healthcare, Trust in healthcare providers, patient Expectations and Needs) Model of Trauma-Informed Healthcare could be of use by nurses, while providing effective treatment during stressful and/or potentially traumatic patient encounters.

Relevance of Existing Practice Theories

As early as 1964, Wald and Leonard (1964) were the first to argue for a 'practice theory' to guide nursing actions. They maintained that theory should emanate from practice, be used and tested in practice and have incorporated causal hypotheses within it. In other words, with practice theory, a nurse should be able to say, 'If I do this, then the following will happen'. Therefore, practice theory can help APNs to prescribe clinical interventions. An example of a practice theory is Scheel's (2005) theory of interactional nursing.

The view of practice theory being a directive for practice is important for nurses in new roles. For instance, APNs running a pain clinic know that they can reduce the patient's experience of pain by undertaking specific actions, while APNs in the care of the elderly know that pressure area damage can be reduced by turning every two hours. Similarly, preoperative APNs know that postoperative anxiety can be reduced by providing the patient with information before surgery. Because this may not happen every time with every patient, this is not a law. However, since it should have the desired effect with most patients, it represents practice theory. By using practice theory, nurses are going further than simply describing, explaining or predicting a phenomenon; they are prescribing actions that will, all being equal, have positive effects. Therefore, more so than mid-range theory, practice theory provides APNs with a repertoire of practices whereby the outcome is predictable, if not prescribable.

If you recall from Chapter 3, we emphasised the importance and emerging situation-specific theories. Im and Meleis (2021) introduced them as a variant of mid-range theory, while Peterson and Bredow (2020), referencing Jacox, argued they are essentially practice theories. While acknowledging the differences between mid-range, situation-specific and practice theories, we here focus on their relevance to APNs. Examples include Situation-Specific Theory for Health Management in Heart Failure by Hirano et al. (2023), Situation-Specific Theory of Heart Failure Self-Care by Riegel, Dickson and Faulkner (2016), Situation-Specific Theory of Perinatal Loss, Devastating Cyclone by Furtado-Eraso, Marín-Fernández and Escalada-Hernández (2024), Situation-Specific Theory for African American Emerging Adults by Smith et al. (2024), Situation-Specific Theory for Older Adults such as Geropalliative Caring Model (GCM) by Lee (2018) and many others not listed here. These theories may have the potential to guide APNs. However, it is important to note that due to the nature of APN, which includes a variety of patients, situation-specific theories characterised by their focus on sociopolitical, cultural and historical contexts, unique environments and limited generalisation might be challenging to employ. APNs should consider utilising several situation-specific theories to effectively guide their practice, which could cause additional challenges.

To summarise: using the biomedical model as a framework to guide nursing practice in these new roles is no longer relevant. It may be useful to revisit some of the existing nursing theories, in particular mid-range theories, to test their relevance for contemporary nursing practice in new roles. Similarly, the situation-specific theories used by APNs should be identified, articulated and tested to add to the body of nursing knowledge.

Conclusion

Throughout history, the nursing profession has continually evolved to address challenges related to health, society and person-centred care (ICN 2020). As patient populations and healthcare systems change, nursing roles will continue to adapt. To support the optimal use of nursing knowledge and ensure safe patient care, role clarity is essential. Leadership plays a crucial role in establishing professional practice parameters and fostering a culture of collaboration and respect. Leadership is key to establishing professional practice parameters and creating a culture of collaboration and respect (Lankshear et al. 2016).

The increase in new nursing roles worldwide, often encompassing responsibilities previously held by other health professionals, significantly impacts on nurses and the nursing profession. Understanding role theory is crucial to avoid role strain, confusion and conflict.

To meet the demands of dynamic healthcare systems, APNs must be supported and allowed to advance their practice. Conversations that trivialise the role and maintain hierarchical structures must be replaced with discussions recognising the unique contributions of APNs. By doing so, healthcare professionals can move beyond comparisons with medicine and focus on the specific strengths of nursing (Thompson & McNamara 2022). While the role of the APNs builds on and extends beyond traditional nursing, it should remain firmly grounded in 'caring' (Zhang 2024).

Within these new roles, nurses require theories to guide their practice. Because many of the interventions undertaken by nurses in new roles were previously undertaken by physicians, the influence of the biomedical model should be acknowledged. However, a holistic approach is necessary to enhance the role of APNs in delivering comprehensive and compassionate care.

The benefits of grand theories for APNs were discussed, but it is argued that mid-range theories and situation-specific theories (i.e. practice theories) are the most relevant and useful guides for prescribing nursing interventions. Integrating these theoretical frameworks into practice can help nurses meet the complex demands of modern healthcare systems effectively.

Revision Points

- Changes in healthcare, demographics and technology have led to the development of new advanced practice roles in nursing.

- As the healthcare setting is dynamic and changing, some theoretical perspectives were examined as to their utility for these new roles such as role theory, the biomedical model, alternative models and existing nursing theories.

- It was concluded that mid-range and situation-specific theories offered the greatest potential for these new roles.

Further Reading

Butts J.M. & Rich K.L. (eds) (2018) *Philosophies and Theories for Advanced Nursing Practice*, 3rd edition. Burlington: Jones & Bartlett Learning.

Hansen B.S. & Dysvik E. (2022) Expanding the theoretical understanding in advanced practice nursing: framing the future. *Nursing Forum*, **57**(6), 1593–1598.

Zhang Y. (2024) What is nursing in advanced nursing practice? applying theories and models to advanced nursing practice-A discursive review. *Journal of Advanced Nursing*, **80**(12), 1–14.

References

Abdellah F.G., Beland I.L., Martin A. & Matheney R.V. (1960) *Patient Centred Approaches to Nursing*. New York: Macmillan.

Abumaria I.M., Hastings-Tolsma M. & Sakraida T.J. (2015) Levine's conservation model: a framework for advanced gerontology nursing practice. *Nursing Forum*, **50**(3), 179–188.

Adam E.T. (1975) A conceptual model for nursing. *The Canadian Nurse*, **71**, 40–43.

Allen D. (2014) *The Invisible Work of Nurses: Hospitals, Organisation and Healthcare*. London: Routledge.

Bernick L. (2004) Caring for older adults: practice guided by Watson's caring-healing model. *Nursing Science Quarterly*, **17**(2), 128–134.

Biddle B.J. & Thomas E.J. (eds) (1966) *Role Theory: Concepts and Research*. New York: John Wiley & Sons Inc.

Bogdanovic A. (1989) Non-verbal communication. *Nursing Times*, **85**(1), 27–28.

Bridges J., Meyer J., Glynn M., Bentley J. & Reeves S. (2003) Interprofessional care co-ordinators: the benefits and tensions associated with a new role in UK acute health care. *International Journal of Nursing Studies*, **40**, 599–607.

Brownwood I. & Lafortune G. (2024) *Advanced practice nursing in primary care in OECD countries: Recent developments and persisting implementation challenges*, OECD Health Working Papers, No. 165. Paris: OECD Publishing.

Bryczynski K.A. & Mackavey C.L. (2019) Role development of advanced practice nurse. In Tracy M.F. & O'Grady E.T. (eds) *Hamric and Hanson's Advanced Practice Nursing: An Integrative Approach*, 6th edition, pp. 80–107. St. Louis, MO: Elsevier.

Chism L.A. & McLain N. (2022) The essentials of the doctor of nursing practice: a philosophical perspective. In Butts J.M. & Rich K.L. (eds) *Philosophies and Theories for Advanced Nursing Practice*, 4th edition, pp. 47–66. Burlington: Jones & Bartlett Learning.

Choi M. & De Gagne J.C. (2016) Autonomy of nurse practitioners in primary care: an integrative review. *Journal of the American Association of Nurse Practitioners*, **28**(3), 170–174.

Clark J. (1986) A model for health visiting. In Kershaw B. & Salvage J. (eds) *Models for Nursing*, pp. 97–109. Chichester: John Wiley & Sons.

Cooper M.A., McDowell J., Raeside L. & ANP–CNS Group (2019) The similarities and differences between advanced nurse practitioners and clinical nurse specialists. *British Journal of Nursing*, **28**(20), 1308–1314.

Davidson L. (2008) *Recovery: Concepts and Application*. Recovery Devon Group. https://recoverydevon.co.uk/ wp-content/ uploads/ 2010/ 01/ Recovery_Concepts_Laurie_Davidson.pdf – accessed 24 October 2023.

De Leon-Demare K., MacDonald J., Gregory D.M., Katz A. & Halas G. (2015) Articulating nurse practitioner practice using King's theory of goal attainment. *Journal of the American Association of Nurse Practitioners*, **27**(11), 631–636.

Dickoff J. & James P. (1968) A theory of theories: a position paper. *Nursing Research*, **17**(3), 197–203.

Engel G.L. (1977) The need for a new medical model: a challenge for biomedicine. *Science*, **196**(4286), 129–136.

Erickson H., Tomlin E. & Swain M. (1983) *Modelling and Role Modelling*. Lexington, SC: Pine Press.

Falk-Rafael, A., & Betker, C. (2012). The primacy of relationships, a study of public Health Nursing practice from a critical caring perspective. ANS. *Advances in Nursing Science*, **35**(4), 315–332.

Farre A. & Rapley T. (2017) The new old (and old new) medical model: four decades navigating the biomedical and psychosocial understandings of health and illness. *Healthcare*, **5**(4), 88.

Fawcett J. (2022a) Using theory in evidence based advanced nursology practice. In Butts J.M. & Rich K.L. (eds) *Philosophies and Theories for Advanced Nursing Practice*, 4th edition, pp. 531–544. Burlington: Jones & Bartlett Learning.

Fawcett J. (2022b) Theory testing and theory evaluation. In Butts J.M. & Rich K.L. (eds) *Philosophies and Theories for Advanced Nursing Practice*, 4th edition, pp. 517–530. Burlington: Jones & Bartlett Learning.

Fitzpatrick J.J. (1982). In Fitzpatrick J.J., Whall A.L., Johnston R.L. & Floyd J.A. (eds) *Nursing Models: Applications to Psychiatric Mental Health Nursing*. Bowie, MD: Brady & Co.

Friend B. (1990) Working at health. *Nursing Times*, **86**(16), 21.

Furtado-Eraso S., Marín-Fernández B. & Escalada-Hernández P. (2024) Perinatal loss, a devastating cyclone: a situation-specific nursing theory. *Journal of Nursing Scholarship*, 664–677.

Geden E.A., Isaramalai S.A. & Taylor S.G. (2001) Self-care deficit nursing theory and the nurse practitioner's practice in primary care settings. *Nursing Science Quarterly*, **14**(1), 29–33.

Goffman E. (1959) *The Presentation of Self in Everyday Life*. Harmondsworth, Middlesex: Penguin.

Green C. (1988) The development of a conceptual model for mental handicap nursing practice in the UK. *Nurse Education Today*, **8**, 9–17.

Gutiérrez-Rodríguez L., García Mayor S., Cuesta Lozano D., Burgos-Fuentes E., Rodríguez-Gómez S., Sastre-Fullana P. et al. (2019) Competences of specialist nurses and advanced practice nurses. *Enfermería ClíNica (English Edition)*, **29**(6), 328–335.

Hall L. (1959) *Nursing – What Is It?* Virginia: Virginia State Nurses Association. Winter.

Hamric A.B. & Tracy M.F. (2019) A definition of advanced practice nursing. In Tracy M.F. & O'Grady E.T. (eds) *Hamric and Hanson's Advanced Practice Nursing: An Integrative Approach*, 6th edition, pp. 61–79. St. Louis: Elsevier.

Hansen B.S. & Dysvik E. (2022) Expanding the theoretical understanding in advanced practice nursing: framing the future. *Nursing Forum*, **57**(6), 1593–1598.

Harris M. & Fallot R.D. (2001) Envisioning a trauma-informed service system: a vital paradigm shift. *New Directions for Mental Health Services*, **89**, 3–22.

Hindin M.J. (2007) Role theory. In Ritzer G. (ed.) *The Blackwell Encyclopedia of Sociology*, pp. 3959–3962. Oxford: Blackwell.

Hirano G.S.B., de Barros A.L.B.L. & da Silva V.M. (2023) Situation-specific theory for health management in heart failure. *Nursing Science Quarterly*, **36**(3), 264–272.

Horner D.K. (2020) Mentoring: positively influencing job satisfaction and retention of new hire nurse practitioners. *Plastic Surgical Nursing*, **40**(3), 150–165.

Im E.O. & Meleis A.I. (2021) *Situation Specific Theories: Development, Utilization, and Evaluation in Nursing*. Cham: Springer.

International Council of Nurses (ICN) (2020) *Guidelines on Advanced Practice Nursing 2020*. Switzerland: International Council of Nurses.

Johnson D.E. (1959) The nature of a science of nursing. *Nursing Outlook*, **7**, 291–294.

King I. (1968) A conceptual frame of reference for nursing. *Nursing Research*, **17**(1), 27–31.

Lankshear S., Rush J., Weeres A. & Martin D. (2016) Enhancing role clarity for the practical nurse: a leadership imperative. *Journal of Nursing Administration*, **46**(6), 300–307.

Lee S.M. (2018) Lee geropalliative caring model: a situation-specific theory for older adults. *Advances in Nursing Science*, **41**(2), 161–173.

Leininger M.M. (1978) *Transcultural Nursing: Concepts, Theories, and Practices*. New York: John Wiley & Sons Inc.

Levine M.E. (1966) Adaptation and assessment: a rationale for nursing intervention. *American Journal of Nursing*, **66**(11), 2450–2453.

Lewis C.L., Langhinrichsen-Rohling J., Selwyn C.N. & Lathan E.C. (2019) Once BITTEN, twice shy: an applied trauma-informed healthcare model. *Nursing Science Quarterly*, **32**(4), 291–298.

Locsin R.C. (2015) Technological competency as caring. Knowing as process and tecnological knowing as practice. In Smith M.C. & Parker M.E. (eds) *Nursing theories and nursing practice*, 4th edition, pp. 449–459. Philadelphia: F.A. Davis Company.

Lusk B., Cockerham A.Z. & Keeling A.W. (2019) Historical and developmental aspects of advanced practice nursing. In Tracy M.F. & O'Grady E.T. (eds) *Hamric and Hanson's Advanced Practice Nursing: An Integrative Approach*, 6th edition, pp. 1–24. St. Louis, MO: Elsevier.

Maier C., Aiken L. & Busse R. (2017) *Nurses in advanced roles in primary care: Policy levers for implementation*", OECD Health Working Papers, No. 98. Paris: OECD Publishing.

McFarland M.M. & Eipperle M.K. (2008) Culture care theory: a proposed practice theory guide for nurse practitioners in primary care settings. *Contemporary Nurse*, **28**(1–2), 48–63.

McFarlane J.K. (1982) Nursing: A Paradigm of Caring. Unpublished paper. Ethical Issues in Caring. University of Manchester, UK.

McKenna H.P. (2004) 'Role drift' to unlicensed assistants: risks to quality and safety. *Editorial. Quality and Safety in Health Care*, **13**(6), 410–411.

McKenna H.P., Keeney S. & Bradley M. (2003) Generic and specialist nursing roles in the community: an investigation of professional and lay views. *Health & Social Care in the Community*, **11**(6), 537–545.

McKenna H.P., Hasson F. & Keeney S. (2004) Patient safety and quality of care: the role of the health care assistant. *Journal of Nursing Management*, **12**(6), 452–459.

McKenna H.P., Keeney S.R., Hasson F., Richey R., Sinclair M. & Poulton B. (2005) *Innovative Roles in Nursing and Midwifery*. Belfast: Northern Ireland Practice and Education Council for Nursing and Midwifery.

Meleis A.I. (ed.) (2010) *Transitions Theory: Middle-Range and Situation-Specific Theories in Nursing Research and Practice*. New York, NY: Springer.

Merton R.K. (1966) Instability and articulation in the role-set. In Biddle B.J. & Thomas E.J. (eds) *Role Theory: Concepts and Research*. New York: John Wiley & Sons Inc.

Minshull J., Ross K. & Turner J. (1986) The human needs model of nursing. *Journal of Advanced Nursing*, **11**, 643–649.

Neuman B. & Young R.J. (1972) A model for teaching total person approach to patient problems. *Nursing Research*, **21**(3), 264.

Newcomb P. (2010) Using symptom management theory to explain how nurse practitioners care for children with asthma. *Journal of Theory Construction & Testing*, **14**(2), 2924–2933.

Newman M.A. (1979) *Theory Development in Nursing*, 3rd edition. Philadelphia, PA: F.A. Davis.

Nightingale F. (1859/1980) *Notes on Nursing: What It Is and What It Is Not*. Edinburgh: Churchill Livingstone.

Noyes A.L. (2022) Navigating the hierarchy: communicating power relationships in collaborative health care groups. *Management Communication Quarterly*, **36**(1), 62–91.

Orem D.E. (1971) *Nursing Concepts of Practice*, 1st edition. New York: McGraw Hill.

Orlando I. (1961) *The Dynamic Nurse Patient Relationship. Function, Process, and Principles*. New York: G.P. Putnam & Sons.

Oulton J.A. & Caldwell P. (2017) Nurses. *International Encyclopedia of Public Health*, **5**, 264–270.

Pajnkihar M., Petek Š.M., Betlehem J. & Vrbnjak D. (2021) Report on activity C2: deliverable D5 (V2): analysis of training needs for nurses working in primary care, development of a curriculum for an advanced practice nurse (APN) special license course and recommendations for improving the legislative and licensing framework for APN. In Švab I., Homar V. & Arvidsson E. (eds) *Support for the Development of the Primary Care System in Hungary*, pp. 259–396. Ljubljana: Institute for Development of Family Medicine.

Parse R.R. (1981) *Man-Living-Health: A Theory of Nursing*. New York: John Wiley & Sons.

Parsons T. (1952) *The Social System*. London: Tavistock Publications.

Paterson J.G. & Zderad L.T. (1976) *Humanistic Nursing*. New York: John Wiley & Sons.

Peplau E.H. (1952) *Interpersonal Relations in Nursing: A Conceptual Frame of Reference for Psychodynamic Nursing*. New York: G.P. Putnam & Sons.

Peterson S.J. & Bredow T.S. (2020) *Middle Range Theories: Application to Nursing Research and Practice*, 5th edition. Philadelphia, PA: Wolters Kluwer.

Ray M. (2018) Theory of bureaucratic caring. In Smith M.J. & Liehr P. (eds) *Middle range theory for nursing*, 4th edition, pp. 107–117. New York: Springer Publishing Company.

Riegel B., Dickson V.V. & Faulkner K.M. (2016) The situation-specific theory of heart failure self-care: revised and updated. *Journal of Cardiovascular Nursing*, **31**(3), 226–235.

Riehl J.P. (1974) The Riehl interactional model. In Riehl J.P. & Roy C. (eds) *Conceptual Models in Nursing Practice*, pp. 125–146. New York: Appleton-Century-Crofts.

Rocca E. & Anjum R.L. (2020) Complexity, reductionism and the biomedical model. In Anjum R.L., Copeland S. & Rocca E. (eds) *Rethinking Causality, Complexity and Evidence for the Unique Patient*, pp. 75–94. Cham: Springer.

Rodríguez C., Archibald D., Grad R., Loban K. & Kilpatrick K. (2024) Professional identity work of nurse practitioners and family physicians in primary care in Quebec and Ontario - a study protocol. *BMC Primary Care*, **25**(1), 178.

Rogers M.E. (1970) *An Introduction to a Theoretical Basis of Nursing*, 1st edition. Philadelphia, PA: F.A. Davis.

Roper N., Logan N. & Tierney A. (1983) *Using a Model for Nursing*. Edinburgh: Churchill-Livingstone.

Roy C. (1970) Adaptation: a conceptual framework for nursing. *Nursing Outlook*, **18**(3), 42–45.

Sangster-Gormley E., Frisch N. & Schreiber R. (2013) Articulating new outcomes of nurse practitioner practice. *Journal of the American Association of Nurse Practitioners*, **25**(12), 653–658.

Scheel M.E. (2005) *Interaktionel sygeplejepraksis*, 3rd edition. København: Munksgaard.

Slevin O. (1995) Theories and models. In Bashford P. & Slevin O. (eds) *Theory and Practice in Nursing*. Edinburgh: Campion Press.

Smith S.B., Abshire D.A., Magwood G.S., Herbert L.L., Tavakoli A.S. & Jenerette C. (2024) Unlocking population-specific treatments to render equitable approaches and management in cardiovascular disease: development of a situation-specific theory for African American emerging adults. *Journal of Cardiovascular Nursing*, **39**(4), E103–E114.

State of Victoria, Department of Health (2011) *Framework for Recovery-Oriented Practice: Guide for Practitioners and Providers*. Melbourne, Victoria: Mental Health, Drugs and Regions Division, Victorian Government Department of Health.

Stockwell F. (1985) *The Nursing Process in Psychiatric Nursing*. London: Croom Helm.

Sullivan H.S. (1953) *The Interpersonal Theory of Psychiatry*. London: Routledge.

Swanson K.M. (1991) Empirical development of a middle range theory of caring. *Nursing Research*, **40**(3), 161–166.

Thompson W. & McNamara M. (2022) Constructing the advanced nurse practitioner identity in the healthcare system: a discourse analysis. *Journal of Advanced Nursing*, **78**(3), 834–846.

Torrens C., Campbell P., Hoskins G., Strachan H., Wells M., Cunningham M. et al. (2020) Barriers and facilitators to the implementation of the advanced nurse practitioner role in primary care settings: a scoping review. *International Journal of Nursing Studies*, **104**, 103443.

Tracey M.F. (2019) Competencies of advanced practice nursing. In Tracy M.F. & O'Grady E.T. (eds) *Hamric and Hanson's Advanced Practice Nursing: An Integrative Approach*, 6th edition, pp. 143–178. St. Louis: Elsevier.

Travelbee J. (1966) *Interpersonal Aspects of Nursing*. Philadelphia, PA: F.A. Davis.

Wade D.T. & Halligan P.W. (2017) The biopsychosocial model of illness: a model whose time has come. *Clinical Rehabilitation*, **31**(8), 995–1004.

Wald F.S. & Leonard R.C. (1964) Towards the development of nursing practice theory. *Nursing Research*, **13**(4), 309–313.

Watson J. (1979) *Nursing: The Philosophy and Science of Caring*. Boston, MA: Little, Brown.

Wheeler K.J., Miller M., Pulcini J., Gray D., Ladd E. & Rayens M.K. (2022) Advanced practice nursing roles, regulation, education, and practice: a global study. *Annals of Global Health*, **88**(1), 42.

Wiedenbach E. (1964) *Clinical Nursing: a Helping Art*. New York: Springer Publication Company.

Wood S.K. (2020) Keeping the nurse in the nurse practitioner: returning to our disciplinary roots of knowing in nursing. *Advances in Nursing Science*, **43**(1), 50–61.

Wright S.G. (1986) *Building and Using a Model of Nursing*. London: Edward Arnold.

Yip J.Y.C. (2021) theory-based advanced nursing practice: a practice update on the application of Orem's self-care deficit nursing theory. *SAGE Open Nursing*, **7**, 23779608211011993.

Yoo K.H. (1991) Expectation and evaluation of occupational health nursing services, as perceived by occupational health nurses, employees and employers in the United Kingdom. University of Ulster, Unpublished PhD thesis.

Zhang Y. (2024) What is nursing in advanced nursing practice? Applying theories and models to advanced nursing practice – A discursive review. *Journal of Advanced Nursing*, **80**(12), 4842–4855.

CHAPTER 5

Nursing Theories or Nursing Models

Outline of Content

In the previous chapter, we described how new nursing roles and nursing theories have evolved and the importance of grand theory, mid-range theory, situation-specific theory and practice theory for guiding practice within these new roles. Invariably, situation-specific theories are referred to in the literature as practice theories. In other words, they are very narrow in their scope and can inform practice. Until now in the chapters, we have tried to reflect on and discuss the role of theory in nursing, including its impact on theory-based practice, research and the professional and disciplinary status of nursing. In this chapter, we will further explain the construction of theory, discuss the often controversial relationship between theories and models and show how models can lead to the development of theory. In the following section, we will build on what was described and discussed in previous chapters. We will finish by outlining in detail the advantages and disadvantages of nursing theories.

Learning Outcomes

At the end of this chapter, you should be able to:

1. Explain the reasons for the development of nursing theory

2. Define nursing 'theory' and 'model'

3. Explain the basic parts of the theory

4. Differentiate between nursing theories and nursing models

5. Discuss theory classification

6. Explain the main paradigms used in theoretical nursing

7. Describe the elements of the metaparadigm

8. Outline the benefits and the main criticisms of nursing theories

Fundamentals of Nursing Models, Theories and Practice, Third Edition. Hugh P. McKenna, Majda Pajnkihar and Dominika Vrbnjak.
© 2025 John Wiley & Sons Ltd. Published 2025 by John Wiley & Sons Ltd.
Companion website: www.wiley.com/go/nursingmodels3e

Introduction

In Chapters 1 and 3, we explained that there are numerous definitions of nursing theories. You will have seen that the terms grand theory and model are used interchangeably. You saw that one of the most important features of a grand theory/model seems to be its abstract nature (Fawcett 2005a; Fawcett & DeSanto-Madeya 2013; Meleis 2012, 2018); mid-range theories are, by contrast, narrower in scope and less abstract. In the last decade, there have been descriptions of situation-specific theories that were introduced by Im and Meleis (1999). Meleis (2018) described the main characteristic of situation-specific theories as their focus on sociopolitical, cultural and historical contexts, but pointing out that they are less abstract and generalisable.

Theories are always in the process of development, and the differences between the terms theory and model are, at best, tentative, semantic and unclear. We have stated on numerous occasions that nurses employ theories in their everyday work, using different types of theories to help describe, explain, predict and, as Dickoff and James (1968) pointed out, prescribe nursing care. It is also important to bear in mind that different authors have different views on the level of abstraction of their own and others' theories. One way of classifying nursing theories is according to their level of abstraction (McKenna 1997; Meleis 2012, 2018); another is by reference to the range of the theory (Marriner Tomey 1998). But first, let us explain the reasons for nursing theory development.

Reasons for Historical Nursing Theory Evolution

In Chapter 1, it was noted that all the early 20th-century nursing theories originated from the United States. The United Kingdom started developing its own theories about 20 years later (see Reflective Exercise 5.1). Florence Nightingale's theory was an exception to this timeline. You saw in Chapter 3 how, in the late 1950s, other American nursing theories were developed. These theories aimed to distinguish nursing from other health professions and define nurses as professionals with specific responsibilities to patient care. In the previous chapters, we pointed out the ongoing development of nursing education, refining and development theories, and their application in practice and research.

In the 1950s, nurse graduate and postgraduate education programmes were increasingly being delivered, not in schools of nursing on isolated hospital sites but in universities. This transition to the academy reflected a growing recognition that nursing needed to demonstrate its own distinct knowledge base and scientific approaches to studying nursing. With the development of postgraduate education and the consequent higher level of nurses' knowledge, we can also observe the development of nursing practice grounded in theory and research and the support of theory in research. Theories at all levels of development have contributed to and influenced the disciplinary and professional status of nursing in healthcare and society. In addition, Rodgers (2022) discussed the role of Doctor of Nursing Practice (DNP)-prepared nurses in leadership, public engagement, collaboration with researchers to identify needs and innovations, and the development of nursing knowledge, highlighting the challenges and responsibilities associated with their advanced degree. Through the evolution of theory, Alligood (2018a) described the role of theory in nursing, the impact of theory-based practice, research and the professional and disciplinary status of nursing.

It is important that the nursing profession and discipline are supported by nursing theories. Otherwise, the lectures would be based on a variant of the biomedical model and theories from other disciplines. You will recall that the basic structure of the biomedical model was discussed in Chapter 4. The reasons why theorising started in the 1950s in America and much later flourished on a global scene were therefore as follows:

- In America, the inclusion of nursing study programmes within the universities much earlier than in other parts of the world, meant a shift from vocational to university education.
- The advent of university education for nurses and an increased number of graduate and postgraduate study programmes MSc and PhD, and later professional doctorates (DNP) and advanced practice nurses (APN) facilitated the development of concepts, theories and a body of knowledge derived from practice for practice.
- Nurses and patients began rejecting the biomedical model used in practice and education, moving away from traditional approaches and focusing on nursing theories (knowledge) and their application.

- There was growth in the development of mid-range and situation-specific theories, as well as refinements, testing, application and utilisation for patient safety, effectiveness and quality of practice.
- There was a quest for recognition and acknowledgement of nursing's disciplinary and professional status, aiming to define the boundaries of nursing and nurses' work.
- Postgraduate education resulted in increased research and publication activity.
- There emerged theoretical and methodological diversity and plurality in nursing.
- Women's increased contribution to the Second World War effort sparked debates about the female role in work and education.

In Chapter 4, you were introduced to the names of theorists who developed their theories in America in the 1960s and 1970s. Interestingly, many were reluctant to claim theoretical status for their work. Such reluctance was no longer common in the 1980s and 1990s. For example, in 1959, Orem published her first publication, and in 1971, she published her book *Nursing: Concepts of Practice*, with subsequent editions in 1980, 1985, 1991 and 1995. She worked alone and with colleagues on the continued conceptual development of the self-care deficit nursing theory. The fifth edition is organised into two parts: nursing as a unique field of knowledge and nursing as a practical science. In the 1980s, some theorists also tried to revise their earlier work in line with some of the criticisms made by meta-theorists (Pajnkihar 2003). Orem developed her theory with the help of theory analysis and evaluation and according to the changes and needs in practice.

Reflective Exercise 5.1

Reasons for the Evolution of Theories

In Chapter 4, you saw a long list of theories that were developed in the United States and a shorter list of those developed in the United Kingdom. Form a small group with your fellow students and consider whether the reasons for their emergence were the same in each country and why the times and places were important.

Also, consider the reasons why there was a slowing down in the development of nursing theories in the United States in the 1980s and in the United Kingdom in the 1990s.

The so-called 'caring theories' first appeared in the 1980s, and Meleis (2018) stated that caring theories have a lot of similarities with interaction theories and were influenced by existential philosophy. Perhaps the most famous was that of Jean Watson, who said that caring is the moral ideal of nursing. In an environment like central Europe, where the essence of nursing, that is, caring, is stressed, Jean Watson's theory is integrated at various levels in the curricula. Emphasising caring awareness starts with graduate students and analysis and evaluation of the theory with master students. PhD students often choose Watson's theory as a theoretical framework for their research. The theory delivers an essential message: caring, which people need in everyday life and when we get sick. Leininger's theory is also a well-known theory of caring, but it also incorporates cultural characteristics relevant to healthcare in an increasingly multicultural society. In 1998, Tracey et al. wrote that Watson's framework was still being taught in numerous baccalaureate nursing curricula in the United States and that these concepts were also widely used in nursing programmes in many countries, including the United Kingdom, Slovenia and Croatia. Morris (1996) also noted that Watson's human care theory was used as the basis for doctoral nursing programmes in the United States and Canada. The incorporation of this theory into nursing curricula added a new dimension to nursing as a whole (Pajnkihar 2003). In addition, Watson's theory is tightly connected with education and practice through the Watson Caring Science Institute that promotes caring science.

In the 1980s, most theorists generally accepted that a qualitative research methodology with a historicist paradigm (see Chapter 2) was the basic methodology for nursing. Consequently, many nursing theorists started to revise their work, leading to an increase in mid-range theories (Pajnkihar 2003). Meleis introduced situation-specific theories in 1999. As a result, the 1990s saw numerous research studies aiming to test nursing theories (George 1995b), which further expanded the number of mid-range theories.

The stimuli for the development of theories in the United Kingdom in the 1980s are interesting. These may have followed from the perception that American theories were not suitable for practice in the United Kingdom. As with the United States, the introduction in the United Kingdom of university education for nurses in the late 1970s forced many lecturers and students to look at how knowledge unique to their discipline might be developed and taught. A similar trend can be seen in other European countries and in Australia, where nursing programmes were being incorporated into academia. In addition, as had happened previously with their American counterparts, UK nurses began to examine the biomedical model and found it an inappropriate framework to guide nursing care. The biomedical model was also questioned in some other European countries but much later. Alligood (2018a) stated that philosophies, models, theories and mid-range and situation-specific theories are being used in nursing education, practice, research and nursing administration in many countries. In addition, she says, theory-based research in nursing contributes to evidence-based practice and the global recognition of the diverse nursing values found in models and theories.

Model

In Chapter 4, readers saw that the term model, in the eyes of most meta-theorists (apart from Jacqueline Fawcett), is synonymous with grand theory. In the literature, the term conceptual model is often shortened to model. Perhaps the difference between conceptual model and theory is best explained by Fawcett and DeSanto-Madeya (2013: 15) in their definition of the theory. They stated, 'one or more relatively concrete and specific concepts that are derived from a conceptual model, the propositions that narrowly described these concepts, and the propositions, that state relatively concrete and specific relations between two or more of the concepts'. In the literature, however, there are many views on the differences and similarities between theories and models.

This often depends on the authors or on the users, and when referring to the term model, most are speaking about grand theory. Another explanation of the conceptual model and its benefits is provided by Butts (2022), who maintained that conceptual models shape the propositions and empirically testable hypotheses. According to Butts, they inform the development or refinement of mid-range theories because everyone perceives the world through a specific frame of reference, known as a conceptual model. However, the term conceptual model continues to be referred to in both literature and practice.

In the following, we provide a classification and an example of a theorist from Alligood (2018b). She defined nursing as a systematically organised body of knowledge from different theorists within philosophies (Watson), conceptual models (Orem), theories and grand theories (Meleis), and mid-range theories (Swanson). In contrast, Fawcett (2021) distinguished grand theories from conceptual models. Practising nurses often refer to Orem's model or Roper, Logan and Tierney's model, but seldom refer to these conceptualisations as theories. Therefore, in this short section, we will discuss what is meant by models. You can decide for yourself if you think that the designation 'model' or 'theory' is the best way to describe the work of the various theorists.

The term 'model' has been defined by Chinn et al. (2022: 156) as:

A symbolic representation of an empiric experience in the form of words, pictorial or graphic diagrams, mathematical notations, or physical material.

Some of the simplest definitions of a model describe it as a representation of reality (McFarlane 1986) or a simplified way of organising a complex phenomenon (Stockwell 1985). Other authors have elaborated on both these descriptions. Fawcett (2006) stated that a model comprises a set of concepts and the assumptions that integrate them into a meaningful configuration. The discoverers of DNA, Watson and Crick, did not fully comprehend its structure and function until they built the three-dimensional double helix model. Therefore, models are tools that enable users to understand more complex phenomena in a simple way.

McKenna (1994) suggested that a nursing model is a mental or diagrammatic representation of care that is systematically constructed and assists practitioners in organising their thinking about what they do. In addition, transferring their thinking into practice benefits the patient and the profession. Perhaps the term 'model' brings to users a more practical connotation through their experiences in life, for example, model toys, or in nursing, 'model simulators'.

We can define models as describing nursing phenomena and assumptions in very abstract yet logical ways. They can then be presented and organised using nursing language, words, mental pictures, diagrams, drawings or logical structures to help understand what is observed in practice. In this way, models assist in organising and understanding situations in practice and in conceptualising their reality. Models are very abstract tools used in all disciplines and everyday life, such as model airplanes, dolls' house or diagrammatic instructions for putting together a new bookshelf.

Theory

In Chapter 1, we explained that there are numerous definitions of nursing theories. The theories enable nurses to describe, explain, predict and, according to Dickoff and James, prescribe nursing care to help patients, families or society at large, and support practice, education and research (see Reflective Exercise 5.2).

Reflective Exercise 5.2

Defining Theory

Refer to Chapter 1 to review the different definitions of nursing theory that were identified.

Goodson (2022) put it very well when she wrote that it is difficult to understand what a theory is, how it can help with research and how to decide which theory to use. She outlined that the allure of theory is found in its sophisticated complexity, which is like the enchanting intricacies seen in a kaleidoscope, a fractal pattern or the internal mechanisms of the human body. Each is a unique system, rich in detail and complexity, contained within its own distinct framework. It is not necessary to reiterate the various descriptions of theory here, but the following section will show there that is still some confusion as to whether the work of a theorist is a model, a conceptual model, a grand theory or a paradigm. Readers should select the view they feel comfortable with and know that not everyone will agree.

McKenna (1997) suggested that nurses selected the term model rather than theory because of their lack of confidence as a profession. At the time, they had only just entered the hallowed surroundings of the university, so how could they suddenly come up with all these theories. To call them models on a continuum towards theory building was more acceptable. However, Rodgers (2022) stated that as nurses have attained higher levels of education, especially those with doctorates, there has been an even greater need to understand the core nursing knowledge (see Reflective Exercise 5.3).

Reflective Exercise 5.3

Model or Theory – You Decide

In Chapter 1, you were introduced to the theory and its working elements of concepts, propositions and assumptions. In this chapter, the term model has been described. Think of those theorists whose work you are most familiar with and decide whether you think 'model' or 'theory' is the best descriptor.

Discuss your thinking with a fellow student or colleague – remember, they may not agree with you, but that does not mean you are wrong.

Theory or Model?

Peplau published her theory of *Interpersonal Relations in Nursing* in 1952. You will learn more about her work in Chapter 6. She was the first nurse, since Nightingale (1859/1980), to develop an explicit nursing theory. She worked in psychiatric nursing practice in New Jersey, USA, and observed that building interpersonal relationships was important but often lacking in patient care. So, in her theory, she described the importance of the therapeutic interrelationship between nurses and patients. Peplau has left a remarkable legacy because 70 years later interpersonal relationships are still at the heart of nursing, valued by staff and patients alike, and they will continue to be.

With no obvious explanation, she called it a 'partial theory for the practice of nursing'. A second edition of the book appeared in 1988 with little change. The aim of the theory, as Peplau (1952: xiii) said, was 'helping nurses to understand the relationship of nurse personalities to these functions'. Later, the meta-theorist Marriner Tomey (1998) classified Peplau's work as a mid-range theory, Butts (2022) categorised it as a descriptive mid-range theory, George (1995a) described it as a theory and Alligood (2018b) described it as philosophy. In contrast, Reed (1996) referred to it as a practice theory (Pajnkihar 2003). More recently, and shortly before her death, Peplau (1995a) did explicitly refer to her work as a theory.

Analyses of Orem's theory are awash with controversy. Meleis (1997: 398) asserted that it is a descriptive theory, while Feathers (1989) maintained that Orem developed a complete descriptive theory, adding some elements of explanatory theory. More recently, Marriner Tomey (1998) and Pajnkihar (2003) both viewed Orem's work as a grand theory.

Watson (1988: 1, 2012: 4) asserted that her work on caring is 'not hard scientific theory' but is still a theory – a descriptive theory. Her explanation for this assertion was not forthcoming. Nonetheless, Marriner Tomey (1998) and Alligood (2018b) classified it as a philosophy, while Smith and Parker (2015) and Pajnkihar et al. (2017) argued that it is a grand theory.

Readers may be frustrated in the lack of agreement among authors on what to call these conceptualisations. However, this is the current status of theoretical evolution within the profession. The theory–model debate may best be understood by looking at the views of these chief protagonists. Jacqueline Fawcett firmly believes in differentiating models, conceptual models, from theories. In the opposite corner is Afaf Meleis, who has a determined view that all these conceptualisations are theories. Both are highly respected meta-theorists; let us examine their arguments.

According to Fawcett (2005a), models are more abstract than their theoretical counterparts. They present a generalised, broad and abstract view of phenomena. To underpin her strong views Fawcett wrote several editions of two distinct books, one on nursing theories and the other on conceptual modes. She maintained that theories are more specific and precise, containing more clearly defined concepts with a narrower focus. So, as we have seen in earlier chapters, the difference is one of abstraction, explication and application. Let us refer to this argument as 'position A' (Figure 5.1).

This differentiation would appear to clear up the confusion, but Meleis (2007, 2018) argued that it matters little what we call these 'things'. She believed that much time has been wasted debating the differences between models, theories

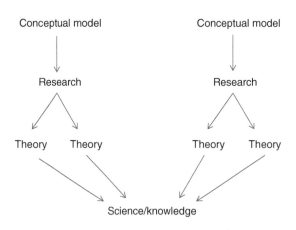

FIGURE 5.1   The theory–model controversy: position A.

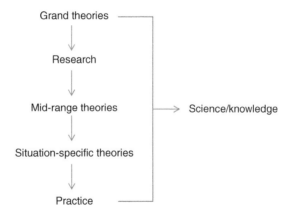

FIGURE 5.2 The theory–model controversy: position B.

and paradigms. Rather, she maintains that time would be better spent evaluating the effects of these conceptualisations on patient care.

Meleis based her argument on her desire to concentrate on content and not on labels. She asserted that theory exists at different stages of development, from the most primitive to the most sophisticated form, and therefore even the simplest conceptualisation is a theory. Her stance would be that models are theories, but at a more abstract level than the theories developed through research. The most primitive may be referred to as grand (or broad) theories, while the most sophisticated are referred to as mid-range or practice theories. We will refer to this view as 'position B' (Figure 5.2).

However, for the purpose of this book, you will have detected that the term we will use throughout will be theory (position B). The basis for this decision lies with Meleis's call for professionals to concentrate on substance (content) rather than structure (terminology). When theories are mentioned in this book, we will be referring to position B, unless otherwise specified (see Key Concepts 5.1 and Reflective Exercise 5.4).

It is important that both theories and models present phenomena in systematic ways that help to organise the work of nurses both in practice and in education and develop the body of nursing knowledge and science.

Key Concepts 5.1

Theory and Model

Theory exists at different stages of development and a conceptual model is an early stage on the way to becoming a theory.

Reflective Exercise 5.4

Position A or Position B?

Both positions can be supported by referring to various bodies of literature. We would urge you to view both approaches as worthy of consideration. However, for the purposes of this exercise, consider which position you are attracted to. Think of those theorists whose work you are most familiar with and decide whether you think models or theories are the best descriptors. Write down the pros and cons of each and your justification for selecting your favoured position.

Discuss your thinking with a fellow student or colleague – remember, they may not agree with you, but that does not mean you are wrong. Check if they have identified the same or different advantages and disadvantages.

The Classification of Theories

Since the mid-1970s, there have been various attempts to categorise a large number of grand theories into a number of common types. Aggleton and Chalmers (2000) believed that this trend would help nurses to make some preliminary decisions about the choice of theory that was most appropriate for a particular clinical setting. This grouping of theories by some specific trait also leads to understanding the various schools of thought underpinning each theory. Systems of cataloguing theories often arise when the editors of a book try to arrange them into some orderly scheme.

In Chapter 3, we described another classification of theories and now will make a short summary. Mid-range theories in nursing are classified into specific types that help structure various aspects of nursing knowledge. McKenna and Slevin (2008) identify four main categorisations: descriptive, explanatory, predictive and prescriptive. According to the authors, we can say that descriptive theories (describe phenomena), explanatory theories (describe phenomena and explain relationships), predictive theories (describe, explain and forecast cause and effect relationships among concepts) and prescriptive theories (describe, explain and forecast cause-and-effect relationship among concepts, apply knowledge in practice). Other slight variations on types of theory exist as well. For instance, Meleis (2007, 2018) described them in two categories: descriptive and predictive.

The following section gives some examples of theory classification. Different authors classified theories according to the level of use that can be made of them in describing, explaining, predicting or (according to Dickoff & James 1968) prescribing (McKenna 1997; Meleis 2012, 2018). Within the classification this means that descriptive theory is the least developed theory because it has no explanatory, predictive or prescriptive power (Pajnkihar 2003).

Meleis (2007, 2018) organised theories into those that 'describe what we do'; 'those that describe how we do it'; and 'those that describe the why of practice'. She also classified them into four schools of thought: needs, interaction, outcome and caring/becoming. In contrast, Stevens-Barnum (1998) used the following classifications: intervention, conservation, substitution, sustenance and enhancement. Alligood and Marriner Tomey (2006) sorted theories into humanistic, interpersonal, systems and energy fields. Fawcett (2012b) talks about empirical, aesthetic, ethical theories, sociopolitical or emancipatory theories, and theories of personal knowledge. She differentiated theories according to organisational and individual factors that influenced evidence-based nursing practice.

Marrs and Lowry (2006) proposed an expanded hierarchy of nursing knowledge in which theories are classified. They sort components of nursing knowledge by the level of abstraction: meta paradigm as the most abstract component, followed by philosophies, conceptual models, grand theories, mid-range theories, practice theories and empirical indicators as the most concrete, and we can add situation-specific theories.

Colley (2003) classified nursing theories based on the philosophical underpinnings of the theories (need, interaction, outcome and humanistic theories) and, according to Polit et al. (2001), on the generalisability of their principles (meta-theory, grand theory, mid-range theory and practice theory) and function (descriptive, explanatory, predictive and prescriptive). Also, McEwen (2019) saw theories according to their purpose as descriptive, explanatory, predictive and prescriptive.

To summaries this section, the most common classification of theories is first, the level of abstraction. Therefore, Walker and Avant (2019) and McEwen (2019) classify them as meta-theories, grand theories, mid-range theories and practice theories. Im and Meleis (2021) categorise them into grand theories, mid-range theories and situation-specific theories. Fawcett (2021) delineates four levels: conceptual models, grand theories, mid-range theories and situation-specific theories.

In Chapter 3, we described a meta-theory, and here we wish to summarise the classification. In the hierarchy of nursing knowledge, grand, mid-range and situation-specific theories are the primary categories discussed. Meta-theory and practice theory, although not explicitly named in Fawcett's framework, are introduced to help Advanced Practice Nurses (APNs) understand their roles and perspectives in theoretical discussions. Meta-theory, often seen as the highest level of theoretical abstraction, involves a philosophical examination of theory itself. It is concerned with the methods and processes of theory creation and evaluation. Unlike theorists who create specific theories and content, meta-theorists engage in discussions and analyses that aim to unify and advance the discipline's theoretical foundations.

🔍 Key Concepts 5.2

Classification of Theories

Theories can be classified according to the level of use or function, their generalisability, level of development, philosophical underpinnings and their paradigmatic roots.

Classification of Theories According to Their Paradigm Roots

As you can see from the preceding section, theories are classified in many different ways. One of the most popular is a categorisation according to their paradigmatic roots (see Key Concepts 5.2). Smith and Parker (2015) claimed that the concept of a paradigm is useful for grasping nursing knowledge. A paradigm is a broad framework consisting of assumptions about critical aspects of the discipline, as agreed upon by its members for its development. Paradigms represent specific viewpoints within the metaparadigm or disciplinary domain. The paradigms that have been identified as relevant to nursing theories are 'systems', 'interactional', 'developmental' and 'behavioural'. You will recall from Chapter 1 that a paradigm represents a broad worldview.

Systems Paradigms

These theories are largely based on the 'general systems' paradigm put forward by von Bertalanffy (1951). Put simply, a system is a collection of parts that function as a whole entity for a particular purpose. The parts within a particular system are connected and interrelated. These interrelationships may form 'subsystems' within the parent system. Similarly, the system itself may form part of an overall 'suprasystem'. If the system has permeable boundaries, it is called an 'open system'. If not, it is referred to as a closed system. In system theories, the patient is often referred to as an 'open system' (see Reflective Exercise 5.5). The work of Johnson (1959), Roy (1970), Parse (1981), Neuman (1982) and Fitzpatrick and Whall (1983) may be grouped under the systems paradigm.

Reflective Exercise 5.5

Systems

A system is made up of subsystems. Think of the human body as a system, with subsystems including the mind, the respiratory system, the cardiac system and so on. But systems exist in a larger supra-system (e.g. family and class grouping). The 'human body' system interacts with other systems and has permeable boundaries because there are inputs into the system (e.g. knowledge, food and water) and outputs (e.g. waste, speech and perspiration). Therefore, it is an open system.

Think of a hospital ward as a system. What subsystems could exist in that system? What supra-system is the ward part of and what are the inputs and outputs to the system? What are the permeable boundaries that exist between this system and other similar systems?

Identify two other things that may be conceptualised as a system.

Interactional Paradigms

Interactional theories have their origin in the symbolic interactionist paradigm (Blumer 1969). This paradigm emphasises the relationships between people and the roles they play in society. Nursing activities are perceived as interactional processes between practitioners and patients. Among the better-known interactional theories are those of Orlando (1961), Levine (1966), Riehl (1974), Paterson and Zderad (1976) and King (1968).

Take the example of a nurse assessing a patient. Here, an interaction is taking place in which there is a transaction of information. The interaction and its results may be influenced by the various roles played by the nurse and the patient. The nurse also reacts to the patient's interaction and vice versa, and both may alter their own interactional processes as a result of reactions from each other. This demonstrates how the interactional theories can be applied to practice situations (see Reflective Exercise 5.6).

Reflective Exercise 5.6

Interactional Paradigms

Interaction theorists focus their attention on the relationship between the patient and the nurse and these theories can be applied to practice situations.

Think about a particular patient with whom you have worked. Think of the interaction that took place. Was it two-way or just one-way? How did you react to the patient's interaction and how did the patient react to your interaction? Was it an equal interaction or was one of you taking the lead?

Developmental Paradigms

The developmental paradigm originated from the work of Freud (1949) and Sullivan (1953). The central themes are growth, development, maturation and change. It is argued that human beings are constantly developing, whether this be physiologically, socially, psychologically or spiritually. Development is seen as an ongoing process in which the person must pass through various stages. The nurse's role is to encourage positive development and discourage the formation of barriers to natural development. The works of Peplau (1952), Travelbee (1966) and Newman (1979) are often perceived as having their foundations in developmental theory. Some of these theories will be discussed in greater detail in Chapter 6.

Within a developmental paradigm, nurses are often encouraging growth and development, much as a gardener would do with plants, encouraging maturation and removing barriers to development such as weeds or parasites. The patient may have had a stroke and have to live with a new disability or be a mother who has given birth to a disabled child. Initially, care will be required for these patients to learn new attitudes, knowledge and skills in order to mature in the new situation in which they find themselves. The nurse will also discourage thoughts of hopelessness and anxiety. Hopefully, their care will reach a point where they will no longer require the support and presence of the nurse because they will have changed to a higher level of growth within the limits of the disabilities.

Behavioural Paradigms

These theories owe much to the theoretical formulations of Maslow (1954). Because of this, they are often referred to as 'human needs theories' (Webb 1986). Behavioural theories assume that individuals normally exist and survive by meeting their own needs. Included in this category is the work of Orem (1959), Wiedenbach (1964), Henderson (1966), Roper et al. (1980) and Minshull et al. (1986) (see Reflective Exercise 5.7).

Reflective Exercise 5.7

Behavioural Paradigms

You will recall from previous chapters that Roper, Logan and Tierney's theory focuses on 12 activities of daily living (ADLs), and Orem's work focuses on self-care. In each case, the nurse's role is to identify the patient's needs. In the former case, the needs are those where the patient is dependent on some of their ADLs; in the latter, the needs result from the fact that the patient cannot self-care.

In the United Kingdom, the most popular nursing theories in use in clinical settings are those of Roper et al. and Orem. Discuss with fellow students why human needs theories are so popular.

An easily understood article on human needs is that of Minshull et al. (1986). Read it and decide whether you see validity in this approach to theorising.

Because there are no rigid criteria available to place theories into these paradigmatic classifications, it will not surprise you that there are disagreements among authors as to which group a particular theory belongs. For instance, Orem's work has been seen as having its basis in the systems paradigm by Suppe and Jacox (1985), in the interactional paradigm by Greaves (1984), in the developmental paradigm by McFarlane (1986), and in the behavioural paradigm by Chapman (1985). Despite these disagreements, this method of classification has been considered a valid one for categorising nursing theories.

Current Trends in Nursing Theories

Nursing theories are crucial to the development of nursing as a professional discipline and profession. They support and inform practice and education and provide a theoretical framework for research. Theories at all levels of abstraction and development have clearly become integral to the complexity of nursing by supporting complex knowledge. Mid-range and situation-specific theories are gaining special recognition. With literature analyses, we noticed a large amount of published literature about scientific development in nursing, closing practice–theory gap and a new focus on less abstract theories. Furthermore, McEwen and Wills (2019) noticed a continuous review of trends in nursing theory and nursing science, highlighting a growing focus on mid-range and situation-specific theories.

Critiques of nursing theories are a useful endeavour. Theofanidis and Fountouki (2008) noticed that if a theory is adopted too rigidly, the care becomes vague. Nonetheless, even if theories are weak, there is still value in them because they may stimulate discussion and debate. Despite all that has been written, Schmenner et al. (2009) claimed that we cannot just criticise existing notions of theory and models without offering feasible alternatives. Nurses must appreciate different types of theories and critique them, and in this way contribute to the continued development of nursing (Colley 2003). Smith and Parker (2015) supported the idea that nursing theory is driven by questions and curiosities that emerge from nursing practice.

What is important for the future development of theories is reflection on practice needs and to take into account situations in healthcare systems where interdisciplinary knowledge is needed. The point is not to develop new theories for their own ends, but to analyse, evaluate, test and apply current theories in practice to assess their usefulness. More attention is needed to develop clear criteria for theory analysis and evaluation. This will be explored further in Chapter 9.

The Nursing Metaparadigm

Regardless of how theories are categorised, there is a consensus that each must specify certain central concepts. These 'essential elements' have been referred to as the 'metaparadigm' of nursing (Fawcett 2005a). Metaparadigm represents the broadest global consensus in nursing. In theory, it shows the essence of the theorist's conceptualisation, the theorist's view of nursing and how the theorist views the (largely included) four always abstract concepts of metaparadigm, namely, person, nursing, health and environment (see Key Concepts 5.3).

Key Concepts 5.3

The Metaparadigm abstract components to cover practice phenomena, which usually include four essential elements – person, nursing, health and environment (see Appendix A).

For Hardy (1978: 89), a metaparadigm is the 'broadest consensus within a discipline' or 'a gestalt or total view within a discipline'. Hardy also calls it the 'prevailing paradigm', presenting 'a general orientation or total worldview that holds the commitment and consensus of the scientists in a particular discipline'. Fawcett pointed out that every discipline singles out certain named phenomena (broad concepts) with which it will deal uniquely and such phenomena combine to form the metaparadigm for that discipline. The metaparadigm acts as a vital unit or framework within which the more specific structures develop. Most professions have a single metaparadigm from which numerous theories emerge; contemporary nursing appears to have reached this level of theoretical sophistication.

During the 1970s and 1980s, authors wrote extensively about the importance of the essential concepts of nursing science. The argument was put forward that if a nursing theory did not include assumptions about 'nursing', 'health', 'person' and 'environment', it could not be considered to be a theory (see Reflective Exercise 5.8).

Reflective Exercise 5.8

The Metaparadigm

Get three or four of your colleagues together and spend 15 minutes considering how each of you describes 'nursing', 'health', 'person' and 'environment'. Write one sentence on each and try to refrain from using quotations from well-known theorists. Once you've all done this, compare what you have all written and then, as a group, attempt to categorise the views in one or more of the systems, interactional, developmental or behavioural paradigms (see Appendix A).

However, the complete four-concept metaparadigm has its dissenters. For example, Stevens-Barnum (1998) excluded 'environment' and Kim (1983) excluded 'health'. Some authors believe that 'nursing' should be omitted as a concept, maintaining that its inclusion is a redundancy in terms and that instead the term 'caring' should be included (Leininger, cited in Huch 1995). Plummer and Molzahn (2009) found, from a review of the theories of Peplau, Rogers, Leininger, King and Parse, that health could be replaced by quality of life as a metaparadigm element. Schim et al. (2007) explored community and public health nursing in urban settings and suggested the inclusion of social justice as a fifth element of the nursing metaparadigm.

Kao et al. (2006) explored the Western nursing four-element metaparadigm through a Chinese lens. Shattell (2006) commented that this provided nurses with theoretical knowledge of other ways of viewing the nursing metaparadigm by giving a refreshing look at an 'alternative' way of seeing the world. There is a wide debate in the literature on the topic of metaparadigm.

O'Rourke and Fawcett (2024) continue their discussion about metaparadigm concept culture and subcultures and clearly state why they reject the subculture. The impact of rejecting the concept of subcultures on broader cultural metaparadigm emphasises its significance for human diversity, global health and nursing practices. In the article, Fawcett (2024) introduced the new metaparadigm concept of culture and also described all metaparadigm concepts with relational propositions.

Fawcett (2023), in defining nursology, complemented the concepts of the metaparadigm by including:

- Human beings: Encompassing all cultures of the world, including families, communities and groups.
- Global environment: Encompassing the internal and external environments of human beings, including local, regional and global cultures, as well as social, political and economic conditions that affect human beings.
- Planetary health: Recognising that human beings and the planet continue to evolve towards well-being, encompassing the processes of living and dying.
- Activities of nursing psychologists: Highlighting the interaction process between nurses and participants.

Later she added:

- Culture: To learn about, explain and predict people's life pathways over time and in different environments. Culture emerges from beliefs, attitudes, religious practices, language, art, music, values, morals, behavioural patterns and dietary customs (Leininger 2006; Fawcett 2024a).

She changed 'environment' to 'global environment' and 'health' to 'planetary health' to emphasise the contemporary focus on all countries and the health of all human beings of our planet and to capture the effects of climate change, peace and war and global interpersonal violence on the well-being of all people and the planet.

As the metaparadigm represents the foundation stones for various theories, one would expect each theory to outline its beliefs and assumptions regarding the 'person', to present an identification of the person's 'environment', to define what 'nursing' (and/or midwifery) is and to discuss the theorist's views on 'health'.

Although each grand nursing theory conceptualises the four essential concepts of the metaparadigm, they tend to view them from different perspectives. Therefore, how nursing, health, person and environment are described and defined varies greatly from theorist to theorist. So, while theorists consider the same metaparadigmatic elements, they may emphasise different aspects and see them in different relations to one another. Such a rich diversity of assumptions concerning the same factors can only enrich the nursing profession (see Reflective Exercise 5.9).

Reflective Exercise 5.9

Metaparadigms in Different Professions

Each profession has its own metaparadigm, which encapsulates the central elements of that discipline. For architecture, they could be structure, design, aestheticism and materials. For the legal profession a metaparadigm might include, law, crime and justice.

Think about the professions of teaching and religion. For each one, identify what you believed the metaparadigm elements would be. You may want to compare these with what other students or colleagues thought.

How Different Theorists Viewed the Metaparadigm

In the following, we extract the metaparadigm concepts from the works of Peplau (1952), Henderson (1966), Watson (1988) and Orem (1991, 1995) (see Appendix A).

Person
- Henderson (1966, 1991) believed that body and mind are inseparable and viewed the patient as a person who needs help with basic life activities and achieving health and independence, or to die peacefully.
- Orem (1991: 181) described a person or human being as 'a unity that can be viewed as functioning biologically, symbolically, and socially'.
- Watson (1988: 45) viewed the person as 'a being in the world' who is the locus of human existence. A person exists as a living and growing gestalt and possesses the three dimensions of being – mind, body and soul – which exist in harmony in good health, where the essence of the person is the soul, which is 'spirit, or a higher sense of self'.
- Peplau (1952: 82) defined humans as organisms that live in an unstable equilibrium (i.e. physiological, psychological and social fluidity). She asserted that all individuals have physical, psychological and social needs, and that in an unstable environment, they constantly meet new situations and new problems.

Nursing
- Henderson (1966) described nursing as a profession that helps people, sick or well, in the performance of the 14 basic life activities that contribute to health or its recovery (or to a peaceful death) that they would perform unaided if they had the necessary strength, will or knowledge.
- Orem (1995) described nursing as a specialised human service to society. She characterised nursing as action and assistance with the goal of helping people meet their own demands for self-care on a therapeutic and continuous basis.
- Watson (1988: 73) asserted that caring is essential to nursing and is 'a moral ideal that includes concepts such as a phenomenal field, an actual caring occasion, and transpersonal caring', which are central to her theory. She saw

nursing as both a science and an art. Watson (1988: 54) defined nursing as 'a human science of persons and human health-illness experiences that are mediated by professional, personal, scientific, aesthetic, and ethical human care transactions'. Watson (1988: 17) further explained that in this view of nursing as a human science, nursing can combine and integrate science with beauty, art, ethics and aesthetics of the human-to-human care process.

- Peplau (1952) defined nursing as a significant, therapeutic, interpersonal process. It functions cooperatively with other processes that make health possible for people and communities. 'Nursing is an educative instrument, a maturing force, that aims to promote forward movement of personality in the direction of creative, constructive, productive, personal, and community living'.

Health

- Henderson (1966, 1991) did not specifically define her own concept of health, but she sees it as the ability of people to function independently by reference to the 14 basic life activities. Therefore, health relates to independence.
- Orem (1995: 96) suggested that the 'term health has considerable general utility in describing the state of wholeness or integrity of human beings'. Orem (1995: 101) explained that well-being is used in the sense of an individual's 'perceived condition of existence'. The nursing domain concerning health involves the promotion and maintenance of health and protection against specific diseases and injuries.
- Watson (1988: 48) referred to health as 'unity and harmony within the mind, body, and soul'. To her, health is associated with 'the degree of congruence between the self as perceived and the self as experienced'. A person becomes ill when there is conscious or unconscious disharmony between these. 'Illness is not necessarily disease'.
- Peplau (1952: 12) maintained that health 'is a word symbol that implies forward movement of personality and other ongoing human processes in the direction of creative, constructive, productive, personal, and community living'. She saw health as a process whereby an individual has a quality of life that enables the contribution to personal and community living.

Environment

- Henderson (1966, 1991) did not explicitly define the environment, but through her explanation of what a patient is, it is evident that she was concerned with the influences affecting the life and health of patients, especially the family and cultural influences.
- For Orem (1991: 38), the person and the environment are in constant interaction and the nurse must consider the human environment, analysing and understanding the various 'physical, chemical, biological, and social features'.
- Watson (1988: 75) did not explicitly define environment, but the environment is specifically used in her 10 carative factors (in later refinements she changed to caritas processes), in particular, the promotion of a 'supportive, protective, and/or corrective mental, physical, societal, and spiritual environment'. Nurses must recognise the influence of internal and external environments on the health and illness of individuals and also the need to support and protect individuals.
- Peplau (1952: 14) defined the environment as forces existing 'outside the organism and in the context of the culture'.

In recent decades, we have been concerned about the environment at a global level, given climate change, poverty, unrest, wars and migration, which bring with them sociocultural and economic changes in societies and have an impact on the health environment as well. Kalogirou, Olson and Davidson (2020) explained the reasons for nursing's delayed response to climate change and the shift towards a planetary health perspective. Fawcett (2022) discusses the impact of the external environment on the nursing discipline and its context of theoretical models. She goes on to say that interest in the environment has broadened to include environmental security and climate change and she asks how we can change our understanding of the environment as it relates to human well-being and disease. Fawcett (2024b) continued these discussions about an environment with the evolution of nursing's focus from immediate surroundings to a global environmental perspective.

Students often have problems differentiating between concepts of metaparadigms and basic concepts of theory and their interactions (see Reflective Exercise 5.10). Basic concepts of the theory are always synchronised and well connected with concepts of the metaparadigm. For example, the central concepts of Watson's theory are human care, transpersonal care relationships, the self, the phenomenal field, events, actual caring occasions and caritas processes.

Reflective Exercise 5.10

Differentiation Between Concepts of Metaparadigms and Basic Concepts of Theory

Go to the library or online and read up on Swanson's (1991) mid-range theory of caring. She explicated her beliefs about the four metaparadigm elements of concern to the discipline of nursing (nursing, person/client, health and environment) and defined the main concept of her theory: caring and five concepts of the caring process.

Consider whether nursing, health, environment and person capture the essence of nursing. Would you change any of these or add anything?

Benefits of Nursing Theories

Nursing theories offer frameworks and concepts that establish the role of nursing within healthcare. These theories provide nurses with perspectives for collaborating with professionals from other disciplines to deliver human services. There are significant expectations placed on nursing theories (Smith & Parker 2015). Those who advocate the use of theories do so for a number of reasons. The two distinct benefits are the substitution of the biomedical model for delivering care and the understanding that theories lead to the development of nursing knowledge. These have already been discussed. However, the literature highlights several other equally favourable advantages. Hardin (2018) stated that scientific progress is based on the review and validation of theoretical knowledge by the scientific community. Smith and Parker (2015) noticed a growing body of literature and evidence that theories have become linked to and underpin practice.

Alligood (2010a) highlighted the significant benefits of theories from both patients' and professionals' perspectives, considering them a systematic approach to person-oriented care. According to Marrs and Lowry (2006), nurses who use nursing theories establish a theoretical foundation for their practice. Pajnkihar (2003) argued that nursing as a profession and as a discipline needs a unique body of knowledge and that nursing theory provides an organised, systematic, empirical and logical view of the knowledge that nurses need for everyday practice, education and research to benefit their patients. However, we need to be aware of the allures, uniqueness and complexity of each theory. As Goodson (2022) pointed out, the allure of theory is found in its sophisticated complexity – a unique system, rich in detail and complexity, contained within its own distinct framework. Considering the breadth of theoretical publications, it is indisputable that theories are derived from practice and returned to support practice. This creates a never-ending cycle of interaction between practice, research and theory.

A Guide to Practice

Evidence clearly shows that as the science and discipline of nursing have developed, theories are being applied to underpin practice (Smith & Parker 2015). Colley (2003: 33) wrote that: 'ideally, nursing theory should provide the principles that underpin practice'. Although British nurses have been introduced to theories, they have been wrestling with the nursing process for some decades. There is a consensus of opinion that the implementation of the nursing process without a theory to underpin it is an empty exercise akin to 'practising in the dark' (Aggleton & Chalmers 2000). It could be argued that they have put the 'cart before the horse'. By providing a systematic basis for assessment, planning, implementing and evaluating, theories offer a way to 'revitalise' the nursing process.

In many instances, the nursing process was also introduced in many European countries before an understanding of nursing theories. Therefore, nurses knew that they had to assess but did not always know what to assess; they knew they had to plan but did not always know how to plan; and they knew they had to intervene but did not always know what interventions to use. Nursing theories would have provided them with the missing details (McKenna 1997; Pajnkihar 2003).

In order to be implemented successfully and to have meaning for practitioners, the nursing process as a problem-solving exercise must be framed within a theory. Nursing theories also stress the importance of the wholeness and integrity of the person, thereby enhancing the practitioner's ability to provide individualised care. Theories are essential guides for practice, and as such they help to bring theory and the process of practice closer together. Butts (2022) asserted that the construction and categorisation of related theories play a crucial role in advanced practice nursing, emphasising the deliberate application of appropriate theory.

The usefulness of these frameworks has also been recognised in the areas of nursing education, administration and research (Nicholl 1992). American nursing theories were first adapted for European countries and were used in nursing education rather than in practice. When nursing education accepted theories, there was not enough knowledge in practice to deal with them. A nurse who took part in a research project observed: 'Practical work is not possible without theories, but many of them are hard to understand and the nurses' level of knowledge does not allow them to use the theories' (Pajnkihar 2003). In addition, in the era of digitalisation in healthcare, faster, more complex and individualised approaches to interdisciplinary patient management are expected. Nursing theories have shown and demonstrated that they can be implemented into electronic health records, supporting more efficient and personalised patient care.

Education

Education has a key influence on the understanding and acceptance of theories, research and practice. It is imperative that theories are included in undergraduate and postgraduate degree programmes to understand the historical development of the profession and discipline. Although the dichotomy between the classroom and the ward is well documented (Meleis 2007; Smith & Liehr 2018) and much was made of the theory–practice gap in earlier chapters, there is evidence to suggest that the structuring of an education programme around a theory is extremely beneficial for students and as a result, theory and practice may eventually meet. Alligood (2011) stated that nursing theories provide important frameworks for nurse educators. To ensure a strong theory–practice relationship, we have to incorporate theory into the curricula (Donohue-Porter et al. 2011).

However, if theories are only taught in the classroom and if students do not come across them in practice, theories will remain 'academic'. It can be difficult for students to understand and see the usefulness of theories when they cannot see those theories they learned in the classroom playing a part in how care is delivered in practice. Nurses have become aware that practice based on theory shapes their professional work. For example, Pajnkihar et al. (2020, 2023) found that implementing caring theories in nursing curricula is essential for cultivating a caring culture among students. Positive faculty role modelling and creating caring environments enhanced students' caring behaviours and values. This approach ensured that future nurses embody caring values in their professional practice.

Professionalisation

Johnson (1959: 212) stated that 'no profession can exist for long without making explicit its theoretical basis for practice'. Later, Smith (1986) maintained that nursing can achieve full professional status comparable with other professions by basing its practice on theories. It is important to have the mindset that nursing is a professional discipline based on care and caring, and it needs to be based on nursing knowledge from nursing philosophies, theories, concepts and research evidence to support practice (Walker & Avant 2019). On the other hand, McEwen (2019) claimed that nursing is a profession, academic discipline and science. Theories were also seen as indicators of autonomy, responsibility and leading to professional accountability (Meleis 2007, 2018). Pajnkihar (2011) argued that without care, there is no medical treatment, and without theory, there is no nursing, no profession and no discipline. Contemporaneously, Bond et al. (2011: 404) stressed that 'a meaningful triadic relationship in theory, research and practice is essential for nursing to be recognised as a profession'. Nursing cannot claim to be a profession if its scientific knowledge is not developed and applied to clients' benefit. Theory helps to develop the discipline and profession of nursing. A typical interviewee's convictions about the usefulness of nursing theories are as follows (Pajnkihar 2003):

Nursing theories are the basis of the profession. We need them if we want nursing care to be acknowledged publicly. Theories are our groundwork; we build on them. Without nursing theory and history, there is no profession. If we fail to see that, we fail to acknowledge our status and our profession.

Quality of Care

The quality, safety and effectiveness of patient care are linked to the core knowledge that theories contribute. In his research, McKenna (1994) found that the quality of care given by a practitioner using a theory is high because practice is built on a systematic knowledge base. The quality of service cannot be assessed unless there are standards against which an appraisal can be made. Quality of care evaluation in contemporary practice is becoming increasingly related to cost-effectiveness. If used appropriately, nursing theories can demonstrate cost-effectiveness through reducing dependency, encouraging self-care and the early detection of patients' problems. A nursing theory also allows staff a greater articulation of health goals, hence identifying more efficiently the resources and skills needed to achieve them.

For example, the introduction of caring theories of nursing has a positive impact on quality of care. Pajnkihar et al. (2017) found that when patients perceived caring behaviours from nursing staff, they reported greater satisfaction with the care received during their hospital stay. Vrbnjak (2017) and Vrbnjak et al. (2023) also claimed that caring is a foundation for safety and quality. Research showed that medication error reporting is influenced by caring culture and perceptions of Caritas processes.

Perceived benefits of theories for practice are shown in Table 5.1.

TABLE 5.1   Perceived benefits of theories for practice.

- Assist student learning
- Help to structure patient assessment
- Permit meaningful communication between nurses with professional language, values and beliefs
- Improve critical thinking and problem-solving with practical actions
- Increase patients' and nurses' satisfaction
- Identify the goals of practice and theory-guided practice and education
- Substantially improve quality of care
- Clarify nurses' realm of accountability
- Focus observations on important phenomena
- Guide and justify actions on the basis of valid knowledge
- Clarify thinking among nurses about practice and linking theory to practice
- Provide others with a rationale for nurses' work
- Direct research into clinical needs
- Help to establish more holistic, compassionate, person-centred and individualised care

Limitations of Nursing Theories

We touched a little bit on the benefits and limitations of nursing theories in Chapters 1 and 3. However, the following sections offer an overview of the disadvantages (see Table 5.2). It will not surprise you that nursing theories have a number of well-publicised limitations, although the number of published benefits of theories is growing. There is no theory that can be right for all environments or fit into all nursing fields, or simply be the perfect one. Meleis (2018, 2021) elaborated on this by pointing out that many nursing theories fail to account for the complexities of individual patient experiences. They often do not sufficiently address the cultural, social and economic factors that significantly influence patient outcomes. This gap can lead to a disconnect between theories and the realities of nursing care.

Chinn (2021) criticised some nursing theories for their lack of interdisciplinary perspectives. In today's healthcare environment, where teamworking and collaborative care are crucial, the insular nature of some nursing theories can limit their effectiveness and relevance. This isolation can prevent the integration of nursing theory into the broader healthcare context, where interprofessional collaboration is often necessary for optimal patient care. Smith (2018) identified another significant limitation: the evolution of healthcare and nursing roles. Many nursing theories were developed decades ago and do not fully reflect current healthcare practices or the evolving scope of nursing responsibilities.

Fawcett (2021) highlighted that one major limitation of many nursing theories is their often abstract nature, which can result in difficulties in their practical application. Nurses at the bedside may find these theories too theoretical, making it challenging for them to apply theories directly to clinical practice. Research carried out in Slovenia saw that nurses who wanted to use nursing theories found that there were too many of them and they were too hard to understand (Pajnkihar 2003).

Theories are also not part of everyday practice, are too generalised and complicate patient care (Colley 2003). The perceived weaknesses presented in Table 5.2 are largely reduced or, for the most part, no longer present difficulties in understanding theories. In Chapter 3, we suggested that undergraduate and postgraduate education has provided nurses with a core of knowledge to develop, refine, evaluate and apply theories to practice, education and research. Notwithstanding the limitations of nursing theory, we agree with Goodson (2022) that separating theory from practice is an artificial distinction. The fusion of pertinent questions with accurate answers is invaluable, enlightening and empowering. It enhances understanding, refines professional practice, and sharpens awareness, firmly linking relevant theoretical thinking to practical application.

TABLE 5.2   Perceived limitations of theories for practice.

• Do not always prepare nurses for the reality of practice
• Offer little guidance for action
• Too abstract, academic, idealistic and irrelevant
• Are not responsible for any change in practice
• Lead to premature closure on ideas
• Their application is a criticism of current practice
• Provide only tentative ideas about practice
• Unable to cope with multiple clinical foci
• Not always empirically tested or evaluated in practice
• In some cases, they demand more staff than are available

To conclude this section, while nursing theories provide a valuable theoretical base for nursing practice, their limitations must be acknowledged and addressed (see Reflective Exercise 5.11). These include challenges in applicability, failure to encompass patient diversity and complexity, lack of interdisciplinary integration and their occasionally outdated nature. Addressing these limitations is crucial for advancing nursing practice and improving patient care outcomes.

Reflective Exercise 5.11

Limitations of Theories – What Do Others Think?

The main limitations of nursing theories have been outlined here. Can you think of any others that we have not identified? To help you to consider this, we would like you to take the views of patients, family members and other healthcare professionals into account. Write down what you believe they would think of all these nursing theories.

Webb (1986) differentiated between low- and high-level criticisms, the former being more easily overcome than the latter.

Low-Level Criticisms

Documentation

Global efforts are needed to formalise and integrate nursing knowledge into electronic health records (EHRs). This will make nursing care visible in patient outcomes and emphasise the critical role of nurses in patient care (Queirós et al. 2023). By incorporating nursing theories into EHRs, nurses can more effectively translate theory into practice at the bedside. However, challenges may arise due to differences in terminologies used in various nursing theories, impacting the standardisation of these terms in EHRs (Ali & Sieloff 2017). When healthcare facilities incorporate nursing theory, nurse administrators must ensure that tools are available for nursing staff to document the theory in daily practice. Reviewing and improving current documentation systems to incorporate standardised terminology will assist in expressing the patient experience within the context of the applied theory. When the necessary terminology does not exist within current taxonomies, nurse leaders should take an active role in developing and supporting new terminology as needed (Rosenberg 2006).

Jargon or Specific Terminology Used in Theories

Most of the available theories are characterised by elaborate and abstruse language. This has been referred to as 'abstract jargon' (Wright 1985) and 'semantic confusion' (Hardy 1986). This contributes much to the unmanageability of theories in practice. There is also the danger that the use of this 'jargonese' will lead to widespread confusion not only among practising nurses but also among the public and multidisciplinary colleagues. One of the criticisms of nursing theories is that they overcomplicate practice with very complex terminology, which means that nurses end up spending too much time trying to understand the new concepts and, as a result, overlook their relevance to practice. Inconsistent and interchangeable use of terminology in nursing theory aggravates poor communication in nursing and across multidisciplinary teams (Colley 2003). In addition, Butts (2022) noticed that graduate nursing students, delving deeper into nursing knowledge and theory, often struggle with the varied terminology used by different authors.

Although Rogers (1970) is quoted as emphasising the need to avoid jargon, she wrote that the environment was 'a four-dimensional negatrophic energy field identified by pattern and organisation, and encompassing all that is outside any given human field'. Similarly, 'adaptation' in Roy's (1970) theory means something totally different from 'adaptation' in Levine's (1966) theory. A 'stressor' is viewed as a negative stimulus by Roy (1971a), while it is defined as a positive force by Neuman (1982). As Bartle (1991) noted, theory is complex, and great effort is required to understand the specific language. If the reader needs to use a glossary or dictionary to understand typical terms included in the theory, the theory lacks semantic clarity, creating difficulties in practice and education (Pajnkihar 2003).

Although acknowledging the over-use of jargon in theories, Aggleton and Chalmers (2000) believed that singling it out as a major criticism was unduly cynical. Modern nursing is highly complex so theory must have complexity to be significant. The problem is not reserved for theories within nursing: remember that Freud's theory introduced the terms ego, superego, id, Oedipus complex and Electra complex, while Jung's theory introduced extrovert and introvert! You will find more on clarity and simplicity of language use in Chapter 9, where the focus is on description, analysis and evaluation of theory.

High-Level Criticisms

Conceptual Substance

Many theories have been criticised for adopting a restricted view of nursing. Some authors believe that theorists have trodden a narrow path in their efforts to theorise. Elsewhere in this book, we castigated the biomedical model for its emphasis on reductionism. However, the theories of Roper et al., Roy, Henderson, King and Orem could also be ridiculed for being reductionist – after all, they reduce the patient to a list of activities, needs or modes of adapting or to a set of self-care needs.

There are also contrasting accusations that, in an attempt to be all-inclusive, nursing theories provide inadequate guidance for practice. The belief that grand theories are general statements about care has led some nurses to think that a theory can be used in a wide range of settings. A blanket application of one theory may, according to Hardy (1986), be unwise and even dangerous. Theofanidis and Fountouki (2008) suggest that models do not imply a uniform worldview for everyone. If a theory were to encompass all existing worldviews, it would need to be as vast as the world itself.

Ideal Concepts Versus Practical Reality

Most theories deal with how practice ought to be, rather than how it is in reality. However, if we do not know what nursing is, how can we work in the real world of practice? In considering this problem, Meleis (2007, 2018) felt that theorists were becoming more competent in articulating what theory is, rather than what is the substance of the practice itself. McCrae (2012) observed that regardless of how well-constructed a theory is, it quickly becomes irrelevant if it does not resonate with practitioners.

Watson (1988) explained that in formulating her theory, she used knowledge from other disciplines and philosophies, as well as from Eastern philosophy. For European nurses, it may be difficult to understand nursing theories that have roots in a different culture, Eastern philosophy, a different healthcare structure or a different nurse education system. The need to be familiar with Eastern philosophy and to have a liberal arts background may be asking too much (Pajnkihar 2003; Pajnkihar et al. 2017). However, Watson continues to refine her theory, with the evolution of these refinements evident in her publications.

Conclusions

Theories and models have numerous definitions and mean different things to different people; thus, a model is often seen as interchangeable with a theory. Fawcett (2005a) saw models as more abstract than theories because they present a more generalised and abstract view of phenomena, but when they are tested by research, they could lead to the formation of theory. From Meleis's (2018) perspective, theories exist at different stages of development, and therefore models are also theories, but at a lower level of construction and abstraction.

It is important to bear in mind that each theory also says something about the essential elements of metaparadigm. A metaparadigm in nursing is the global consensus that refers to the foundation elements of the profession and generally includes the 'person', 'nursing', 'health' and the 'environment'. It also explains the theorist's view on the conceptualisations, perspectives and relationships among the four elements that cover the field of nursing (Pajnkihar 2003).

There are also numerous different classifications of nursing theories. We suggest considering the classification according to the abstraction and development of the theory. However, it is more important to concentrate on the use of the theory and its testing in practice. Nursing does not exist without theories, although not all authors agree on this. Some believe that theory has no relevance to practice and therefore to nursing. The limitations and benefits of theories have been questioned.

Compared with other professions, such as law, medicine and religion, the development of scientific knowledge in nursing is still in its early stages and has depended a great deal on knowledge from other disciplines. Despite a vast array of publications on developing and refining theories, and the increasing evidence supporting these theories in practice and education, there is still potential for further integration of these theories into daily practice and their acceptance among students.

Revision Points

- We have different definitions for nursing theories and nursing models, and sometimes the terms are used interchangeably.

- A theory is a creative and scientific practice-based text that describes, explains and predicts specific nursing phenomena within the interrelated concepts, definitions and propositions.

- A conceptual model is a stage of development on the way to becoming a theory: grand or mid-range theory.

- Theories can be classified according to the level of use or function, their generalisability, level of development, philosophical underpinnings and their paradigmatic roots.

- Theories are classified into grand theory, mid-range theory and situation-specific theory (i.e. practice theory).

- Theories can have their basis in one or more paradigms: system, behavioural, development or interactional.

- The consensus is that nursing's metaparadigm includes the concepts of person, health, environment and nursing.

- The benefits of nursing theories are as follows: a replacement for the biomedical model, a guide for practice, education and research, development for the nursing profession, discipline and science of nursing. The greatest benefit is that theories help nurses to provide individual, humane and patient-oriented care. Nursing theories help with nursing science and the art of nursing in everyday practice and can make nurses' work more satisfying and respected.

- The main limitation of nursing theories is that there is a gap between theory and practice; however, the gap is closing because of postgraduate study programmes (master, APN and DNP) and nurses in practice have higher levels of knowledge development

- Criticisms of nursing theories relate to the following: documentation, the suitability of American nursing theories to other countries, the jargon used by theorists, nurses in practice and their (lack of) theoretical knowledge, the conceptual substance of the theory and what kind of theory we are looking for, ideal or practical reality.

Additional Reading

Fawcett J. (2022) Thoughts about environment. *Nursing Science Quarterly*, **35**(2), 267–269.

Fawcett, J. (2023) Evolution of one version of our disciplinary metaparadigm. Blog. https://nursology.net/2023/01/17/evolution-of-one-version-of-our-disciplinary-metaparadigm/

Fawcett J. (2024a) More thoughts about the evolution of the metaparadigm of nursing: addition of culture as another metaparadigm concept and definitions of all the concepts. *Nursing Science Quarterly*, **37**(2), 183–184.

Fawcett J. (2024b) More thoughts about environment. *Nursing Science Quarterly*, **37**(1), 89–91.

References

Aggleton P. & Chalmers C. (2000) *Nursing Models and Nursing Practice*, 2nd edition. Basingstoke: Palgrave.

Ali S. & Sieloff C.L. (2017) Nurse's use of power to standardise nursing terminology in electronic health records. *Journal of Nursing Management*, **25**(5), 346–353.

Alligood M.R. (2010a) Introduction to nursing theory: its history, significance, and analysis. In Alligood M.R. & Marriner Tomey A. (eds) *Nursing Theorists and Their Work*, 7th edition, pp. 3–15. St. Louis, MO: Mosby, Inc.

Alligood M.R. (2011) The power of theoretical knowledge. *Nursing Science Quarterly*, **24**(4), 304–305.

Alligood M.R. (2018b) *Nursing Theorists and Their Work*, 9th edition. St. Louis, MO: Elsevier.

Alligood M.R. (2018a) Introduction to nursing theory: its history and significance. In Alligood M.R. (ed.) *Nursing Theorists and Their Work*, 9th edition, pp. 2–10. St. Louis, MO: Elsevier.

Alligood M.R. & Marriner Tomey A. (2006) *Nursing Theory: Utilization and Application*, 2nd edition. St Louis, MO: Mosby Inc.

Bartle J. (1991) Caring in relation to Orem's theory. *Nursing Standard*, 5(37), 33–36.

Blumer H. (1969) *Symbolic Interactionism: Perspective and Method*. Englewood Cliffs, NJ: Prentice Hall.

Bond A.E., Eshah N.F., Bani-Khaled M., Hamad A.O., Habashneh S., Kataua H. et al. (2011) Who uses nursing theory? A univariate descriptive analysis of five years' research articles. *Scandinavian Journal of Caring Sciences*, 25(2), 404–409.

Butts J.B. (2022) Components and Levels of Abstraction in Nursing Knowledge. In Butts J.M. & Rich K.L. (eds) *Philosophies and Theories for Advanced Nursing Practice*, 4th edition, pp. 81–98. Jones & Bartlett Learning: Burlington.

Chapman C.M. (1985) *Theory of Nursing: Practical Application*. London: Harper & Row.

Chinn P.L. (2021) Equity and social justice in developing theories. In Im E.O. & Meleis A.I. (eds) *Situation Specific Theories: Development, Utilization, and Evaluation in Nursing*, pp. 29–37. Cham: Springer.

Chinn P.L., Kramer M.K. & Sitzman K. (2022) i StartKnowledge Development in Nursing: Theory and Processi End, 10th edition. St. Louis: Elsevier.

Colley S. (2003) Nursing theory: its importance to practice. *Nursing Standard*, **17**(4), 33–37.

Dickoff J. & James P. (1968) A theory of theories: a position paper. *Nursing Research*, **17**(3), 197–203.

Donohue-Porter P., Forbes M.O. & White J.H. (2011) Nursing theory in curricula today: challenges for faculty at all levels of education.

Fawcett J. (2005a) *Contemporary Nursing Knowledge: Analysis and Evaluation of Nursing Models and Theories*, 2nd edition. Philadelphia, PA: F.A. Davis.

Fawcett J. (2006) *Conceptual Models, Theories, and Research*. Jordanstown, Northern Ireland: Lecture Delivered at University of Ulster.

Fawcett J. (2012b) Thoughts about evidence-based nursing practice. *Nursing Science Quarterly*, **25**(2), 199–200.

Fawcett J. (2021) Empirical indicators: conceptual and theoretical origins. *Aquichan*, **4**, e2144.

Fawcett J. (2022) Thoughts about environment. *Nursing Science Quarterly*, **35**(2), 267–269.

Fawcett, J. (2023) Evolution of one version of our disciplinary metaparadigm. Blog. https://nursology.net/2023/01/17/evolution-of-one-version-of-our-disciplinary-metaparadigm/

Fawcett J. (2024a) More thoughts about the evolution of the metaparadigm of nursing: addition of culture as another metaparadigm concept and definitions of all the concepts. *Nursing Science Quarterly*, **37**(2), 183–184.

Fawcett J. (2024b) More thoughts about environment. *Nursing Science Quarterly*, **37**(1), 89–91.

Fawcett J. & DeSanto-Madeya S. (2013) *Contemporary Nursing Knowledge: Analysis and Evaluation of Nursing Models and Theories*, 3rd edition. Philadelphia, PA: F.A. Davis.

Feathers R.L. (1989) Orem's self-care nursing theory. In Riehl-Sisca J. (ed.) *Conceptual Models For Nursing Practice*, 3rd edition. Norwalk: Appleton & Lange.

Fitzpatrick J.J. & Whall A.L. (1983) *Conceptual Models of Nursing: Analysis and Application*. Bowie, MD: Brady & Co.

Freud S. (1949) *An Outline of Psychoanalysis*. New York: W.W. Norton.

Goodson P. (2022) Theory as practice. In Butts J.M. & Rich K.L. (eds) *Philosophies and Theories for Advanced Nursing Practice*, 4th edition. Burlington: Jones & Bartlett Learning.

George J.B. (1995a) Interpersonal Relations in Nursing: Hildegard E. Peplau. In George J.B. (ed.) *Pearson New International Edition, Nursing Theories: The Base for Professional Nursing Practice*, 6th edition, pp. 77–100. California: Pearson.

George J.B. (1995b) An introduction to nursing theory. In George J.B. (ed.) *Pearson New International Edition, Nursing Theories: The Base for Professional Nursing Practice*, 6th edition, pp. 13–34. California: Pearson.

Greaves F. (1984) *Nurse Education and The Curriculum: A Curricular Model*. London: Croom Helm.

Hardin S.S. (2018) Theory development process. In Alligood M.R. (ed.) *Nursing Theorists and Their Work*, 9th edition, pp. 35–43. St. Louis, MO: Elsevier.

Hardy M.E. (1978) Perspectives on nursing theory. *Advances in Nursing Science*, **1**, 37–48.

Hardy L.K. (1986) Janforum. Identifying the place of theoretical frameworks in an evolving discipline. *Journal of Advanced Nursing*, 11, 103–107.

Henderson V. (1966) *The Nature of Nursing: A Definition and its Implications for Practice, Education and Research*. London: Collier Macmillan.

Henderson V.A. (1991) *The Nature of Nursing. Reflections after 25 Years*. New York: National League for Nursing.

Huch M.H. (1995) Nursing and the next millennium. *Nursing Science Quarterly*, **8**(1), 38–44.

Im E.O. & Meleis A.I. (1999 Dec) Situation-specific theories: philosophical roots, properties, and approach. *Advances in Nursing Science*, 22(2), 11–24. DOI: 10.1097/00012272-199912000-00003 PMID: 10634184

Im E.O. & Meleis A.I. (2021) *Situation Specific Theories: Development, Utilization, and Evaluation in Nursing*. Cham: Springer.

Johnson D.E. (1959) The nature of a science of nursing. *Nursing Outlook*, **7**, 291–294.

Kalogirou M.R., Olson J. & Davidson S. (2020) Nursing's metaparadigm, climate change and planetary health. *Nursing Inquiry*, **27**(3), e12356.

Kao H.F., Reeder F.M., Hsu M.T. & Cheng S.F. (2006) A Chinese view of the Western nursing metaparadigm. *Journal of Holistic Nursing*, **24**(2), 92–101.

King I. (1968) A conceptual frame of reference for nursing. *Nursing Research*, **17**(1), 27–31.

Kim H.S. (1983) *The Nature of Theoretical Thinking in Nursing*. Norwalk, CT: Appleton-Century-Crofts.

Leininger M.M. (2006) Culture care theory and uses in nursing administration. In Leininger M.M. & McFarland M.R. (eds) *Culture care diversity and universality: A worldwide nursing theory*, 2nd edition, pp. 365–379. Sudbury, MA: Jones & Bartlett.

Levine M.E. (1966) Adaptation and assessment: a rationale for nursing intervention. *American Journal of Nursing*, **66**(11), 2450–2453.

Marriner Tomey A. (1998) Introduction to analysis of nursing theories. In Marriner Tomey A. & Alligood M.R. (eds) *Nursing Theorists and Their Work*, 4th edition. St Louis, MO: Mosby Year Book.

Marrs J.A. & Lowry L.W. (2006) Nursing theory and practice: connecting the dots. *Nursing Science Quarterly*, **19**(1), 44–50.

Maslow A.H. (1954) *Motivation and Personality*. New York: Harper & Row.

McCrae N. (2012) Whither nursing models? the value of nursing theory in the context of evidence-based practice and multidisciplinary health care. *Journal of Advanced Nursing*, 68(1), 222–229.

McFarlane J.K. (1986) The value of models of care. In Kershaw B. & Salvage J. (eds) *Models for Nursing*. Chichester: John Wiley & Sons.

McKenna H.P. (1994) *Nursing Theories and Quality of Care*. Aldershot: Avebury Press.

McKenna H. (1997) *Nursing Theories and Models*. London: Routledge.

McKenna H.P. & Slevin O.D. (2008) *Nursing Models, Theories and Practice. Vital Notes for Nurses*. Oxford: Blackwell Publishing.

McEwen M. (2018) Overview of theory in nursing. In McEwen M. & Wills E.M. (eds) *Theoretical Basis for Nursing*, 5th edition, pp. 49–71. Philadelphia: Wolters Kluwer.

McEwen M. & Wills E.M. (eds) (2019) *Theoretical Basis for Nursing*, 5th edition. Philadelphia: Wolters Kluwer.

Meleis A.I. (1997) *Theoretical Nursing: Development and Progress*, 3rd edition. Philadelphia, PA: Lippincott.

Meleis A.I. (2007) *Theoretical Nursing: Development and Progress*, 4th edition. Philadelphia, PA: Lippincott Williams & Wilkins.

Meleis A.I. (ed.) (2012) *Theoretical Nursing: Development and Progress*, 5th edition. Philadelphia, PA: Wolters Kluwer/Lippincott Williams & Wilkins.

Meleis A.I. (2018) *Theoretical Nursing: Development and Progress*, 6th edition. Philadelphia, PA: Wolters Kluwer/Lippincott Williams & Wilkins.

Meleis A.I. (2021) Development of situation-specific theories: an integrative approach. In Im E.O. & Meleis A.I. (eds) *Situation Specific Theories: Development, Utilization, and Evaluation in Nursing*, pp. 49–65. Cham: Springer.

Minshull J., Ross K. & Turner J. (1986) The human needs model of nursing. *Journal of Advanced Nursing*, **11**, 643–649.

Morris D.L. (1996) Watson's theory of caring. In Fitzpatrick J.J. & Whall A.L. (eds) *Conceptual Models of Nursing, Analysis and Application*, 3rd edition. Stamford: Appleton & Lange.

Neuman B. (1982) *The Neuman Systems Model: Application to Nursing Education and Practice*. Norwalk, CT: Appleton & Lange.

Newman M.A. (1979) *Theory Development in Nursing*, 3rd edition. Philadelphia, PA: F.A. Davis.

Nicholl L.H. (1992) *Perspectives on Nursing Theory*, 2nd edition. Boston, MA: Little Brown & Co.

Nightingale F. (1859/1980) *Notes on Nursing: What It Is and What It Is Not*. Edinburgh: Churchill Livingstone.

Orem D.E. (1959) *Guides for Development of Curriculae for the Education of Practical Nurses*. Washington, DC: US Department of Health, Education and Welfare.

Orem D.E. (1991) *Nursing Concepts of Practice*, 4th edition. St. Louis: Mosby.

Orem D.E. (1995) *Nursing Concepts of Practice*, 5th edition. St. Louis, MO: Mosby, Inc.

Orlando I. (1961) *The Dynamic Nurse Patient Relationship. Function, Process, and Principles*. New York: G.P. Putnam & Sons.

O'Rourke M.W. & Fawcett J. (2024) More thoughts about culture as a metaparadigm concept: rejection of the reality of subcultures. *Nursing Science Quarterly*, **37**(3), 297–298.

Pajnkihar M. (2003) Theory development for nursing in Slovenia. PhD thesis. Manchester: University of Manchester, Faculty of Medicine, Dentistry, Nursing and Pharmacy.

Pajnkihar M. (2011) Teorija v praksi zdravstvene nege. Theory in nursing practice. *Utrip*, **19**(2), 4–5. (in Slovene)

Pajnkihar M., McKenna H.P., Štiglic G. & Vrbnjak D. (2017) Fit for practice: analysis and evaluation of Watson's theory of human caring. *Nursing Science Quarterly*, **30**(3), 243–252.

Pajnkihar M., Kocbek P., Musović K., Tao Y., Kasimovskaya N., Štiglic G. et al. (2020) An international cross-cultural study of nursing students' perceptions of caring. *Nurse Educ Today*, **84**, 104214.

Pajnkihar M., Vrbnjak D., Štiglic G., Kocbek P., Smith M.C. & Musović K. (2023) Fit for practice: assessing faculty nurse caring behaviours. In Čuček-Trifkovič K. et al. (eds) *Innovative Nursing Care: Education and Research*, pp. 1833–1195. Berlin; Boston: De Gruyter.

Paterson J.G. & Zderad L.T. (1976) *Humanistic Nursing*. New York: John Wiley & Sons.

Peplau H.E. (1995a) *Schizophrenia*. Conference Presentation, Annual Conference, University of Ulster, N. Ireland.

Parse R.R. (1981) *Man-Living-Health: A Theory of Nursing*. New York: John Wiley & Sons.

Polit B., Beck C.T. & Hungler R. (2001) *Essentials of Nursing Research: Methods, Appraisal and Utilization*. Philadelphia, PA: Lippincott Williams & Wilkins.

Plummer M. & Molzahn A.E. (2009) Quality of life in contemporary nursing theory: a concept analysis. *Nursing Science Quarterly*, **22**(2), 134–140.

Reed P.G. (1996) Peplau's interpersonal relations model. In Fitzpatrick J.J. & Whall A.L. (eds) *Conceptual Models of Nursing, Analysis and Application*, 3rd edition, pp. 55–76. Stamford: Appleton & Lange.

Riehl J.P. (1974) The Riehl interactional model. In Riehl J.P. & Roy C. (eds) *Conceptual Models in Nursing Practice*. New York: Appleton-Century-Crofts.

Rodgers B.L. (2022) The evolution of nursing science. In Butts J.M. & Rich K.L. (eds) *Philosophies and Theories for Advanced Nursing Practice*, 4th edition, pp. 17–46. Burlington: Jones & Bartlett Learning.

Rogers M.E. (1970) *An Introduction to a Theoretical Basis of Nursing*, 1st edition. Philadelphia, PA: F.A. Davis.

Roper N., Logan N. & Tierney A. (1980) *Elements of Nursing*, 1st edition. Edinburgh: Churchill Livingstone.

Rosenberg S. (2006) Utilizing the language of jean Watson's caring theory within a computerized clinical documentation system. *Computers, Informatics, Nursing*, **24**(1), 53–56.

Roy C. (1970) Adaptation: a conceptual framework for nursing. *Nursing Outlook*, **18**(3), 42–45.

Roy C. (1971a) Adaptation: a conceptual framework for nursing. *Nursing Outlook*, **18**(3), 42–45.

Queirós C., Paiva E., Silva M.A.T.C., Gomes J., Neves H., Cruz I. et al. (2023) Self-care nursing interventions: a qualitative study into electronic health records' contents. *International Nursing Review*, **70**(3), 383–393.

Schim S.M., Benkert R., Bell S.E., Walker D.S. & Danford C.A. (2007) Social justice: added metaparadigm concept for urban health nursing. *Public Health Nursing*, **24**(1), 73–80.

Schmenner R.W., Wassenhove L.V., Ketokivi M., Heyl J. & Lusch R.F. (2009) Too much theory, not enough understanding. *Journal of Operations Management*, **27**, 339–343.

Shattell M.M. (2006) Commentary on "a Chinese view of the Western nursing metaparadigm". *Journal of Holistic Nursing*, **24**(2), 102.

Smith L. (1986) Issues raised by the use of nursing models in psychiatry. *Nurse Education Today*, **6**, 69–75.

Smith M.C. (2018) Disciplinary perspectives linked to middle range theory. In Smith M.J. & Liehr P.R. (eds) *Middle Range Theory for Nursing*, 4th edition, pp. 3–13. New York: Springer Publications.

Smith M.J. & Liehr P.R. (2018) *Middle Range Theory for Nursing*, 4th edition. New York: Springer Publications.

Smith M.C. & Parker M.E. (eds) (2015) *Nursing Theories and Nursing Practice*, 4th edition. Philadelphia, PA: F.A. Davis.

Stevens-Barnum B. (1998) *Nursing Theory: Analysis, Application, Evaluation*, 5th edition. New York: Lippincott Williams & Wilkins.

Stockwell F. (1985) *The Nursing Process in Psychiatric Nursing*. London: Croom Helm.

Sullivan H.S. (1953) *The Interpersonal Theory of Psychiatry*, 1st edition. London: Routledge. DOI: 10.4324/9781315014029

Suppe F. & Jacox A. (1985) Philosophy of science and development of nursing theory. *Annual Review of Nursing Research*, **3**, 241–267.

Swanson K.M. (1991) Empirical development of a middle range theory of caring. *Nursing Research*, **40**(3), 161–166.

Theofanidis D. & Fountouki A. (2008) Nursing theory a discussion on an ambiguous concept. *International Journal of Caring Sciences*, **1**(1), 15–20.

Travelbee J. (1966) *Interpersonal Aspects of Nursing*. Philadelphia, PA: F.A. Davis.

von Bertalanffy L. (1951) Theoretical models in biology and psychology. *Journal of Personality*, **20**(1), 24–38.

Vrbnjak D. (2017) Skrb za pacienta in varnost pri dajanju zdravil v zdravstveni negi / Caring for Patient and Safety in Medication Administration in Nursing. Doctoral thesis. Maribor: University of Maribor Faculty of Medicine.

Vrbnjak D., Pahor D. & Pajnkihar M. (2023) The relationship between perceptions of caring relationships, person-centred climate, and medication administration in nursing: a mixed-methods study. In Čuček-Trifkovič K. et al. (eds) *Innovative Nursing Care: Education and Research*, pp. 45–60. Berlin; Boston: De Gruyter.

Walker L.O. & Avant K.C. (2019) *Strategies for Theory Construction in Nursing*, 6th edition. Boston, MA: Pearson.

Watson J. (1988) *Nursing: Human Science and Human Care. A Theory of Nursing*, 2nd printing. New York: National League for Nursing.

Watson J. (2012) *Human Caring Science: A Theory of Nursing*, 2nd edition. Sudbury, Ontario, Canada: Jones & Bartlett Learning.

Webb C. (ed.) (1986) *Using Nursing Models Series: Women's Health, Midwifery and Gynecological Nursing*. London: Hodder & Stoughton.

Wiedenbach E. (1964) *Clinical Nursing: a Helping Art*. New York: Springer Publication Company.

Wright S.G. (1985) It's all right in theory. *Nursing Times*, **81**(34), 19–20.

McEwen M. & Wills E.M. (eds) (2019) *Theoretical Basis for Nursing*, 5th edition. Philadelphia: Wolters Kluwer.

CHAPTER 6

Interpersonal Relationships: The Essence of Nursing Models and Theories

Outline of Content

Interpersonal relationships are crucial in nursing, with caring as the foundation for these relationships. Without such relationships, one could argue that nursing would not exist. Even in intensive care units, where most of the patients are unconscious, there is a relationship between the intensive care nurses and those they look after. This chapter will describe the uniqueness of interpersonal relationships in nursing and how they differ from those in general society. It will also introduce nursing theories with interpersonal relationships and caring at their core and identify factors that help or hinder forming therapeutic interpersonal relationships.

We need to be aware that interpersonal relations and caring have been integral since the beginning of modern nursing. Dunphy (2015) described Florence Nightingale's legacy of connecting caring with activism, noting that this tradition continues. Nightingale's views on nursing as both an art and a science are consistent with this caring foundation.

Learning Outcomes

At the end of this chapter, you should be able to:

1. Understand and accept that living has interpersonal relationships as its core

2. Differentiate between therapeutic interpersonal relationships and therapeutic relationships generally

3. Recognise that interpersonal relationships in nursing are different from those between individuals generally

4. Understand how a number of nursing theories describe the building and developing of interpersonal and caring relationships

5. Identify the facilitators of and barriers to the formation of therapeutic interpersonal relationships

Introduction

The following quote by Albert Camus (1913–1960) illustrates the centrality of interpersonal relationships with others:

Human relationships always help us to carry on because they always presuppose further developments, a future – and also because we live as if our only task was precisely to have relationships with other people.

Camus, an existentialist, suggested that this is why we exist as human beings. As a philosophy, existentialism holds that the experiences of the individual affect their existence and development. We spend our daily lives connecting with others, whether with family, friends, neighbours, work colleagues or briefly interacting with members of the community. Therefore, being human is about having interpersonal contact with other human beings. Such contacts can evoke the full range of human emotions and behaviour, such as laughter, tears, hope, anger and despair. To paraphrase Mahatma Gandhi, we would argue that interpersonal relationships affect our beliefs, which affect our thoughts, which affect our actions, which affect our values and which affect our destiny.

People need other people. Much is written about the negative effects of being isolated for long periods. The Anxiety Support Network (2011) outlined the toxic effects of isolation. These include increased anxiety, depression if the isolation continues over the long term, low self-esteem and perhaps, in extreme cases, suicide. The COVID-19 pandemic provided us with additional evidence on how social isolation led to loneliness and significantly impacted the mental health of populations worldwide (Ernst et al. 2022) (see Reflective Exercise 6.1).

Reflective Exercise 6.1

Impact of Social Isolation During the COVID-19 Pandemic

Reflect on the impact of social isolation during the COVID-19 pandemic. What did you miss the most during lockdowns and periods of quarantine? Was it objects, activities or interactions with others? If it was interactions with others, what aspects of these interactions did you miss the most? Write down your thoughts and reflect on how social isolation impacted your interpersonal relations with others.

Types of Interpersonal Relationships

There are different types of isolation. Nurses often encounter people who are isolated within their own communities. They, too, can experience the symptoms described in the preceding section. For instance, Jordan et al. (2012) investigated the experiences of suicidal young men in Northern Ireland. They found that many of these young men felt isolated and struggled to maintain meaningful social and interpersonal relationships, even when they appeared to have numerous family and friends. While people can derive satisfaction from interpersonal relationships, the absence of meaningful connections can lead to loneliness, even within a social network.

Interpersonal relationships are only one dimension of human functioning. Hoff et al. (2009) argued that a crisis, such as illness, can only be resolved if mediating factors are present. These factors include intrapersonal, interpersonal and extrapersonal elements. Intrapersonal factors are internal, like an individual's perception of the crisis, past experiences and emotional and physical health. Interpersonal factors include family networks, professional input, and social support. Extrapersonal factors encompass the timing and duration of the crisis, financial resources and competing family and work obligations. This chapter focuses on interpersonal factors and how models and theories help us understand these relationships.

The term interpersonal relations was first coined by psychiatrist Jacob Moreno in 1941, who is also known for founding psychodrama. The phrase, interpersonal relations, was later defined more precisely by the American psychoanalyst, Harry Stack Sullivan (1953). Born to Catholic Irish immigrants and raised in an anti-Catholic town in New York State, Sullivan often experienced social isolation. Unlike Freud, Sullivan's form of psychoanalysis was based on observation, making his methodology more interactional than interpsyche. He observed that understanding a person's web of relationships was key to understanding the individual.

In 2013, the renowned psychiatrist Robert Spitzer made the following statement (Reisz 2013: 22):

The thing I took from that and that has never left me is that psychiatry is utterly based in and dependent on a relationship. It is not a secondary, luxury add-on. It is the core of the activity. What I feel anxious about in modern psychiatry is that we have become quite preoccupied with the technology and, certainly in our writings, downplay the importance of continuity of care and relationships.

Professionals who work in the field of mental health nursing often witness how poor and unstable interpersonal relationships lead to psychiatric problems. Conversely, they also observe that developing stable interpersonal relationships can help individuals regain mental health. In the Northern Ireland suicide study mentioned earlier, Cutcliffe et al. (2012) found that interpersonal relationships often played a crucial role in helping respondents survive suicide attempts. We would assert that most emotional problems stem from interpersonal relationship difficulties. But helping people to establish or re-establish interpersonal relationships is not just important for mental health professionals; it is a core element of the caring repertoires of all health professionals (see Key Concepts 6.1).

Nurses must care for and care about clients as holistic human beings because care is the essence of nursing and of an equal partner-like relationship between the nurse and the client. Nurses are responsible for establishing interpersonal relationships with their clients through sensitive, empathic and intellectual responses to clients' beliefs, needs and problems. This approach encourages respect, trust, safety and dignity, helping clients regain their independence and integrity in mind, body and soul. Research and supporting literature suggest that equal partner-like relationships include both artistic and scientific knowledge elements. In such relationships, clients are treated as equal partners, informed and supported with knowledge and skills to make their own decisions, fostering self-responsibility and autonomy (Pajnkihar 2003).

Key Concepts 6.1

Interpersonal relationships form the basic building blocks for good nursing.

In McCaughan and McSorley's (2007b) research on patients diagnosed with cancer, it was noted that good-quality care occurred within a very specific interpersonal atmosphere. Participants in the study felt a sense of relief by being able to discuss their feelings, thoughts and experiences within a therapeutic relationship. In such a relationship, they felt free to express themselves, leading to feelings of security and emancipation. Interestingly, though, there was something qualitatively different about the patients' relationship with the nurse, as opposed to their relationship with family and friends. While patients expressed their feelings sparingly with family and friends to avoid causing pain or distress, they felt able to express their feelings and fears more freely with nurses. This supports Hildegard Peplau's assertion that the relationship between nurses and patients is not the same as the more common social relationships that other people have with each other. Peplau (1992: 14) stated that:

The nurse patient relationship is a particular kind of interaction. It is not a social relationship of friend to friend. It is not a clerk to customer relationship. Nor is it a master to servant relationship. Rather, the nurse is a professional, which means a person having a definable expertise. That expertise pertains to reliable interventions which have been research tested and therefore have predictable known outcomes.

This differentiates interpersonal relationships generally from therapeutic interpersonal relationships. There is an element of treatment in the latter. If we accept Peplau's statement, we cannot ignore the fact that the caring process that underpins the craft of nursing has therapeutic interpersonal relationships as its core. Living our lives will always be about humans interacting with humans, and caring is about doing this in a mutually respectful partnership where there are clear therapeutic objectives.

In research by Sharkiya (2023), it was found that the quality of care received by patients was related to the quality of the interpersonal relationships they had with nurses. Patients value interpersonal relationships very highly, which often leads to high patient satisfaction (see Key Concepts 6.2).

Key Concepts 6.2

Building interpersonal relationships and caring is pivotal to nursing.

By contrast, negative interpersonal relationships are reflected in concepts such as such as distrust, anger, disrespect, disapproval and dislike. The role of health professionals generally and nurses specifically is to encourage the formation of positive interpersonal relationships and eliminate or discourage the formation of those that are negative (see Reflective Exercise 6.2).

Reflective Exercise 6.2

What Are Interpersonal Relationships?

Many people and organisations pride themselves on having good interpersonal relationships with those with whom they come into contact. Tour guides or hotel workers who look after you when you are on holiday see their role as being about forming positive interpersonal relationships, as do shop assistants, police officers, doctors and firefighters.

Using your learning and library resources, look up interpersonal relations. You may wish to consult the work of Harry Stack Sullivan, Clara Thompson, Karen Horney, Erich Fromm, Otto Allen Will, Jr, Erik H. Erikson or Frieda Fromm-Reichmann.

Once you have read some work on this topic, write a page on whether or not you believe the interpersonal relationships formed by nurses are different from those in the other occupations discussed.

Several well-known nursing theories act as guides to show how best to do this. However, before exploring these, it is important to first revisit the concept of personal knowing.

Personal Knowing

You will recall from Chapter 2 that Barbara Carper (1978) identified *personal knowing* as one of the four ways that nurses know. This is pertinent for this chapter. Personal knowing, as explained by Chinn et al. (2022), is awareness of self and others, and 'personal knowing of the self is what makes therapeutic use of self in nursing practice possible' (7). It involves nurses bringing their selves to their practice and developing self-awareness through critical reflection on their caring practices. Personal knowing incorporates experience, self-encounter and actualisation, emphasising personal maturity and freedom, potentially including spiritual and metaphysical dimensions. It is subjective, focusing on self-consciousness, personal awareness and empathy, which are essential for developing meaningful interpersonal relationships (Carper 1978; McEwen 2019).

Personal knowing is subjective – it is about nurses knowing themselves and how they relate to others. In other words, you cannot develop a meaningful interpersonal relationship with another person if you do not know yourself. Here, personal knowing represents knowledge that focuses on self-consciousness, personal awareness and empathy. It requires self-regard and active empathic participation on the part of the nurse (see Key Concepts 6.3).

Key Concepts 6.3

Personal knowing: an essential prerequisite to being able to develop interpersonal relationships with others.

Why is personal knowing so important in the context of this chapter? Well, if we accept that nursing is an interpersonal process, then we must understand our own strengths and weaknesses to interact meaningfully with those requiring care. As stressed in a previous chapter, most nurses do not possess a case full of medications or an arsenal of surgical instruments: what we have is ourselves, and we can use ourselves therapeutically to make a difference to patients. The requirement to know ourselves before we can know our patients is highlighted in a number of nursing theories.

Research by Hasson et al. (2012) would lend some credence to this. In their study on the nursing assistant's role, they found that because registered nurses were too busy at the nurses' station on administration tasks, most of the 'hands on' care was undertaken by students and nursing assistants. The conclusion here is that if nurses cannot find time or space to develop meaningful interpersonal relationships with patients, they will indeed be perceived as uncaring and perhaps they cannot justifiably retain the title nurse. This supports the view that 'the nurse–patient relationship is the essence of caring' (Meleis 2012: 93) (see Reflective Exercise 6.3).

Reflective Exercise 6.3

Returning to the Metaparadigm

In Chapter 5, you were asked to undertake an exercise on the metaparadigm. You will recall that the metaparadigm of nursing is composed of four essential elements: nursing, health, person and environment. You were asked to consider adding essential elements that you felt were important.

Did you or any of your fellow students or colleagues add interpersonal relationships? Did you think it was already covered in the 'nursing' element? (See Appendix A.)

Research by McKenna (1997) noted that there were over 50 grand nursing theories. He studied each of these in some depth and found, to a greater or lesser extent, that all of them refer to interaction between nurses and patients. This is not surprising, of course, since a nursing theory that does not refer to such interactions would not be worthy of the title 'nursing theory' (see Key Concepts 6.4). Nonetheless, some theories place a greater emphasis on nurse–patient interaction than others.

Key Concepts 6.4

All nursing theories refer, to some extent, to human-to-human interactions and interpersonal relationships.

Classifications of Interaction Theories According to Different Authors

As already established by this chapter, theories are classified differently. In this section, we will explore how interaction theories are classified according to several authors.

1. The first is the complex classification of Meleis (2018), where she classified theories according to four schools of thought:
   - *First school of thought: Needs* – theories that focus on describing the functions and roles of nurses. These theories are also closely tied to the biomedical model, as they prominently address physical and medical needs. Meleis included theories such as Henderson (1964), Abdellah (1969), Minshull et al. (1986) and Orem (1995) in this group.
   - *Second school of thought: Interaction* – theories that focus on the interaction process to answer how nurses do whatever it is they do. Peplau, who considered nurses–patient relationships to be fundamental to nursing practice, was the pioneer in that group. Other interaction theorists are Orlando (1961), Wiedenbach (1964), Travelbee (1966), King (1968) and Paterson and Zderad (1976).
   - *Third school of thought: Outcomes* – theories that conceptualise the outcomes of nursing care and describe the recipient of care. Johnson (1959), Levine (1966), Rogers (1970) and Roy (1970) are included here.
   - *Fourth school of thought: Caring/becoming* – theories that focus on act of caring in interactive situations and have many similarities to interaction theories. Watson (1979) and Parse (1992) are included in this group.

2. The second is the classification of Nelson (2022), who categorised theories focused on interpersonal relationships in the following way:
   - *Interpersonal relationships:* theories that emphasise nurse–patient interactions. Key theorists include Peplau (1952), Orlando (1961) and Travelbee (1966).
   - *Humanism/caring:* theories that focus on humanism and caring. Notable theorists are Paterson and Zderard (1976).
   - *Existentialism/phenomenology:* theories that explore the existential and phenomenological aspects of nursing. Key theorists include Watson (1979), Newman (1979) and Parse (1992).

3. The third is classification by Wills (2019), who ordered grand theories into four categories of focus:
   - *Human needs:* theories focus on meeting clients' needs for nursing care. Notable theorists include Orem (1959), Johnson (1959), Nightingale (1859/1980), Henderson (1966), Abdellah (1969) and Neuman (1982).
   - *Interactive process:* theories that view humans as holistic beings who interact with and adapt to the situations they encounter. Notable theorists include King (1968), Roy (1970), Watson (1979), Erickson, Tomlin and Swain (1983) and Artinian (1983).
   - *Unitary process:* theories that reflect the newer views of science in their complexity and view the human as an energy field, as intentional, as dynamic, limitless and unpredictable. Notable theorists include Rogers (1970), Newman (1979) and Parse (1992).

4. The fourth is classification by Smith and Parker (2015), who also saw grand theories as belonging to four categories:
   - *Grand theories on nurse–patient relationships:* focus on the dynamics and processes of the nurse–patient relationship. Notable theorists include Peplau (1952), Orlando (1961) and Travelbee (1966).
   - *Grand theories in the integrative–interactive paradigm:* view persons as integrated systems interacting with larger environmental systems. Key theorists include Johnson (1959), Orem (1959), King (1968), Roy (1970), Neuman (1982), Erickson, Tomlin and Swain (1983) and Dossey (2008).
   - *Grand theories in the unitary-transformative paradigm:* conceptualise the human being and environment as irreducible fields, open to the environment. Prominent theorists include Rogers (1970), Parse (1992) and Newman (1979).
   - *Grand theories about care and caring:* focus on the phenomenon of care or caring within nursing practice. Notable theorists in this category include Leininger (1978), Watson (1979) and Boykin and Schoenhofer (1993).

All of these classify theories on interpersonal relationships and caring. Considering Smith and Parker's (2015) classification, we will present two important theories from the categories *Nurse–patient relationships* (Peplau) and *Care and caring* (Watson).

First, we will describe Peplau's theory. The main reason for this is that her theory was the first to be formulated (1952). From our perspective, she can rightly be regarded as the mother of interaction theories in nursing. Peplau's theory was the first contemporary theory in nursing generally and in psychiatric nursing in particular. Her writings in the 1950s greatly influenced others who later used interpersonal relationships as a basis for their theories.

From her long and distinguished experience as a psychiatric nurse, Hildegard Peplau realised that people who have good mental health often have good interpersonal relationships with others such as their family, friends and work colleagues. Conversely, she noted that people who were emotionally unwell invariably had poor interpersonal skills and had difficulty communicating appropriately with others.

As discussed in Chapter 2, theories can be formulated in three main ways: induction, deduction or retroduction. To remind you, induction involves building a theory directly from what is observed and understood in practice. By contrast, theories can be formulated from other existing theories through a process of deduction. Retroduction is an amalgamation of both induction and deduction (see Key Concepts 6.6).

🔍 Key Concepts 6.6

Peplau developed her theory retroductively – inductively and deductively.

Peplau's studied interpersonal relations over many years and began to develop her theory deductively due to the influence of Henry Stack Sullivan's (1953) interpersonal relations theory. However, through induction, she reflected on her clinical experience in psychiatric nursing. It is noteworthy that Peplau never actually used the term 'interpersonal relationships', preferring instead to use 'interpersonal relations'. This may be due simply to her respect for Harry Stack Sullivan's theory.

Peplau (1952) defined nursing as a therapeutic interpersonal process through which nurses facilitate growth and development among patients. She saw the relationship as reciprocal, with both the nurse and the patient participating in and contributing to it.

If you remember, Chapter 1 pointed out that all theories often have a number of assumptions. As you saw, these are simply statements that we accept as true, even though they may not have been tested and proved (see Key Concepts 6.7).

🔍 Key Concepts 6.7

Theories are composed of assumptions, which are statements that you assume to be true, even though they may not have been tested.

Consider the following assumptions from Peplau (see also Reflective Exercise 6.5):

- People need relationships with other people (Peplau 1987: 166).
- Relationships constitute the social fabric of life (Peplau 1987: 116).
- Interpersonal relationships are important throughout the life span (Peplau 1994: 13).
- Interpersonal relationships are the bedrock of quality of life (Peplau 1994: 13).
- In every nurse–patient contact, there is the possibility of working towards common understandings and goals (Peplau 1952: 10).
- The nurse and patient come to know and to respect each other as persons who are alike and yet different, as persons who share in the solution of problems (Peplau 1952: 9).
- Each patient–nurse relationship is unique in terms of process and outcome (Peplau 1962: 5).

- Interpersonal relationships are person-to-person interactions that have structure and content and are situation dependent (Peplau 1994: 10).
- At their best, interpersonal relationships confirm self-worth, provide a sense of connectedness with others and support self-esteem (Peplau 1987: 166).

Reflective Exercise 6.5

Testing Assumptions

Read the list of Peplau's assumptions carefully and see if you can agree with them without them being tested scientifically. If you disagree with any of them, explain why.

As these assumptions were formulated in the early 1950s, check their validity with fellow students, family or friends to see if they stand the test of time in the 21st century. Again, identify any that do not gain agreement and determine the reasons why.

See if you can think up some more assumptions around interpersonal relations that you could add to Peplau's list.

Peplau (1952: 17) identifies four distinct phases in the development of the nurse–patient relationship: orientation, identification, exploitation and resolution (see Table 6.1). Each phase is characterised by overlapping roles and functions related to health problems, as the nurse and patient learn to work cooperatively to resolve difficulties. These phases facilitate the therapeutic process and help in building a strong, supportive relationship between the nurse and the patient. The orientation phase involves the patient's initial reaction to illness and the recognition of a need for assistance. The patient experiences a 'felt need' and seeks 'professional assistance' that is perceived as beneficial. This phase is the beginning of a dynamic learning experience with the potential for constructive personal and social growth. In the identification phase, the patient identifies with those who can help and determines their role in the process. Peplau emphasises the importance of allowing patients to express their feelings while receiving the required nursing care. This process helps patients reorient their feelings and strengthens positive personality traits. The exploitation phase occurs when the patient fully identifies with the nurse, who can recognise and understand the interpersonal relations involved in the situation. The patient uses the nurse's expertise to navigate their health challenges effectively. The resolution phase is the final phase and involves the patient meeting their own needs and achieving independence. In this phase, old goals are gradually replaced by new ones. The resolution phase is a freeing process that depends on the successful progression through the earlier phases (Peplau 1952).

Peplau (1952) also identified six roles of nursing within the interpersonal process:

- *Stranger:* Initially, nurses and patients are strangers. In this role, the nurse demonstrates respect and positive interest, establishing the foundation for a trusting relationship.
- *Resource person:* Nurses provide essential health information, viewing themselves as sources of knowledge and technical procedures to enhance patient and community health.
- *Teacher:* This role combines various roles, focusing on what the patient already knows and their interest in new information, thereby facilitating learning and understanding.
- *Surrogate:* Patients may cast nurses into roles based on their perceptions, seeing the nurse as someone else, which requires the nurse to navigate these perceptions carefully.
- *Counsellor:* The extent to which nurses fulfil this role depends on the development of the nurse–patient relationship. It involves promoting health experiences, helping patients become aware of conditions necessary for health and aiding them in identifying health threats.
- *Leader:* Nurses guide the patient through the health journey, providing support and direction as needed (Peplau 1952; Pajnkihar 2003).

125

By adopting these roles, nurses rely more on guiding, supporting, teaching and helping patients to find meaning in their situations – and less on doing and functioning (see Reflective Exercise 6.6).

Reflective Exercise 6.6

Peplau's Theory?

Study Table 6.1 carefully. A nurse could be considered a resource person if the patient or patient's family wanted health promotion information or literature. On the other hand, if showing a diabetic patient how to administer insulin, the nurse is adopting the role of teacher.

Identify three situations in which a nurse would adopt each of the roles in the working phase of the theory.

The second theory we describe is Jean Watson's theory. Her first book, *Nursing: The Philosophy and Science of Caring*, was published in 1979, and she refers to it as a treatise. Watson described caring as fundamental to nursing, framing it as both a human science and an art. She emphasised the importance of transpersonal caring relationships, highlighting a unique form of professional and human-to-human interaction (Pajnkihar et al. 2017b).

Watson's theory posits that nursing is fundamentally about transpersonal communication of human caring. It involves transpersonal processes aimed at helping individuals find meaning in illness and existence, and to achieve self-knowledge, self-control and self-care while maintaining inner harmony and independence. The patient is seen as a co-participant in this process. The relationship between the nurse and the patient is warm and genuine, with a focus on the patient's dignity and humanity. Nurses are encouraged to be sensitive to themselves and others within a helping–trusting relationship to protect and enhance dignity. Holistic care, according to Watson, empowers nurses in caring partnerships with individuals, fostering freedom, autonomy and professional responsibility (Pajnkihar 2003).

Watson's theory can be similarly classified as retroductive, much like Peplau's, because it draws from her views on nursing, her own research in practice and education and the work of various authors. These include Erikson, Heidegger, Maslow, Rogers, Selye and Lazarus as well as the traditional nursing knowledge of Nightingale, Henderson, Leininger, Krueter and Hall (Watson 1988).

TABLE 6.1   **Phases and roles within a significant, therapeutic, interpersonal process in Peplau's theory.**

Phases in relationship	Orientation phase	Identification phase	Exploitation phase	Resolution phase
Patient's role	Patient's 'felt need' and relates to the 'professional assistance'.	A patient identifies with people who are able to help him/her and assist in determining what role they will play in the process.	A patient has identified him/herself with the nurse capable of recognising and understanding the interpersonal relations in the situation.	The patient meets his/her own needs and becomes independent. in this phase, old goals are gradually put aside, and new goals are adopted.
Nurse's role: Stranger Resource person Teacher Surrogate Counsellor Leader	The nurse's role changes through different phases of interpersonal relations in the situation.	The nurse's role changes through different phases as they interact with patients.	The nurse's role changes through different phases as they interact with patients.	The nurse relies more on guiding, supporting, teaching and helping patients to find meaning in their situations – and less on doing and functioning.

Adapted from Peplau (1952).

Watson's clearly described three out of four metaparadigm concepts, which are described in Chapter 5, and we encourage you to read their definitions again. The assumptions related to human care and the values of human caring in nursing can be traced back to Watson's early works (Watson 1979, 1985). Wills (2019) listed assumptions that were derived from Watson's (2005) theory as:

- 'An ontologic assumption of oneness, wholeness, unity, relatedness, and connectedness.
- An epistemologic assumption that there are multiple ways of knowing.
- Diversity of knowing assumes all, and various forms of evidence can be included.
- A caring science model makes these diverse perspectives explicitly and directly.
- Moral-metaphysical integration with science evokes spirit; this orientation is possible and necessary for our science, humanity, society-civilisation, and world-planet.
- A caring science emergence, founded on new assumptions, makes explicit an expanding unitary, energetic worldview with a relational human caring ethic and ontology as its starting point'. (Willis 2019: 180)

Central concepts of Watson's theory are the transpersonal caring relationship, which has three dimensions: self, the phenomenal field and intersubjectivity; caring moments/caring occasions; caring (healing) consciousness and Caritas processes™ (Fawcett 2005a; Pajnkihar et al. 2017b).

Both the patient and nurse engage in a transpersonal caring relationship, transforming an event into an actual caring occasion. This involves two individuals coming together with their unique life histories, creating a unique phenomenal field that transcends time and space, leading to healing through self-awareness and self-discovery (Watson 1999). This actual caring occasion ultimately fosters self-discovery. The nurse's entire caring consciousness is embedded within a single caring moment or occasion, extending beyond the physical moment itself (Watson 2015). Consciousness, intentionality and authentic presence are essential to develop and sustain a trusting relationship and caring moment. Caring-healing modalities, or nursing therapeutics, are related to the human-caring-healing process (Watson 2012). The Caritas processes (previously called carative factors) facilitate healing, honour wholeness and contribute to the evolution of humanity by fostering a deeper connection and understanding between nurse and patient (Watson 2008).

Watson's descriptions of the relationship show it as one of mutuality in which the whole nurse and patient are engaged and each of them brings his/her own experiences and meaning to an actual caring occasion, recognising the value and importance of both the clients' and nurses' subjectivity. However, the ideal of the nurse as a professional engaged in caring relationships with many patients or clients and sharing such personal values, meaning, self and spirit with another unknown person, is difficult, may be even impossible, to achieve (Pajnkihar 2003).

To summarise, Peplau's theory emphasises the importance of therapeutic interpersonal relationships, focusing on the phases of the nurse–patient interaction and nurses' roles in facilitating patient growth and healing. Watson's theory centres on transpersonal caring relationships, highlighting the spiritual and holistic aspects of care, where both the nurse and the patient engage in a shared human experience to achieve healing and self-discovery. In the literature, readers will find applications of both Peplau's and Watson's theories in practice, education and research. These theories underscore the importance of interpersonal relationships and caring in nursing. Other theories that emphasise interpersonal relationships and caring also contribute significantly to the field.

Implications for Nurse Practice, Research and Education

It is a given that all disciplines are underpinned by theories. These theories help us to describe, explain and predict the elements of our professions. Pokorny (2018) referenced various authors and research studies based on Peplau's theory. These highlight several key areas: the impact of communication on nurse–patient relationships, empathy among nurses, holistic communication training for nursing students with older adults and the application of Peplau's theory in simulation training for undergraduates. Additional research focuses on nurses' roles in home care for children with complex needs, best practices for children of incarcerated parents, identity issues in adolescent dating violence, evaluating advanced practice nurses (APNs) models in Australia, and interactions between home health nurses and homebound geriatric patients with depression and disability. Collectively, these studies demonstrate the extensive applicability of Peplau's theory in enhancing nursing practices and patient care.

Wei et al. (2019) synthesised research studies based on Watson's theory and identified 19 articles that included caring interventions directed towards patients, nurses and nursing students. The primary aims of these caring interventions were to enhance patients' perceptions of nurse caring, improve patient–nurse relationships, increase patient satisfaction, reduce surgery-related pain and anxiety and improve psychological health. Interventions directed towards nurses included in-service education sessions designed to improve both patient and nurse outcomes. Caring interventions for nursing students also applied Watson's caring theory processes to their education.

In the last three decades of the 20th century, all nurse education programmes in the western world had classes on nursing models or theories, with many programmes using them as frameworks for their curricula. Considering their centrality to nursing, you would expect as much. Because of their relationship with caring, interpersonal relationship theories were particularly valued. In particular, many psychiatric, mental health nursing programmes were underpinned by these theories.

However, Turkel et al. (2018) expressed some concerns that contemporary nursing programmes are not firmly based on nursing theories. There seems to be a greater focus on interprofessional practice than on nursing theory-driven practice with less emphasis on nursing conceptual models and theories in the curricula (see Key Concepts 6.8).

🔍 Key Concepts 6.8

While their importance is recognised, interpersonal theories are not a central part of nurse education curricula today.

Earlier in this chapter, we noted the prevailing view that new nursing graduates lack fundamental caring skills and that many hard-pressed clinical nurses do not have the time to develop interpersonal relationships with patients or their families. A cynic might argue that interpersonal relationship theories belonged to when there was no shortage of nurses and patients remained in the hospital for prolonged periods – even for minor procedures. We assert that in a busy technological healthcare setting, interpersonal theories are needed more than ever.

Evidence in the literature shows that caring theories in nursing curricula effectively improve students' caring behaviours, empower students' confidence, enhance teamwork capabilities and foster a caring attitude toward themselves and others. Educating and training students in caring attitudes and behaviours can prepare them to face challenges in their first nursing jobs, increase problem-solving skills and provide quality patient care. Nursing is a profession that combines scientific knowledge and interpersonal caring skills as one unity (Wei et al. 2019).

We recommend that nurse educators address this gap and foster an interpersonal culture in education. Within such a culture, nurses should learn to:

- acknowledge that interpersonal relationships are foundational to caring;
- recognise themselves and the ways in which they talk to each other and to patients as part of the therapeutic process;
- accept interpersonal responsibility and encourage open, sensitive personal relations and strong feelings of interpersonal trust;
- develop their personal knowing so that they have a good understanding of their own values, attitudes and knowledge, as this will determine the extent to which they can understand the situation confronting the patient;
- be sensitive to the human problems faced by patients and cultivate relationships that help address these challenges.

Social Capital

Another way to view interpersonal relations is through the concept of social capital (Ferragina 2012). There are three kinds of capital: economic, human and social. In the context of this chapter, social capital is the most important type. Pierre Bourdieu first used this term in 1972 in 'Outline of a Theory of Practice' (see Bourdieu 1977). One way to understand this concept is to consider the two words that comprise the term, 'social', meaning relating to humans, and 'capital', meaning wealth. Within the context of interpersonal relationships, nurses must be educated to become expert in developing this social wealth in themselves and in their patients.

According to Cohen and Prusak (2001: 4): 'Social capital consists of the stock of active connections among people: the trust, mutual understanding, and shared values and behaviors that bind the members of human networks and communities and make cooperative action possible'. Therefore, social capital represents the values and norms individuals share, which facilitate the development of interpersonal relationships (see Key Concepts 6.9).

Generating social capital in nursing benefits patients and enhances multidisciplinary teamwork. Modern healthcare is primarily provided through multiprofessional teams, with each member bringing unique skills and competencies to clinical situations. Interpersonal relationship skills are crucial for effective teamwork. If team members share the same theoretical foundations, it strengthens the team, makes it more cohesive and reduces confusion for patients.

Key Concepts 6.9

Social capital: the values and norms that individuals share with others that permit relationship building.

Conversely, a lack of team cohesion harms interpersonal relationships between professional colleagues and between nurses and patients. One way to address this issue is by encouraging interprofessional learning, where different healthcare disciplines are educated together from the start. This approach teaches that no single professional group 'owns' the patient or their problems. As nursing education has become established in universities, opportunities for interprofessional learning have increased, though this does not necessarily mean these opportunities have been fully exploited.

The educational challenge is to equip students with the skills to work both individually and in teams, to be creative and imaginative problem solvers, to communicate clearly and effectively and to excel in developing interpersonal relationships. Many of these competencies are not directly taught in the classroom but are influenced by the overall ethos of the university environment.

Challenges to the Development of Interpersonal Relationships in Nursing and the Use of Interpersonal Theories

Nurses are being criticised in the media and in journal articles for becoming less caring and less able to develop meaningful relationships with patients and their families (see Key Concepts 6.10). We will now outline some of the reasons for this situation.

Key Concepts 6.10

In modern nursing, there are a number of challenges to using interpersonal theory in practice.

Pace of Modern Healthcare

Some readers can remember when healthcare delivery was a much more relaxed endeavour. More than 30 years ago, patients often spent weeks in hospital, and as they improved, they assisted nurses in tasks such as the distribution of meals, feeding of other patients and making beds. Nurses had time to get to know their patients and their patients' families.

However, in the 21st century, nursing has become 'intensified' – there is less time to 'nurse' than was previously the case. Patient throughput has increased, and new treatments and technologies have made healthcare more complex. Hospitals now function almost like large intensive care units where, as soon as patients pass the acute stage of their illness, they are discharged home or to community care. This has implications for the theories that nurses are taught and, as mentioned earlier, some cynics question whether detailed interpersonal theories are still relevant today.

Measuring Interpersonal Relationships and Caring

Healthcare managers and policymakers are fixated on measurement, adhering to the adage that 'if it cannot be measured, it cannot be costed'. Because of the decline in the study of theories in the curriculum, nurses are not good at explaining what they do and providing evidence of effectiveness. For instance, a health service manager who sees a nurse talking to a patient in a busy clinical setting may perceive this as an example of inefficiency. Although the nurse may be establishing a therapeutic interpersonal relationship with the patient, to the untrained eye the nurse is simply talking to the patient – a task that, the manager may judge, less expensive, untrained staff could do just as well. Interpersonal relationships are difficult to measure and thus not easily subjected to rigorous studies of effectiveness. Watson (2006) also stated that caring and economics are often in conflict with each other. However, there is vast evidence that caring positively impacts patient outcomes and healthcare organisations. Creating and sustaining a caring culture is closely linked to healthcare organisations' financial viability and sustainability. Even though it is hard to estimate the exact value of creating a caring culture, healthcare organisations can benefit from improved patient experiences and satisfied employees (Wei et al. 2019). In 2024, researchers at Penn Nursing found that a 10% reduction in hospital nurses could lead to patients having a 7% higher odds of dying and an increase in preventable readmissions. This has obvious cost implications.

Increased Technology

Many people start a career in nursing because they want to help others directly and tangibly. Traditionally, nursing is perceived as a high 'touch' profession that values personal interaction. The development of interpersonal relationships with patients involves attention to touch, facial expressions, body language and tone of voice. This is crucial but presents significant challenges to education when there is a greater emphasis on e-learning and distance learning.

Increasingly, technological gateways are replacing face-to-face teaching. Nurses who value human contact can easily become frustrated because they are geographically removed and unable to physically connect with their instructors or fellow students (see Reflective Exercise 6.7).

Reflective Exercise 6.7

Connected Health

In today's healthcare systems and in the future, the emphasis on AI, telemedicine, telehealth, telenursing and remote monitoring will increase. This revolution in connected health means that from a distance, patients can be monitored in their own homes through digital videoconferencing. Vital signs will be recorded remotely through a smart patch applied to the patient's chest.

Consider in two paragraphs what this will do to interpersonal relationships between nurses and patients. What effect will it have on nursing theories that emphasise such relationships?

The same can apply in clinical situations. In the early 1960s, Isobel Menzies claimed that nurses were engaging in low-level non-nursing tasks as a means of distancing themselves from the stress of dealing directly with patients' problems. Peplau (1962) called this 'busywork' and it kept the nurse away from direct contact with the patient. We believe that 'busywork' to distract nurses is still in existence today, but that it takes the form of computer technology and administration paperwork. While the distractions have altered, they can still keep nurses away from direct contact with patients and, as Menzies intimated, it may be what some nurses subconsciously want.

While advances in technology can impact human health and enable nurses to perform their work efficiently and safely, when introducing and using technology in nursing, there is a danger that too much focus is placed on technology over caring for patients (Krel et al. 2022). Nurse educators must ensure that new graduates are not enticed towards technologies as a means of isolating them physically from patients or emotionally from patients' problems. Nursing theories have an important role in guiding practice and maintaining the focus on caring and person-centred care. There has been an increase in the number of AI supported robots to support the care of older people. Such robots can bring many benefits to the caring situation but it is difficult for these to interact therapeutically with patients and something as simple as human touch is missing.

Role Drift

In Chapter 4, we discussed the increase in the number and type of new roles in nursing and role theory. We argued that many new roles nurses undertake require expertise in interpersonal relationships. This underscores the centrality of the nurse–patient relationship and highlights the importance of skilled communication and interprofessional skills, which are essential for APNs to engage patients, assess their needs and provide personalised, evidence-based care. Arslanian-Engoren (2019) described the development and sustainment of therapeutic relationships and partnerships with patients (individual, family or group) and other professionals to facilitate optimal care and patient outcomes as an essential competence of APNs. However, APNs face challenges in their role transition and in terms of relationships. There is a shift in the nature of their relationships with patients and conversations as they move from facilitating understanding of the information provided by physicians to directly imparting information about diagnoses, prognoses, and exploring goals of care (Stein et al. 2022).

In a climate of a global shortage of registered nurses and demands for them to undertake more medical duties, there is also an increasing reliance on assistants to fill the gaps in care (Hasson et al. 2012). As a result, duties and workload are shifting from doctors to nurses and from nurses to healthcare assistants. The majority of healthcare assistants are caring and conscientious individuals who are often pressured to go beyond their level of competence to perform duties for which they are not qualified or trained, potentially endangering the safety of patients and the quality of care (McKenna et al. 2004).

Some of the duties undertaken by healthcare assistants that were once the remit of nurses include catheter care, wound dressing, venepuncture, formulating patient care plans, setting up and monitoring diagnostic machines, setting up infusion feeds, giving injections, taking charge of shifts, monitoring, providing advice on parenting skills and breast-feeding. According to the literature, much of this work is unsupervised (Hasson & McKenna 2011). Therefore, while many nursing roles are becoming medicalised, healthcare assistants, because of their increasing numbers and their visibility in the clinical setting, are becoming more involved in developing interpersonal relationships with patients and their families (see Key Concepts 6.11 and Reflective Exercise 6.8) Crucially, they lack and theoretical knowledge.

Key Concepts 6.11

Nurses have to be placed in the best position clinically and strategically to develop therapeutic relationships with patients, families and communities.

It is time to re-humanise nursing and ensure that nurses are optimally positioned clinically and strategically to develop caring, therapeutic interpersonal relationships with patients, families and communities. A range of well-tested nursing theories can guide and support this effort.

Reflective Exercise 6.8

Barriers to Nurses Developing Interpersonal Relationships with Patients

Can you think of any other reasons why clinical nurses may have difficulty developing interpersonal relationships with their patients?

If you cannot think of any, ask your fellow students. If you get the opportunity, ask healthcare assistants for their views on this.

Conclusion

The focus of this chapter has been on the importance of interpersonal relationships and caring in nursing and how different theories deal with this issue. From this chapter, we can be certain about five things: interpersonal relationships are at the core of nursing; life generally is about interpersonal relationships; the development of positive interpersonal relationships can be therapeutic; there are nursing theories that guide the development of therapeutic interpersonal relationships; and nurse education has a central role to play in ensuring that nurses have the knowledge and skills necessary to develop caring and interpersonal relationships with others. There are a number of threats to nursing's centrality in interpersonal relationships with patients, including the pace of modern healthcare, increased technology, the challenges of measuring interpersonal relationships and caring and role drift. Peplau's and Watson's theories have inspired a range of research across different aspects of nursing and their use clinically can help remove some of these threats.

Revision Points

- The focus of many nursing theories is on interpersonal relationships, but each of these theories deals with it differently. (See Appendix A)

- Interpersonal relationships are at the core of nursing and caring is the foundation of interpersonal relationships.

- Life generally is about interpersonal relationships.

- The development of positive interpersonal relationships can be therapeutic.

- There are nursing-specific nursing theories that guide the development of therapeutic and caring interpersonal relationships.

- Nurse education has a central role to play in ensuring that nurses have the knowledge and skills necessary to develop interpersonal relationships with others.

- There are a number of threats to nursing's centrality in interpersonal relationships with patients, including the pace of modern healthcare, increased technology, the challenge of measuring interpersonal relationships and role drift.

Additional Reading

Carper B.A. (1978) Fundamental patterns of knowing in nursing. *Advances in Nursing Science*, **1**(1), 13–23.

Pajnkihar M., McKenna H.P., Štiglic G. & Vrbnjak D. (2017) Fit for practice: analysis and evaluation of Watson's theory of human caring. *Nursing Science Quarterly*, **30**(3), 243–252.

Peplau H.E. (1952) *Interpersonal Relations in Nursing*. New York: G.P. Putnam & Sons.

Watson J. (2012) *Human Caring Science: A Theory of Nursing*, 2nd edition. Sudbury, Ontario, Canada: Jones & Bartlett Learning.

Wei H., Fazzone P.A., Sitzman K. & Hardin S.R. (2019) The current intervention studies based on Watson's theory of human caring: a systematic review. *International Journal for Human Caring*, **23**(1), 4–22.

Useful Web Links

http://currentnursing.com/nursing_theory/interpersonal_theory.html
https://nursology.net/nurse-theories/peplaus-theory-of-interpersonal-relations/
https://nursology.net/nurse-theories/watsons-theory-of-human-caring/
https://www.watsoncaringscience.org/

References

Abdellah F. (1969) The nature of nursing science. *Nursing Research*, **18**(5), 390–393.

Arslanian-Engoren C. (2019) Conceptualizations of advanced practice nursing. In Tracy M.F. & O'Grady E.T. (eds) *Hamric and Hanson's Advanced Practice Nursing: An Integrative Approach*, 6th edition, pp. 25–60. St. Louis, MO: Elsevier.

Artinian B.M. (1983) Implementation of the intersystem patient-care model in clinical practice. *Journal of Advanced Nursing*, **8**(2), 117–124.

Bourdieu P. (1977) *Outline of a Theory of Practice* (trans. R. Nice). Cambridge: Cambridge University Press.

Boykin A. & Schoenhofer S.O. (1993) *Nursing as Caring: A Model for Transforming Practice*. New York: National League for Nursing Press.

Carper B.A. (1978) Fundamental patterns of knowing in nursing. *Advances in Nursing Science*, **1**(1), 13–23.

Chinn P.L., Kramer M.K. & Sitzman K. (2022) *Knowledge Development in Nursing: Theory and Process*, 10th edition. St. Louis: Elsevier.

Cohen D. & Prusak L. (2001) *In Good Company: How Social Capital Makes Organizations Work*. Boston, MA: Harvard Business School Press.

Cutcliffe J., McKenna H., Keeney S.R. & Jordan J. (2012) 'Straight from the horse's mouth': rethinking and reconfiguring services in Northern Ireland in response to suicidal young men. *Journal of Psychiatric and Mental Health Nursing*, **20**(5), 466–472.

Dossey B. (2008) Theory of integral nursing. *Advances in Nursing Science*, **31**(1), E52–E73.

Dunphy H.L.M. (2015) Florence Nightingale's legacy of caring and its application. In Smith M.C. & Parker M.E. (eds) *Nursing Theories and Nursing Practice*, 4th edition, pp. 37–54. Philadelphia, PA: F.A. Davis.

Erickson H.C., Tomlin E.M. & Swain M.A.P. (1983) *Modeling and Role-modeling: A Theory and Paradigm for Nursing*. Englewood Cliffs, NJ: Prentice-Hall.

Ernst M., Niederer D., Werner A.M., Czaja S.J., Mikton C., Ong A.D. et al. (2022) Loneliness before and during the COVID-19 pandemic: a systematic review with meta-analysis. *The American Psychologist*, **77**(5), 660–677.

Fawcett J. (2005a) *Contemporary Nursing Knowledge: Analysis and Evaluation of Nursing Models and Theories*, 3rd edition. Philadelphia, PA: F.A. Davis.

Ferragina E. (2012) *Social Capital in Europe: A Comparative Regional Analysis*. Cheltenham: Edward Elgar.

Hasson F. & McKenna H.P. (2011) Greater clarity in roles needed. *British Journal of Healthcare Assistants*, **50**(8), 398–398.

Hasson F., McKenna H.P. & Keeney S.R. (2012) Delegating and supervising unregistered professionals: the student nurse experience. *Nurse Education Today*, **33**, 229–235.

Henderson V. (1964) The nature of nursing. *American Journal of Nursing*, **64**(8), 62–68.

Henderson V. (1966) The Nature of Nursing: A Definition and its Implications for Practice, Education and Research. London: Collier Macmillan.

Hoff L.A., Hallisey B.J. & Hoff M. (2009) *People in Crisis: Clinical and Diversity Perspectives*, 6th edition. London: Routledge.

Johnson D.E. (1959) The nature of a science of nursing. *Nursing Outlook*, **7**, 291–294.

Jordan J., McKenna H.P., Keeney S.R., Cutcliffe J.R., Stephenson C., Slater P. et al. (2012) Providing meaningful care: learning. From the experiences of suicidal young men. *Qualitative Health Research*, **22**(9), 1207–1219.

King I. (1968) A conceptual frame of reference for nursing. *Nursing Research*, **17**(1), 27–31.

Krel C., Vrbnjak D., Bevc S., Štiglic G. & Pajnkihar M. (2022) Technological competency as caring in nursing: a description, analysis and evaluation of the theory. *Zdravstveno Varstvo*, **61**(2), 115–123.

Leininger M.M. (1978) *Transcultural Nursing: Concepts, Theories, and Practices*. New York: John Wiley & Sons Inc.

Levine M.E. (1966) Adaptation and assessment: a rationale for nursing intervention. *American Journal of Nursing*, **66**(11), 2450–2453.

McCaughan E. & McSorley O. (2007b) An exploration of the perceptions of users, nurses and doctors of the service provided by a breast cancer review clinic. *Journal of Advanced Nursing*, **60**(4), 419–426.

McEwen M. (2019) Philosophy, science, and nursing. In McEwen M. & Wills E.M. (eds) *Theoretical Basis for Nursing*, 5th edition, pp. 32–48. Philadelphia, PA: Wolters Kluwer.

McKenna H.P. (1997) Theory and research: a linkage to benefit practice. *International Journal of Nursing Studies*, **34**(6), 431–437.

McKenna H.P., Hasson F. & Keeney S. (2004) Patient safety and quality of care: the role of the health care assistant. *Journal of Nursing Management*, **12**(6), 452–459.

Meleis A.I. (ed.) (2012) *Theoretical Nursing: Development and Progress*, 5th edition. Philadelphia, PA: Wolters Kluwer/Lippincott Williams & Wilkins.

Meleis A.I. (ed.) (2018) *Theoretical Nursing: Development and Progress*, 6th edition. Philadelphia, PA: Wolters Kluwer/Lippincott Williams & Wilkins.

Minshull J., Ross K. & Turner J. (1986) The human needs model of nursing. *Journal of Advanced Nursing*, **11**, 643–649.

Nelson S. (2022) Theories focused on interpersonal relationships. In Butts J.M. & Rich K.L. (eds) *Philosophies and Theories for Advanced Nursing Practice*, 4th edition. Burlington, MA: Jones & Bartlett Learning.

Neuman B. (1982) *The Neuman Systems Model: Application to Nursing Education and Practice*. Norwalk, CT: Appleton & Lange.

Newman M.A. (1979) *Theory Development in Nursing*, 3rd edition. Philadelphia, PA: F.A. Davis.

Nightingale F. (1859/1980) *Notes on Nursing: What It Is and What It Is Not*. Edinburgh: Churchill Livingstone.

Orem D.E. (1959) *Guides for Development of Curriculae for the Education of Practical Nurses*. Washington, DC: US Department of Health, Education and Welfare.

Orem D.E. (1995) *Nursing Concepts of Practice*, 5th edition. St. Louis, MO: Mosby, Inc.

Orlando I. (1961) *The Dynamic Nurse Patient Relationship. Function, Process, and Principles*. New York: G.P. Putnam & Sons.

Pajnkihar M. (2003) Theory development for nursing in Slovenia. PhD thesis. Manchester: University of Manchester, Faculty of Medicine, Dentistry, Nursing and Pharmacy.

Pajnkihar M., McKenna H.P., Štiglic G. & Vrbnjak D. (2017b) Fit for practice: analysis and evaluation of Watson's theory of human caring. *Nursing Science Quarterly*, **30**(3), 243–252.

Parse R.R. (1992) Human becoming: Parse's theory of nursing. *Nursing Science Quarterly*, **5**, 35–42.

Paterson J.G. & Zderad L.T. (1976) *Humanistic Nursing*. New York: John Wiley & Sons.

Peplau E.H. (1952) *Interpersonal Relations in Nursing: A Conceptual Frame of Reference for Psychodynamic Nursing*. New York: G.P. Putnam & Sons.

Peplau H.E. (1962) Interpersonal techniques: the crux of nursing. *American Journal of Nursing*, **62**, 50–54.

Peplau H.E. (1987) Nursing science: a historical perspective. In Parse R.R. (ed.) *Nursing Science: Major Paradigms, Theories and Critiques*. Philadelphia, PA: W.B. Saunders Co.

Peplau H.E. (1994) Quality of life: an interpersonal perspective. *Nursing Science Quarterly*, **7**, 10–15.

Pokorny M.E. (2018) Nursing theorists of historical significance. In Alligood M.R. (ed.) *Nursing Theorists and Their Work*, 9th edition, pp. 12–17. St. Louis, MO: Elsevier.

Reisz M. (2013) Psychiatry. *The Times Higher Education*, 2002, May 23, p. 22.

Rogers M.E. (1970) *An Introduction to a Theoretical Basis of Nursing*, 1st edition. Philadelphia, PA: F.A. Davis.

Roy C. (1970) Adaptation: a conceptual framework for nursing. *Nursing Outlook*, **18**(3), 42–45.

Sharkiya S.H. (2023) Quality communication can improve patient-centred health outcomes among older patients: a rapid review. *BMC Health Services Research*, **23**, 886. DOI: 10.1186/s12913-023-09869-8

Smith M.C. & Parker M.E. (2015) *Nursing Theories and Nursing Practice*, 4th edition. Philadelphia, PA: FA Davis.

Stein D., Cannity K., Weiner R., Hichenberg S., Leon-Nastasi A., Banerjee S. et al. (2022) General and unique communication skills challenges for advanced practice providers: a mixed-methods study. *Journal of the Advanced Practitioner in Oncology*, **13**(1), 32–43.

Sullivan H.S. (1953). In Perry H.S. & Gawel M.L. (eds) *The Interpersonal Theory of Psychiatry*. New York: W.W. Norton & Co. Inc.

The Anxiety Support Network (2011) The toxic effects of isolation. http://www.anxietysupportnetwork.com/articles/the_toxic_effects_of_isolation.php

Travelbee J. (1966) *Interpersonal Aspects of Nursing*. Philadelphia, PA: F.A. Davis.

Turkel M.C., Fawcett J., Amankwaa L., Clarke P.N., Dee V., Eustace R. et al. (2018) Thoughts about nursing curricula: dark clouds and bright lights. *Nursing Science Quarterly*, **31**(2), 185–189.

Watson J. (1979) *Nursing: The Philosophy and Science of Caring*. Boston, MA: Little, Brown & Company.

Watson J. (1985) *Nursing: The Philosophy and Science of Caring*. Colorado: Colorado Associated University Press.

Watson J. (1988) *Nursing: Human Science and Human Care. A Theory of Nursing*, 2nd printing. New York: National League for Nursing.

Watson J. (1999) *Nursing: Human Science and Human Care: A Theory of Nursing*. Boston, MA: Jones & Bartlett Learning.

Watson J. (2005) *Caring Science as Sacred Science*. Philadelphia, PA: F.A. Davis.

Watson J. (2006) Caring theory as an ethical guide to administrative and clinical practices. *Nursing Administration Quarterly*, **30**(1), 48–55.

Watson J. (2008) *Nursing: The Philosophy and Science of Caring*, revised edition. Boulder, CO: University Press of Colorado.

Watson J. (2012) *Human Caring Science: A Theory of Nursing*, 2nd edition. Sudbury, Ontario, Canada: Jones & Bartlett Learning.

Watson J. (2015) Jean Watson's theory of human caring. In Smith M.C. & Parker M.E. (eds) *Nursing Theories and Nursing Practice*, pp. 321–339. Philadelphia, PA: F.A. Davis Company.

Wei H., Fazzone P.A., Sitzman K. & Hardin S.R. (2019) The current intervention studies based on Watson's theory of human caring: a systematic review. *International Journal for Human Caring*, **23**(1), 4–22.

Wiedenbach E. (1964) *Clinical Nursing: a Helping Art*. New York: Springer Publication Company.

Wills E.E. (2019) Unit II: nursing theories. In McEwen M. & Wills E.M. (eds) *Theoretical Basis for Nursing*, 5th edition, pp. 129–203. Philadelphia, PA: Wolters Kluwer.

CHAPTER 7

How to Select a Suitable Model or Theory for Practice

Whenever a theory appears to you as the only possible one. Take this as a sign that you have neither understood the theory nor the problem which it was intended to solve.

(Karl Popper 1989)

Outline of Content

Picture the scenario where you are a clinical nurse and you and your colleagues want to select a nursing theory to guide and underpin clinical practice. This is an exciting endeavour and you set about the task with enthusiasm. After some background reading and a more detailed literature review, you discover that there are around 50 'grand nursing theories' (nursing models) and over 60 mid-range nursing theories. Regardless, how do you decide which one to choose? This chapter will help you do this. It will commence by describing how the selection process has been undertaken in the United Kingdom and the United States. It will then progress to identifying guidelines that you can follow for an appropriate choice in any country. Along the way, it will deal with the challenges you might come across.

Learning Outcomes

When you finish reading this chapter, you should be able to:

1. Describe how nursing theories were introduced in the United Kingdom and the United States

2. Outline the 12 potential problems when selecting a nursing theory for practice

3. Understand the differences between grand and mid-range nursing theories

---

Fundamentals of Nursing Models, Theories and Practice, Third Edition. Hugh P. McKenna, Majda Pajnkihar and Dominika Vrbnjak.
© 2025 John Wiley & Sons Ltd. Published 2025 by John Wiley & Sons Ltd.
Companion website: www.wiley.com/go/nursingmodels3e

4. Identify the criteria used to choose an appropriate nursing theory for practice

5. Discuss the role of the metaparadigm in theory selection

6. Understand who are the best people to select a nursing theory for practice

7. Explain the advantages and disadvantages of borrowing theory from other disciplines

Introduction

You will recall from Chapter 1 that we all use theories in our daily life, sometimes unknowingly. Karl Popper (1989) argued that humans approach everything in the light of a preconceived theory. Our conversations will be underpinned by communication theories or interpersonal theories. Our choice of what to purchase in a shop may be influenced by financial theory or decision theory. Our drive to work will be influenced by theories of motion or theories of geography. Our home life will be affected by theories of family dynamics. It is surprising, then, that in the third decade of the 21st century, many nurses did not accept nursing theories more enthusiastically.

With hindsight, this is perhaps not surprising; in the 1990s, they were often imposed on practising nurses by nurse educators and nurse managers. Nursing theories (at that time they were mostly called nursing models) were the new fashion in nursing; there were dozens of books written about them, and most nursing journals and professional magazines published articles about them (see Key Concepts 7.1). Being so ubiquitous, they were often perceived as a good thing, a means of enhancing our professional practice and our unique body of knowledge. Invariably, clinical settings were seen as not being up to date unless the nurses were using a nursing theory to guide their practice. If another local hospital was using one, we were behind the times if we were not doing so. Nurse managers returned from nursing theory conferences loaded with templates of care plans for one theory or another.

Key Concepts 7.1

Nursing theories: assist nurses in using the nursing process to assess patients' needs, plan care, intervene and evaluate the outcomes of care.

Several years previously, the 'nursing process' had been introduced. By all accounts, it too was the great panacea for patient care. It seemed simple enough: you assessed your patient's needs, planned the care, implemented the care plan and evaluated whether the patient's needs had been met. But for some reason, it too was having difficulty taking root in many clinical settings. Then the proponents of nursing theories spotted what was wrong. To make the nursing process work, a theory was required to give it structure. In fact, it had been argued that the implementation of the nursing process without a theory to underpin it was an empty meaningless approach (McKenna 1997). As a result, nursing theories were perceived as the solution to good care planning, and they were imposed uncritically and, in many cases, artificially, onto hard-pressed clinical nurses.

Reflective Exercise 7.1

Change

If you wish to change someone's behaviour, you need to change their beliefs and attitudes. Otherwise, they will not enthusiastically adopt a new activity or a new way of working.

Consider how you would implement a new evidence-based procedure to change the way nurses in a clinical setting practised. How would you approach the problem? By dictate, by persuasion, by cajoling, by incentive?

You will get some ideas if you read how Everett M. Rodgers (2003) suggested change should happen: http://en.wikipedia.org/wiki/Diffusion_of_Innovations.

137

You will recall from Chapter 2 that Benner's (1984) research identified levels of expertise in nursing from novice to expert. Novice nurses are attracted to guidelines and theories because they provide them with helpful maps to follow in what they see as a complex setting. In contrast, expert nurses find theories and guidelines restricting. They practice aesthetically, seamlessly, and effectively due to many years of experience. A new theory gives these expert nurses a new map to follow and has the result, at least initially, of slowing them down. It is little wonder that such expert nurses did not wholeheartedly embrace nursing theories.

It was not unusual for expert nurses to be informed by managers that they were to introduce a nursing theory to guide their practice by the following week. A common motive for imposing a theory on an unsuspecting workforce was that nurse teachers in the local school of nursing were teaching the specific theory to their students or it underpinned the curriculum. Clinical nurses soon realized that if they had to use nursing theories, it would be better if they could select one that was appropriate for the sort of patients and type of clinical setting within which they worked.

Selecting an Appropriate Nursing Theory

It is surprising that the choice of a nursing theory often took little account of patients' views or the clinical specialism (see Reflective Exercise 7.2). You will recall from the previous chapter that the theories selected most often had more than a passing resemblance to the biomedical model. For instance, Henderson's (1966) and Roper et al.'s (2000) theories were the most popular choices in the United States and the United Kingdom, focusing on activities of living. This was the case regardless of whether the patient population comprised people with mental health problems, women in labour, sick children or older people. This was because such conceptualisations were grand theories, meaning that they were broad and could deal with patient needs across a variety of specialisms. All patients regardless of illness had daily activities such as eating, drinking, elimination, sleeping etc., with which they may have needed help. (See Reflective Exercise 7.2.)

Reflective Exercise 7.2

It is interesting that nurses did not involve patients or patient support groups in the choice of nursing theories. After all, we are supposed to be partners with patients and involve them in decisions about their care. They call this co-design and co-production (discussed later). Think about this and try to understand why patients were not actively engaged in helping nurses to select an appropriate nursing theory. Your answer may reflect the fact that this was the 1980s and 1990s. Another consideration relates to whether patients could understand some of the existing nursing theories, since even many nurses struggled to comprehend them.

Also, ask yourself, should the theory fit the existing nursing practice on a unit or should practice change to fit the theory?

Roskoski (2018: 1) maintained that there is no one universal nursing theory. Previously McKenna et al. (2014) noted that there were over 50 grand theories (models) of nursing and over 60 mid-range theories. Since the assessment of patient needs, the planning of care, the interventions used and the evaluation of care can differ depending on what nursing theory is being used, a new awareness existed as to the necessity of making the right choice. The alternative is to have a nursing theory that does not fit the clinical practice setting.

There is a dearth of research evidence available to help practising nurses decide what theory is best suited for their clinical speciality. For instance, in a psychiatric unit, where the development of interpersonal relationships is important, would Peplau's theory (1992) be most appropriate? But, what about the theories of Orlando (1961), Wiedenbach (1964), Travelbee (1966), King (1968, 1981) and Paterson and Zderad (1976) that also focus on nurse–patient interactions and relationships? So, readers will agree that because it can change how nursing care is provided, choosing the most relevant theory is a daunting task and must be carried out with care.

You will recall from Chapter 3 that grand theories are broad conceptualisations of a discipline. In nursing, they deal with everything from self-care, to adaptation, to nurse–patient interaction, to activities of daily living. As alluded to above, grand theories are so all-encompassing in their scope, they could be applicable in any setting where nursing is taking place. For instance, Orem's self-care theory (Yip 2021) could be used in any setting where the patients were being encouraged to be independent. This would give it wide applicability. Fawcett (2017) suggested that just one theory could be selected for use in all nursing units within a healthcare institution. So, is sorting through theories to find a suitable one a waste of valuable nursing time? Stephens Barnum (2004) did not think so; she asserted that there was a need to employ different theories to suit different patient settings. We concur with this view and argue that the choice of one theory for application throughout an entire hospital is unwise and perhaps even dangerous. We do not believe that patients and staff have to put up with a theory that has a less desirable 'fit' for the sake of organizational conformity for management or educational reasons. Fitting the patient's problems to a theory rather than the theory fitting the patient's problems is a foolish and uncaring exercise.

As stated many times in this book, grand theories are broad frameworks and are often well recognised and publicised (e.g. self-care, adaptation and activities of living). By contrast, mid-range theories are those that have more limited scope and less abstraction, address specific phenomena or concepts and reflect best practice (Peterson & Bredow 2019) (see Key Concepts 7.2). Invariably, they are based on evidence that emerges from research studies. Examples of mid-range theories were given in Chapter 3. Others include mid-range theories of information-seeking behaviour of newly diagnosed cancer patients (McCaughan & McKenna 2007), comfort (Kolcaba 2001), quality caring (Duffy 2008) and self-transcendence (Runquist & Reed 2007). You should refer back to Chapter 3 if you need to update yourself on the difference between grand and mid-range theories. However, regardless of whether we are dealing with grand or mid-range theories, we believe that there are 11 potential problems to acknowledge when selecting an appropriate one for your practice. Some of these reflect the limitations of the theory outlined in Table 5.2 in Chapter 5 (p. 110).

Key Concepts 7.2

Grand theories: broad frameworks that may be widely applicable to most nursing care settings, sometimes referred to as nursing models.

Mid-range theories: these are very specific and are appropriate for a more focused area of care and mainly emanate from research studies.

Potential Problems when Selecting a Nursing Theory

American or UK Nursing Theories?

England and America are two countries separated by a common language.

(George Bernard Shaw 1856–1950)

While the English-born Nightingale (1859) in the 19th century is credited with being the first nurse theorist, most 20th-century nurse theorists were based in the United States (see Reflective Exercise 7.3). We could question whether their nursing theories are transferable to nursing practice in other parts of the world. There is nothing wrong with nurses from different countries exchanging ideas, but the application of one group's practices to another may not always be appropriate. After all, as has been pointed out in earlier chapters, other countries have different healthcare systems from the United States, different nurse education systems and different cultures (see Key Concepts 7.3). Therefore, it is understandable that American nursing theories may not always be the best choice for nursing care in other parts of the world. If nurses in different countries continually look towards America for conceptual guidance, any selected theory will have to be manipulated to fit their local health service. Of the 50 or so well-known grand nursing theories, 38 were formulated in the United States, with about 10 developed in the United Kingdom. By far, the most popular of these latter theories is the Activities of Living Grand Theory by Roper et al. (Holland & Jenkins 2019).

Reflective Exercise 7.3

Why America?

It is a truism that even though the first nursing theory by Nightingale was British, US nurse theorists took the lead in the development of nurse theories. Most of the 50 grand theories and many of the 60 or so mid-range theories are American.

In addition, Peplau developed her interpersonal nursing theory in the 1950s in the United States; this was followed by many other US theories in the 1960s, 1970s and 1980s. By contrast, nursing theories only emerged in the United Kingdom in the 1980s and 1990s.

Think about why this might be the case and why UK nurse theorists were less willing to call their work 'theory' – preferring the word 'model'. Discuss your conclusions with other students and compare views.

Some of the content in Chapter 5 may be helpful for this exercise.

Key Concepts 7.3

American nursing theories: nurses in various parts of the world are attracted to American nursing theories. This may be because they view US nursing as being more advanced; after all university education for nurses in the United States preceded the rest of the world by decades. But, accepting this, it may still be inappropriate to impose a US nursing theory on a non-US healthcare system.

Ethical and Moral Issues

The selection of a nursing theory is value-laden and the choice you make may be right or wrong, good or bad (see Reflective Exercise 7.4). It follows therefore that the choice will be influenced by a nurse's beliefs about and attitude towards the nature of patients, people and healthcare. For instance, Orem's (1995) self-care theory would not be a nurse's first choice if they held the view that patients are dependent and should rest, recuperate and adopt the patient role. On the other hand, if a nurse were to select a theory that encouraged dependency, this could do a great deal of damage to the patient's rehabilitation and self-esteem. It could also mimic the biomedical model's support for the patient adopting the submissive 'sick role', where they are exempt from carrying out some or all of normal social duties and seek and submit to appropriate medical care (Parsons 1951).

Over a number of years, psychologist Lynn (2021) wrote that black people were less intelligent than white people and that men were more intelligent than women. The selection of Lynn's theory to frame policy would have implications for hiring employees, providing educational opportunities and for the self-esteem and respect of many people. This would be highly unethical. Similarly, the rigid application of the theories that the Earth was flat and the Sun orbited the Earth led to people like Galileo Galilei (1564–1642) being imprisoned by Pope Urban Vlll.

Reflective Exercise 7.4

Ethical Considerations

Later in this chapter, we will show that when using a nursing theory, a nurse undertakes a comprehensive and detailed assessment and identifies many actual and potential physical, social and psychological problems. However, in the modern fast-paced healthcare system, the patient will only be in hospital for a short length of stay. Is it fair on patients to have their care based upon an inappropriate nursing assessment or have plans set to meet their needs when they will be discharged home before the plans are implemented?

Write a one-page account of the ethical implications of these issues for nursing care, including any relevant ethical principles such as non-maleficence, justice or fairness.

Length of Patient Stay

Time is an important factor when selecting a nursing theory. For example, a theory used in a care of older people unit may be unsuitable for use in a very rushed emergency room setting. In the former, activities of living theory like that developed by Virginia Henderson (Business Bliss 2018) would be appropriate, whereas the FANCAP theory (fluids, aeration, nutrition, communication, activity and pain) (Baker 2009) would be more appropriate in the rushed environment of the emergency room (Roskoski 2018). Another example is Callista Roy's nursing theory; it has been calculated that 16 A4 pages of a care plan would be required (McKenna et al. 2014). How could nurses in busy emergency settings have times to use this theory?

It was noted in Chapter 6 that the pace of current hospital treatment has increased and that patients are often discharged home once they are over the acute phase of their illness. This has implications for the choice of nursing theory. We should ask ourselves if it is morally correct to put patients through a comprehensive assessment and set goals for nursing interventions when they may not be in the clinical setting long enough to receive the interventions or have the goals of their care plan met. One obvious way to address this is to ensure there is a good discharge plan so that community nurses can pick up the care once the patient has returned home. Of course, this raises another potential complication – if community nursing staff are using a different theory from that used by hospital-based nurses, the chances of confusion and misunderstanding occurring are increased. Important issues could be lost in translation from one theory to another. You were asked to consider the ethical aspects of this example in Reflective Exercise 7.4.

Nurses' Knowledge of Nursing Theories

Nurses' knowledge of different theories will influence their choice, but readers will spot the obvious flaw in this selection process. Is it realistic to expect busy practising nurses to be familiar with any more than a few of the most popular theories from among those available? Their level of knowledge about theories will also be biased depending on what ones they were taught as students, and what ones have the highest profile in the journals and books that they read.

The growth in mid-range theories complicates the selection process. At last count, there were 60 of these (Fawcett & DeSanto-Madeya 2013: 16). It is difficult enough to be up to date with all 50 grand nursing theories, let alone mid-range nursing theories (see the Nursology link at the end of this chapter).

The Implications of a Wrong Choice

Roskoski (2018) argued that the greatest barrier to effective application of any nursing theory is trying to employ the wrong type of theory in a particular nursing situation or to believe that one theory can be applied to all types of patient conditions. It is our belief that the quality of care would be adversely affected by an inappropriate choice of a nursing theory and an early decision on an unsuitable theory could stifle creativity. Therefore, mistakenly selecting a nursing theory that is incompatible with practice may have undesirable consequences. In Chapter 1, we used the analogy of a map. A map will help to direct you to where you want to go and there are different maps according to your specific needs. An underground rail map is different from a street map, which is also different from a map used by airline pilots. An incorrect choice of map could confuse you and get you lost; the same applies to the incorrect choice of a nursing theory. Of course, the map might be the right one, but you have simply misread it or followed it incorrectly. Similarly, the nursing theory may be the right one for your clinical setting, but you may have misunderstood it or implemented it incorrectly. Although an unsuitable choice is regrettable, it is not an insoluble situation: as with an incorrect map, an incorrect theory can be changed for a correct one (see Reflective Exercise 7.5).

Reflective Exercise 7.5

Follow That Map!

Think of the city or town near where you live and identify 10 different maps (above and below ground) that could be used to get around the various terrains. This should make you appreciate why there are so many different nursing theories looking at the same thing – nursing. Consider the problems of getting from A to B armed with the wrong map.

Hybrid Nursing Theories

The idea that different bits (concepts or propositions) can be chosen from several different theories and applied in the clinical area as one amalgamated hybrid theory is supported by some (Fawcett & DeSanto-Madeya 2013). However, there is a danger that such a strategy could lead to the loss of theoretical coherence and rigour, to the introduction of contradiction and to the original theoretical status being compromised. Nurses are conducting more and more research on nursing theories and many of these studies show that particular theories are valid and reliable for guiding practice. For example, Khademian et al. (2020) showed the effectiveness of using Orem's theory with patients who had hypertension, and Roy's theory has shown positive outcomes for patients with cerebral vascular accident (Da Costa et al. 2016). Therefore, if bits and pieces were taken from both these theories and put together to form a blended theory, the validity of the merged theory could be undermined. Furthermore, the effectiveness of the hybrid theory in hypertension and cerebral vascular accident could not be assured (see Reflective Exercise 7.6). While modifications to a theory may be acceptable, the modifications should be acknowledged, and consideration should be given to renaming the theory. Our suggestion is that such a hybrid theory should be retested through robust research.

Reflective Exercise 7.6

A Jig-Saw of Maps and Theories

Consider Reflective Exercise 7.5 where you looked at 10 different maps of your town or city. Imagine taking bits of these maps and putting them together into a collage. You would probably end up with a section of the bus route map, alongside a section of the sewage system map, alongside a section of the electrical grid map, alongside a section of the Ordnance Survey map and so on. In other words, it would be a confused tangle of information. The same principle might apply if you selected bits and pieces of different nursing theories to form a hybrid theory.

Method of Choice

From Chapter 2, readers will recall that experienced nurses know their patients well and through using tacit knowledge (see Chapter 2) they can more or less second-guess their needs. This intuitive knowledge gives them an almost 'gut reaction' when it comes to assessing and providing care. Such intuition, shaped by years of experience, can influence their choice of nursing theory. But should the selection of a theory really be based upon mere 'gut reaction', or should nurses be pursuing the best possible research evidence to choose the most appropriate theory? The former stance was supported in a seminal article by Silva (1986). She urged nurses to value truths arrived at by intuition and introspection as much as those arrived at by scientific research. Again, in Chapter 2, we saw that empiricists would argue that choices must be made on more logical verifiable grounds. However, in support of Silva's assertion, we are aware that in most cases in nursing, the theory exists before the research to test it is conducted. Therefore, if we waited for the research to be completed in all cases, we would have little theoretical creativity or innovation.

Single or Multiple Theories?

Although the selection within one clinical setting of several different theories for different patient groups may be a desirable and recommended stratagem, it leads to complications. For instance, it could take a prolonged period for clinical nurses to be educated about a range of theories and then inducted and trained on how best to employ them all, or a number of them, in practice. Also, if different theories are used in the same setting, there will likely be a need for several different accompanying care planning documents. Furthermore, using a range of different theories could contribute to communication problems. For example, those staff working across a hospital site, such as managers and clinical lecturers, would require a high degree of theoretical sophistication as would bank or agency nurses who work across different units in a hospital. Nurses who are asked to work in a different clinical setting due to staff absences could also be confused. To the uninitiated, such a patient care system may resemble a conceptual 'Tower of Babel'.

Furthermore, communications within and between members of the multiprofessional team could be hampered by such a strategy and patients who are transferred from ward to ward or from ward to outpatient clinic as their condition changes may have trouble understanding or contributing to their care plans. Our medical colleagues, who are guided by the single medical model, would scratch their heads in wonder at what they might perceive as conceptual chaos. It is not surprising therefore that Fawcett and DeSanto-Madeya (2013) noted that all the successful implementation projects reported in the literature tend to focus on the introduction of only one theory, rather than multiple nursing theories (see Key Concepts 7.4).

Key Concepts 7.4

Multiple theories: Theories can be complex, developed over many years and some are continuously evolving. Therefore, the expectation that a clinical nurse can have an in-depth knowledge of many theories and their implementation is an unrealistic one.

Inherent Limitations of Theories

As stressed in Chapter 1, all theories have their own set of assumptions. Remember that assumptions are defined as statements that we can take as true, even though they have never been tested. Obvious ones would be that all humans require sleep to enable them to function, or that humans are bio-psycho-social beings. Assumptions are the distinguishing marks of a theory. However, it could be argued that each theory is limited by its assumptions because no one theory will be able to deal with all eventualities. While nurses may want assurance that a so-called 'right choice' of a theory would eliminate all their patient's care problems, it is possible that the limitations inherent in individual theories may burden nurses with too narrow a perspective. For example, we cannot be criticized for failing to emphasize independence in the activities of daily living (Holland & Jenkins 2019) if the theory we are using stresses the manipulation of stimuli to promote adaptation (Roy 2019). Mid-range theories are, by their nature, even more restrictive. There are mid-range theories on such focused phenomena as 'comfort' (Kolcaba 2001) and 'sorrow' (Gaskill Eakes 2019). It is possible that nurses would have to use a number of different mid-range theories, as no single theory on its own will deal with the total needs of all patients in their caseload.

Social and Political Issues

The Austrian philosopher Feyerabend (1977) argued that theory and truth cannot be divorced from the social and political context in which they exist. He maintained that the theory one chooses is a matter of social convenience or political expediency. Therefore, social and political influences have a role to play in the selection of a nursing theory. It could easily be argued that Orem's work (Khademian et al. 2020) is more suitable for the private health insurance sector because of its emphasis on encouraging and enhancing the patient's ability to undertake self-care outside of expensive hospitals. This is also the case in public sector healthcare, where there is a move away from patients staying in hospitals to being cared for in their own homes. This is manifested by everything from early discharge home to the care of families, to workers being encouraged to sign up for private pensions and private health insurance. In addition, the population is getting older, with more chronic conditions, and healthcare costs are spiralling out of control (see Key Concepts 7.5). You will recall from Chapter 6 that 'connected health' is the term used in relation to supporting older and more chronically ill people in their own homes, through the use of modern technology. Artificial intelligence is also being used to support healthcare independence. A self-care theory would fit well into such a digitally connected health world.

Key Concepts 7.5

Nursing and politics: nursing theories have political and social connotations. This will have implications for what ones are selected for practice.

There is another dimension to this political influence. The high-profile cases of healthcare misconduct and gross negligence as documented by Currie et al. (2019) and the Doctors Defence Services (2023) have shaken people's confidence in health professionals. This has also been affected by the easy access to the internet, whereby patients and their families can gain access to the latest information on diagnosis and treatment. We saw this with the COVID-19 pandemic, where health professionals differed in their approach to care (herd immunity or population lockdown). Nurses are more accountable now than they have ever been and members of the public are rightly asking increasingly perceptive questions about their care and treatment. If nurses select a theory that will commit them to promoting adaptation, independence or self-care, could they be held legally accountable by the public for this particular care focus? (See Reflective Exercise 7.7.)

Reflective Exercise 7.7

Biomedical Model

Patients are more aware of their rights and are more prone to complain and litigate than previously. Nurses should welcome being held to account. Let us say a patient wanted to adopt the sick role as described by Parsons (1951, discussed earlier) but the nurse was insisting that they took on more of a self-caring role as advocated in Orem's theory. Could this lead to the patient complaining about their care? How would you deal with such a scenario if you were the nurse in charge, who had facilitated the introduction of Orem's theory onto the unit?

Staff Attitudes

In the introduction to this chapter, we mentioned that there is often a distrust of nursing theories in the clinical setting, and they were perceived as imposed academic exercises. It is highly likely that this dislike has grown out of the aversion to the nursing process. Such negative views can influence the selection of nursing theories for practice. It is a truism that if nurses have a view that theories will add more paperwork to their already busy schedule, for expedience, they will select the simplest theory available and the one that is easiest to introduce and follow.

Furthermore, we stated earlier that the expert nurses as described by Benner (1984) often use tacit knowledge and have a holistic *gestalt* to their practice. The introduction of formal nursing theories mean that such nurses have to unpick their normal intuitive actions and learn a new way of doing and thinking. This could move them from expert to novice, at least temporarily. The next section provides you with the criteria necessary to select an appropriate nursing theory to underpin your practice.

Choosing a Suitable Nursing Theory

The Criteria

Fawcett and DeSanto-Madeya (2013: 35) recommended that nurses should follow four steps when selecting a nursing theory:

1. thoroughly analyse and evaluate several nursing theories;
2. compare the content of each theory with the mission statement of the clinical setting to determine if the theory is appropriate for use with the population of patients served;
3. determine if the philosophical claims underpinning each theory are congruent with the philosophy adopted in the clinical setting;
4. select the theory that most closely matches the mission of the clinical setting and the philosophy of the nursing department.

From the previous section, you will have spotted the obvious flaws in this recommendation. As we stressed earlier, it would be difficult for hard-pressed nurses to analyse and evaluate several nursing theories. In addition, steps 2 and 3 could be counterproductive. For instance, if the pervading philosophy in their unit is the biomedical model, then the nurses will select a theory that matches that way of working and, in doing so, maintain the *status quo*. In addition, we doubt whether all clinical settings have an explicit mission statement or philosophy underpinning their work? Although we are sure that Fawcett and DeSanto-Madeya meant well, their four steps to selecting a theory may inadvertently allow the introduction of an unsuitable nursing theory. Nonetheless, we concur that there needs to be an agreed checklist to allow busy clinicians to decide on the most appropriate theory for their practice. We propose that the following criteria represent such a checklist:

- clinical setting
- origin of the theory
- paradigms as a basis for choice
- simplicity
- patients' needs
- understandability
- costs

These are discussed in more detail in the following sections.

Clinical Setting

This criterion concentrates on contextual factors in the clinical situation. This could be an emergency room, a children's clinic, a community-based nursing home, or a mental health unit. Fawcett and DeSanto-Madeya (2013) recommended that the fit of the theory under consideration should be compared with the philosophy of the nursing environment. Earlier in this chapter, we likened theories to maps that guide our practice and suggested we require a different map to suit the specific terrain in which we find ourselves. This holds true for clinical settings and so staff should only select a theory if it fits well with the structure and function of that setting. As has been alluded to, Peplau's (1992) theory could be appropriate for a mental health setting, whereas FANCAP could be more relevant for a fast high turnover unit like an emergency room. For an example of Peplau being used in psychiatry, see Delaney et al. (2017). To see how FANCAP can be used, check out Schleur (2021). Academic Research Experts (2023) looked at the selection of nursing theories in an intensive care unit. They stated that the choice would be based on the ability of a theory to address one of the aspects of critical care such as patients facing life-threatening conditions or the dynamics of taking care of patients because that is what critical care entails.

Origin of the Theory

In Chapter 2, you will recall that we distinguished between the 'know that' of knowledge and the 'know how' of knowledge. The former refers to deductive cognitive knowledge, whereas the latter concerns inductive practical knowledge. By definition, practising nurses pride themselves on being 'hands on' professionals. Therefore, they may be more attracted to a theory that has emerged from the 'know how' stable. In contrast, a theory formulated by academic 'armchair theorists' who based their work on reasoning alone may be unattractive to many clinical nurses. Moreover, when selecting a theory, nurses should take its origins into account. It is, of course, possible to identify a theory that was developed through 'retroduction', that is, where both induction and deduction played a part (see Chapter 2). You will recall that Peplau (1992) studied the phenomenon of interpersonal relationships in psychiatric clinical settings over many years and began to develop her theory deductively through being influenced by Sullivan's (1953) interpersonal relations theory. But she also developed her theory inductively by reflecting on her years of clinical experience in psychiatric nursing. This gives clinical nurses the best of both worlds – the theory has clinical credibility and is based on previous scholarly work.

Paradigms as a Basis for Choice

In Chapter 5, you were shown that every nursing theory has its roots in one or more of the following paradigms: systems, interactional, developmental and behavioural. These 'world views' could help nurses make some preliminary decisions about the type of theory that is most appropriate for their work. For instance, mental health nurses who support the development of interpersonal relationships with patients (e.g. Peplau 1992) may find interactional theories more attractive than the more mechanical systems theories (e.g. Roy 2019). Similarly, nurses who work with people who have severe dementia may not favour interactional theories (e.g. King 1968, 1981), whereas behavioural theories that focus on meeting human needs such as Henderson (Pinheiro et al. 2016) or Roper, Logan and Tierney (Holland & Jenkins 2019) might attract more support.

Simplicity

It has been mentioned several times in this text that modern nursing is a complex and demanding profession. Patient throughput has increased, and difficult targets have been set for patient outcomes. In such a situation, nurses do not welcome complex theoretical frameworks to overcomplicate the craft of patient care. Simplicity has to be an important selection criterion, as long as this does not reflect a lack of theoretical soundness. The principle of 'Occam's razor' states that 'the simplest theory is to be selected from among all other theories that fit the facts as we know them' (William of Occam 1300–1349) (see Key Concepts 7.6). This traditional belief is synonymous with the modern idea of 'parsimony'. Parsimony dictates that a good theory is one that is stated in the simplest terms possible. Current Nursing (2024) maintained that a nursing theory should have the characteristics of accessibility and clarity. There are complex nursing theories such as that of Rogers (Fawcett 2018) and there are less complex theories such as that of Orem (Yip 2021). There is little reason to select the former if the latter will suit the clinical requirements just as well.

🔍 Key Concepts 7.6

Occam's razor: the principle that we should select the simplest theory that fits the facts as we know them.

Parsimony: the principle that the best theory is the one that is described in the fewest and the simplest terms.

Patients' Needs

When considering theories for practice, nurses should not be too influenced by what theory is the most popular in their hospital, country or region; rather they should be concerned with which is best to meet the needs of their patients. Experienced nurses know their patients and their patients' needs. They are often best placed to be a patient advocate when patients cannot advocate for themselves. Therefore, the choice of any theory must be based on the nurses' knowledge of their patients. In some cases, a patient caseload would have people with varying needs. Therefore, the theory must also be general enough to deal with the many diverse situations the nurse comes across when dealing with a heterogeneous group of patients.

Today, we see a situation where patients are involved more in the decisions about their care and treatment. Some simply call this 'involvement', whereas others use the terms 'co-production' or 'co-design' (McKenna 2021). It is based on the principle that patients are experts through experience and there should be 'no decision about me, without me'. Regardless of the terminology, it is a welcome development. Is it possible and proper that patients should also be involved in deciding on which nursing theory or theories should be used in their care? Of course, the complicated language of some theories could be off-putting. However, if the patients and some nurses have difficulty with a theorist's language, then it is questionable if this is the right theory for that clinical setting. This is dealt with in the next section.

Understandability

Although this concept is closely related to simplicity, it merits separate consideration. A theory must be easily understood if it is to attract the support of busy nurses. In a previous section, we referred to the complexity of Rogers's (1980) work, but we could have been writing about Parse's (1987) theory or Fitzpatrick's (1982) theory, as both grew out of Rogers's theory. Roskoski (2018: 2) worried that many nurses do not have an adequate enough understanding of the types of nursing theories and that this is due to an inadequate educational background and can lead to unsatisfactory patient care. Current Nursing (2024) supported this, claiming that many nurses have not had the training or experience to deal with the abstract concepts presented by nursing theorists.

But, in case we become overly critical of the complexity of theory, we should acknowledge that a theory must have an element of complexity to be significant. To get their unique meaning across, theorists often have to invent new words or use complex terminology (see Reflective Exercise 7.8). For instance, we learned in Chapter 2 that humans could have more than just the three dimensions of height, width and depth. While this is understandable, clinical nurses may hesitate at referring to patients using Rogers's (1980) phrase – four-dimensional beings!

We are not making a case here for complicated cant that seeks to over-intellectualise the science, art and craft of nursing. However, when you take on a new hobby, there is always a lot of new terminology to get used to, be it knitting (purl), photography (shutter speed), sailing (tack) or computing (tetrabyte). Why, then, should we expect the language of theory to be like everyday speech? As Bronowski (2005) stated in *The Ascent of Man*, the language of science cannot be freed from ambiguity any more than poetry can.

Reflective Exercise 7.8

Understandability and Jargon

We have noticed over the years examples of anti-intellectualism among many nurses. They complain about the big words and jargon used in nursing theories and nursing research. However, they appear to be enthusiastically fluent when it comes to knowing and reciting the long and complex names of certain diseases, medical interventions and pharmaceutical products.

Take a few minutes to consider why this is the case and what can be done to change things. Discuss with your fellow students whether this is a realistic observation of nursing behaviour or simply a biased perception on our part.

Is it possible that after years of experience, nurses wrongly perceive nursing to be simple and ordinary, so they view theories as overcomplicating and intellectualising something as basic as caring? Consider in your group whether caring is basic and what the arguments are either way.

Costs

If the selected theory is going to be overly expensive in terms of reconfiguring the unit's care planning software, paperwork, external consultancy or intense training, then the advantages would have to be weighed against such expenditure. Fawcett and DeSanto-Madeya (2013) highlighted that there is very little in the literature on the costs of implementing nursing theories in practice. They pointed out that 'costs most likely vary from institution to institution depending on the staff's current knowledge of theories, existing staff development resources and extent of change to documentation' (Fawcett and DeSanto-Madeya 2013: 35). They noted that most healthcare institutions already allocate funding for staff induction and development but not for the hiring of external consultants to assist with the implementation of a nursing theory. They also suggested that job descriptions and staff appraisal systems may have to be congruent with the theory selected.

Further Supporting Criteria

It has been suggested that a theory will not gain a foothold in a clinical setting or win the 'hearts and minds' of busy clinical nurses if it is not relevant to the patients being cared for and the practice being provided. The following list of questions supports and add to the previous criteria:

- Does the theory have direct relevance for the way in which nursing is practised?
- Does it describe real or ought-to-be care?
- Have its propositions been tried and tested by research?
- Does it deal with the resources that are necessary for good care?
- Does it guide the use of the nursing process?
- Does it provide practising nurses with good direction for clinical actions?

- Are the concepts within the theory too abstract to be applied in practice?
- Is the language of the theory easy to understand?
- Does the theory coincide with the practising nurses' 'know how' knowledge?

On the website Current Nursing (2024), the following questions are posed as a means of selecting a nursing theory:

- Does the theory reflect nursing practice as I know it?
- Will it support what I believe to be excellent nursing practice?
- Can this theory be considered in relation to a wide range of nursing situations?
- Does it reflect personal interests, abilities and experiences?
- What will it be like to think about this nursing theory in our practice?
- Will my work with nursing theory be worth the effort?

Nurses' Own Philosophy as a Basis for Selecting a Theory

If asked, all professionals would have a personal view regarding the central components of their work. This is based on their attitudes, values and beliefs and is borne out of the education and experience they have been exposed to over a number of years. Nurses, if given time to consider, can describe and explain the essence of what they do. Because thoughts, beliefs and attitudes are the parents of behaviour, it is not surprising that clinical practice varies according to the thoughts, beliefs and attitudes of the nurse giving the care. These have been referred to as elsewhere as the nurse's implicit nursing theory (McKenna et al. 2014).

Based on Benner's work (1984), we would argue that each 'expert' clinical nurse has a 'personal theory' that he or she uses as a guide to practice (see Key Concepts 7.7). Fawcett (2018: 15) seemed to support this, stating that 'conceptual models of nursing are the explicit and formal presentation of some nurse's implicit, private images of nursing'. These personal theories incorporate assumptions concerning the four metaparadigm elements of, nursing, health, person and environment (see Chapter 5). The literature informs us that all formal nursing theories are also built around these four elements (Fawcett & DeSanto-Madeya 2013). Therefore, it is not unreasonable to expect that if clinical nurses were able to match their view of these four elements (personal nursing theory) with what an existing nursing theory says about them, they would be closer to identifying a suitable theory for practice (see Appendix A).

Key Concepts 7.7

Although they may not make it explicit, most nurses have a personal theory of nursing that has been developed over many years based on their education and experience.

Take some time to decide on what you think health is, what nursing is, what a person is and what the environment is. See how it differs from some of your colleagues in your group. Ask yourself why there is a difference.

If asked, most nurses are able to reveal these personal theories; they can identify their views on nursing, health, environment and person. However, in the reality of the practice situation, these are seldom articulated. It is not something that nurses talk about during their coffee break. Consequently, they are mostly hidden in the nurse's mind rather than being made explicit.

Some of the problems with this approach to selecting a nursing theory have already been identified. The main one is the perpetuation of the theoretical status quo. If a nurse's personal theory is based only on being educated and experienced in the physical aspects of the biomedical model, this will reflect their choice of theory. Perhaps, this is why many clinical settings in the United Kingdom and the United States have adopted Roper et al.'s (2000) and Henderson's (1966) theories, respectively. They focus on patients' activities of living, many of which are physical and physiological (e.g. breathing, eating, eliminating, mobilizing and sleeping).

There are other limitations to matching a personal theory with an established one. It is possible that 10 expert nurses in the same clinical unit have 10 different personal theories of nursing. Trying to select one to match the values and beliefs of all 10 would be difficult. Also, many of these personal theories could be immature, untested, unreliable or confused. Using Patricia Benner's terminology, would 'expert' nurses in the team have different personal theories to 'novices' or 'beginner' nurses, with whom they work? Furthermore, the internationally recognised nursing theories are by no means 'value free'. They too were initially formulated around the personal views and preferences of their originators. By selecting these nursing theories, practising nurses may simply be exchanging their own biased views with those of a theorist's prejudices.

Nonetheless, in an era where nursing theories are often perceived to be unpopular, choosing one that best reflects a nurse's own perception of nursing may be the best selection strategy. After all, nurses will have difficulty supporting a nursing theory unconditionally if it does not coincide with their deep-rooted views of what they believe is nursing practice.

A Strategy for Choice

From the preceding discussion, we would suggest that all nurses have a personal theory pertaining to how they view the four metaparadigm elements. As highlighted in Chapter 5, all published nursing theories also possess statements about the metaparadigm. This means that practising nurses can choose a theory that best reflects the beliefs and values that they hold about nursing, people, health and their environment.

Therefore, the beliefs held by nurses about these four elements can direct them to look for a theory congruent with these beliefs (see Key Concepts 7.8). It should be possible for nurses to compare what existing nursing theorists say about these with their beliefs and select the one that closely matches them.

If nurses cannot accept the way some concepts are treated within a particular theory, they should reject that theory and choose another one whose concepts are more compatible with their own. In this way, congruence will be reached between the nurse's personal theory and a recognised theory. The final choice will indicate for nurses what they have always believed about their care but could not articulate in as clear and distinct manner as expressed by the selected theorist (see Reflective Exercise 7.9).

Key Concepts 7.8

Nurses' personal theories: are composed of their beliefs and views about nursing, health, person and environment. Established nursing theories also make assumptions about these elements. This can form the basis for matching and selecting.

Reflective Exercise 7.9

Theory Selection

Refer to any one of the following texts:

Fawcett, J. (2018) *Contemporary Nursing Knowledge: Analysis and Evaluation of Nursing Models and Theories*, 2nd edition. F.A. Davis Company, Philadelphia.

Alligood, M.R. (2021). *Nursing Theorists and Their Work*. 10th edition. Elsevier, St. Louis.

Meleis, AI (2017). *Theoretical Nursing: Development and Progress*. Walters Kluwer Publishers, Philadelphia.

Access the following webpage:

Nursology (2023) https://nursology.net/nurse-theories/

Using one or more of these sources, extract from the theories of Orem, Roy, Henderson, Rogers and Peplau what each says about the person, nursing, health and environment (the metaparadigm). Consider these and see which one matches your personal views about these four elements. Check if any others in your group prefer the same or different theory and, if so, why. Which of the metaparadigms from the theories in Appendix A best reflects your own personal views of the four metaparadigm elements?

Who Should Select the Theory?

As mentioned at the start of this chapter, at one time, it was commonplace for nurse educators or nurse managers to select a theory for blanket application across a hospital. This almost guaranteed that it would hold very little weight with experienced clinically based nurses. The case has been made in preceding sections that a nursing theory has a better chance of being adopted and used if practising nurses and patients have been involved in its selection. Although this may be a lengthy process, in the end, the adoption will be longer-lasting if every concerned individual has been party to the decision-making process. A decision on a nursing theory imposed by others often means a short-lived allegiance among those who have to implement it.

A slightly more controversial notion is that the clinical manager of each setting should select the most relevant nursing theory. This may indeed be a valid nomination, considering that this individual should have the most knowledge and influence regarding clinical work orientation and practical expertise in the unit (see Key Concepts 7.9).

We touched on the importance of 'co-production' and 'co-design' earlier. However, there is a general absence of reports in the literature suggesting that the patient should be involved in the theory selection process. This is strange considering the emphasis on the patient as a partner in care. We would argue that when selecting a theory, the beliefs and values of the most important person concerned, the recipient of care, cannot be ignored. However, if some nursing theories are viewed as confusing by many nurses, would patients not find them equally confusing? If the answer is yes, then one can see why there has been little evidence of partnership between nurses and patients in the selection of a theory. However, this may say more about the unnecessary complexity of the theory than about patients' knowledge.

Key Concepts 7.9

Theory co-production: the clinical manager could have a major role in selecting the theory, but the involvement of patients and other nurses who work in that setting would strengthen the commitment to using the theory.

Nursing Theories Versus Theories Developed by Other Disciplines

There is a great deal of scepticism around using non-nursing theories to guide nursing practice (McKenna et al. 2014). If nurses borrow theories from other disciplines, research problems based on these theories could be phrased as questions that have little to do with nursing. For instance, using and testing sociological theories within nursing may do more for the knowledge base of sociology than for nursing. Also, one of the hallmarks of a profession is having a body of knowledge pertaining to itself. This could never happen if nursing relies only on borrowed theories. This situation formed the basis for the explosion in the number of nursing theories that we see today. But is this not too narrow a view? Should we not use whatever theory fits the patient's problem and can best guide practice? (see Key Concepts 7.10). It is useful to note the following definition put forward by Current Nursing (2024). It stated that a nursing theory is:

a set of concepts, definitions, relationships, and assumptions or propositions derived from nursing models **or from other disciplines** *and project a purposive, systematic view of phenomena by designing specific* *inter-relationships among concepts for the purposes of describing, explaining, predicting, and/or prescribing. This shows how conceptualizations from other disciplines can form the basis for nursing theory.*

🔍 Key Concepts 7.10

Borrowed theory may contribute to the quality of patient care but it could also contribute to expanding the knowledge base of the discipline from which it was borrowed.

Remember that the first nursing theories were only developed in the 1950s and 1960s, so we can appreciate why some nurses might have felt threatened by theories from other disciplines. After all, there were very few nursing theories available at that time. The works of Peplau (1952), Henderson (1955), Orem (1958), Hall (1959) and Johnson (1959) were the exceptions. These were followed by around 40 others over subsequent decades. Most of these early nurse theorists seemed to believe that their work was not worthy of the term 'theory'; they referred to their work instead as models or conceptual frameworks. This suggests that while some nurses held theory from other disciplines in great esteem, they did not wish to embolden these early conceptualisations in nursing with the term theory.

However, many of the emerging nursing theories were based on the work of theorists from other discipline, mainly psychology. To name a few – Peplau's (1952) work was based on that of Harry Stack Sullivan (see Chapter 6); Johnson's (1959) model was based on that of B.F. Skinner; and Henderson's (1955) model was based on that of Abraham Maslow.

Considering the plethora of textbooks on nursing theory that are still being published each year, there remain nurses who would rather pursue nursing theories than borrowed theories. There is perhaps some merit in this. Compared with sociology, psychology, medicine, law and many other professions, nursing is still a relatively new discipline in academia. In the United Kingdom, for instance, nursing only moved into the university sector in the mid-1990s. The transition into universities led many of the new nursing academics to realise that they had to develop a body of knowledge that nursing could claim as its own pertaining to its practice.

We would suggest that the choice of home-grown or borrowed theories should not be either/or. Nurses should formulate their own theories, but they should also use and adapt theories from other disciplines to suit nursing's needs. After all, more nurses are working in interdisciplinary teams and leading interdisciplinary research projects, and the best theories are those that best fit the problems to be solved.

To a large extent, this corresponds to the picture in other allied health professions. Social work, for instance, began with an adherence to the biomedical model, only to supplant it with social theories of its own as the discipline evolved. Similarly, occupational therapy, as one of the 'allied health professions', has moved away from the biomedical model to embrace theories relating to activities of living.

In many instances, nurses borrow theories but do not bother to adapt them. This often results in theories that are incomplete and unrepresentative of nursing. To be useful, such borrowed knowledge must be reformulated and revalidated to suit the particular problems and needs of the patients that nurses serve. For example, psychological, educational or organisational theories are not exclusive to nursing, but how they are used can be distinctive. Yet, because borrowed theories may need to undergo intensive reworking to fit nursing's unique perspective, borrowing may not be as simple a process as it first appears – after much work and adapting, we could end up with an invalid and unreliable hybrid theory.

We should not be worried about ownership; theories belong to the scientific community at large, not to one particular discipline. Discovery does not confer the right of ownership. A note of caution is required here: nurses should be careful to avoid the temptation of borrowing from other disciplines without first investigating what those theories have done for their parent disciplines. If a sociological theory of family care has been rejected by sociologists and psychologists, it may be foolish for psychiatric nurses to borrow it for their practice unless careful consideration is given as to why it was rejected by its parent disciplines. The term 'borrowed' suggests that it will be returned to where it came from. In this case, nursing may adapt a borrowed theory and improve upon it. As a result, the adapted theory could also bring back new perspectives for its parent discipline (see Reflective Exercise 7.10).

It may not be long before other healthcare disciplines begin to borrow theories developed by nurses. In fact, as we outlined earlier, there is some evidence to suggest that occupational therapists and physiotherapists are already borrowing and reformulating nursing theories (e.g. self-care and activity of living theories) for their practices.

151

We maintain that there is nothing wrong with selecting a theory from another discipline if it can shed new light or provide a different, beneficial perspective on the provision of patient care. There is no reason why nurses should 'reinvent the wheel', if the wheel already exists. They may, however, need to add a few extra spokes or inflate or deflate the tyres a little to meet different needs. The important question is whether selecting a 'borrowed' theory brings with it benefits for nursing, nurses and the people who rely on us for care.

Reflective Exercise 7.10

Borrowed Theory

Take some time to consider where you work and identify non-nursing theories that you use to do your job. These could be theories of communication, theories of management, theories of hygiene or theories of teaching. See how many you can come up with and then identify any benefits they bring to your role.

Conclusion

Because the choice of a theory will affect how patients are assessed and how care is planned and delivered, selection should not be a process that nurses take lightly. This chapter has identified several issues that must be taken into consideration when an appropriate nursing theory is to be chosen. It has outlined a range of selection criteria nurses may find useful. The issues of who should make the choice and how this should be done are also addressed. In essence, there are many selection approaches available, and nurses should consider these carefully. Not to do so could waste a lot of time and end up with nurses employing an inappropriate theory to guide their practice.

Theories are like maps, and we require a different one depending on the terrain in which we are working. The days should be over when managers and educators choose theories for practice. Patients or their representatives should work alongside nurses in the selection process. If this occurs, the selected theory will be a realistic reflection of what they see as important for quality care and the nurses will be more likely to use it enthusiastically and appropriately. Finally, there are dangers in borrowing theory from other established disciplines for application in nursing. However, if handled correctly, some borrowed theories can bring a great deal of benefit to nursing. They can also be adapted and enhanced and returned to their parent discipline in a more robust form.

152

Revision Points

- Because the choice of a theory will affect how patients are assessed and how care is planned and delivered, selecting an appropriate theory is important.

- There are 12 potential problems that must be considered when selecting a theory:

  - American or UK nursing theories;

  - ethical and moral issues;

  - length of patient stay;

  - nurses' knowledge of nursing theories;

  - the implications of a wrong choice;

- hybrid nursing theories;
- method of choice;
- single or multiple theories;
- nursing theories vs midwifery theories;
- inherent limitations of theories;
- social and political issues;
- staff attitudes.

- There are a number of selection criteria that should be used when considering a suitable theory for practice:
  - clinical setting;
  - origin of the theory;
  - paradigms as a basis for choice;
  - simplicity;
  - patients' needs;
  - understandability;
  - matching the metaparadigm to personal theories (see Appendix A).

- The days should be over when managers and tutors choose theories for practice. Ideally, patients or their representatives should work alongside clinical nurses in the selection process.

- There are dangers and benefits in borrowing theory from other established disciplines for application in nursing, as follows:
  - If practitioners continued to borrow theories from other disciplines, research problems based on these theories will be addressed that have little or no benefit for nursing.
  - Compared with sociology, psychology, medicine, law and many other professions, nursing is still a relatively new discipline. It requires a body of knowledge pertaining to its work – in other words – its own theories.
  - To be useful, such borrowed knowledge must be reformulated and revalidated to suit the particular problems and needs of our patients and our discipline.
  - Borrowing may not be as simple a process as it first appears – after much work and adapting, we could end up with an invalid and unreliable hybrid.
  - Theories belong to the scientific community at large, not to one particular discipline. Discovery does not confer the right of ownership.
  - Nursing may adapt a borrowed theory and improve upon it. As a result, the adapted theory could bestow new perspectives for its parent discipline.
  - There is nothing wrong with selecting a theory from another discipline if it can shed new light or provide a different beneficial perspective on the provision of patient care.

Useful Web Links

https://currentnursing.com/nursing_theory/nursing_theories_overview.html
https://currentnursing.com/nursing_theory/nursing_theorists.html
https://nursekey.com/outline-of-nursing-theories-and-frameworks-of-care/
https://nurseslabs.com/nursing-theories/
https://nursology.net/
https://uk.indeed.com/career-advice/career-development/nursing-theory
https://www.wgu.edu/blog/understanding-nursing-theories2109.html

References

Academic Research Experts (2023). *The Six Criteria Approach for Selecting Nursing Theories*. New York. https://www.academicresearch experts.net/six-criteria-approach-of-selecting-nursing-theories/

Alligood M.R. (2021) *Nursing Theorists and Their Work*, 10th edition. St. Louis: Elsevier.

Baker N. (2009) *Exposing the Complex Realities of Nursing Unresponsive Patients' Pain in Intensive Care*. Doctor of Philosophy, The University of Technology Sydney. https://opus.lib.uts.edu.au/bitstream/10453/35832/2/02Whole.pdf

Benner P. (1984) *From Novice to Expert: Excellence and Power in Clinical Nursing Practice*. Menlo Park, CA: Addison-Wesley.

Bronowski J. (2005) *The Ascent of Man: The Complete Series Digitally Restored*. London: BBC.

Business Bliss (November 2018). *Virginia Henderson Theory of Nursing*. Business Bliss Consultants FZE. https://nursinganswers.net/essays/virginia-henderson-theory-of-nursing-nursing-essay.php?vref=1

Current Nursing (2024). *Nursing Theories: Open Access Articles on Nursing Theories and Models*. https://currentnursing.com/nursing_theory/application_nursing_theories.html

Currie G., Richmond J. & Muzio D. (2019) Professional misconduct in healthcare: setting out a research agenda for work sociology. *Journal of the British Sociological Association.*, **33**(1). DOI: 10.1177/095001701879335

Da Costa V., Passos C., Luz A., Barros M.H., Bezerra F., Kelly A. et al. (2016) Application of the nursing theory of Callista Roy to the patient with cerebral vascular accident. *Journal of Nursing UFPE*, **Supplement 1**, 352–360.

Delaney K.R., Shattell M. & Johnson M.E. (2017) Capturing the interpersonal process of psychiatric nurses: a model for engagement. *Archives of Psychiatric Nursing*, **31**(6), 634–640. DOI: 10.1016/j.apnu.2017.08.003

Doctors Defence Services (2023). https://doctorsdefenceservice.com/misconduct-in-gmc-cases/

Duffy J. (2008) *Quality Caring in Nursing: Applying Theory to Clinical Practice, Education and Leadership*. New York: Springer Publications.

Fawcett J. (2017) *Applying Conceptual Models of Nursing: Quality Improvement, Research, and Practice*. New York: Springer Publishing Company.

Fawcett J. (2018) Rogers' science of unitary human beings. *Nursology*. https://nursology.net/nurse-theories/rogers-science-of-unitary-human-beings/

Fawcett J. & DeSanto-Madeya S. (2013) *Contemporary Nursing Knowledge: Analysis and Evaluation of Nursing Models and Theories*. Philadelphia, PA: FA Davis Co.

Feyerabend P. (1977) Consolidation for the specialist. In Lakatos I. & Musgrave A. (eds) *Criticism and the Growth of Knowledge*, pp. 32–47. Cambridge: Cambridge University Press.

Fitzpatrick J.J. (1982). In Fitzpatrick J.J., Whall A.L., Johnston R.L. & Floyd J.A. (eds) *Nursing Models: Applications to Psychiatric Mental Health Nursing*. Bowie, MD: Brady & Co.

Gaskill Eakes G. (2019) Chronic sorrow. In Peterson S. & Bredow T.S. (eds) *Middle Range Theories: Application to Nursing Research and Practice*, 5th edition, pp. 146–161. Philadelphia, PA: Wolters Kluwer.

Hall L. (1959) *Nursing – What Is It?* Virginia: Virginia State Nurses Association. Winter.

Henderson V. (1955) *The Nature of Nursing: A Definition and its Implications for Practice, Education and Research*. London: Collier Macmillan.

Henderson V. (1966) *The Nature of Nursing: A Definition and its Implications for Practice, Education and Research*. London: Collier Macmillan.

Holland K. & Jenkins J. (eds) (2019) *Applying the Roper-Logan-Tierney Model in Practice*, 3rd edition. Oxford: Elsevier.

Johnson D.E. (1959) The nature of a science of nursing. *Nursing Outlook*, **7**, 291–294.

Khademian Z., Kazemi F. & Gholamzadeh S. (2020) the effect of self care education based on Orem's nursing theory on quality of life and self-efficacy in patients with hypertension: a quasi-experimental study. *Int J Community Based Nurs Midwifery.*, **8**(2), 140–149. DOI: 10.30476/IJCBNM.2020.81690.0

King I. (1968, 1981) *A Theory of Nursing: Systems, Concepts, Process*, 1st and 2nd editions. New York: John Wiley & Sons Inc.

Kolcaba K. (2001) Evolution of the mid-range theory of comfort for outcomes research. *Nursing Outlook*, **49**(2), 86–92.

Lynn R. (2021) *Sex Differences in Intelligence: The Developmental Theory*. Budapest: Arktos Media Limited.

McCaughan E.M. & McKenna H.P. (2007) Never-ending making sense: towards a substantive theory of the information-seeking behaviour of newly diagnosed cancer patients. *Journal of Clinical Nursing*, **16**, 2096–2104.

McKenna H.P. (1997) *Nursing Models and Theories*. London: Routledge.

McKenna H.P. (2021) *Research Impact: Guidance on Advancement, Achievement and Assessment*. New York: Springer Nature.

McKenna H.P., Pajnkihar M. & Murphy F.A. (2014) *Fundamentals of Nursing Models Theories and Practice*. London: Wiley Blackwell.

Meleis A.I. (2017) *Theoretical Nursing: Development and Progress*. Philadelphia, PA: Walters Kluwer Publishers.

Nightingale F. (1859) *Notes on Nursing: What It Is and What It Is Not*. Edinburgh: Churchill Livingstone.

Nursology (2023) https://nursology.net/nurse-theories/

Orem D.E. (1958) *Nursing: Concepts of Practice*. New York: McGraw Hill.

Orem D.E. (1995) *Nursing Concepts of Practice*, 5th edition. St. Louis, MO: Mosby, Inc.

Orlando I. (1961) *The Dynamic Nurse Patient Relationship. Function, Process, and Principles*. New York: G.P. Putnam & Sons.

Parse R.R. (1987) *Nursing Science: Major Paradigms, Theories, and Critiques*. Philadelphia, PA: Saunders.

Parsons T. (1951) *The Social System*. Glencoe, IL: The Free Press.

Paterson J.G. & Zderad L.T. (1976) *Humanistic Nursing*. New York: John Wiley & Sons.

Peplau E.H. (1952) *Interpersonal Relations in Nursing: A Conceptual Frame of Reference for Psychodynamic Nursing*. New York: G.P. Putnam & Sons.

Peplau H.E. (1992) Interpersonal relations: a theoretical framework for application in nursing practice. *Nursing Science Quarterly*, **5**, 13–18.

Peterson S. & Bredow T.S. (2019) *Middle Range Theories: Application to Nursing Research and Practice*, 5th edition. Philadelphia, PA: Wolters Kluwer Pubs.

Pinheiro F.M., Santo F.H.d.E., Chibante C.L.d.P. & Pestana L.C. (2016) Profile of hospitalized elderly according to Virginia Henderson: contributions for nursing care. *Revista de Pesquisa: Cuidado é Fundamental Online*, **8**(3), 4789–4795. DOI: 10.9789/2175-5361.2016.v8i3.4789-4795

Popper K. (1989) *Conjectures and Refutations: The Growth of Scientific Knowledge*, revised edition. London: Routledge.

Rodgers E. (2003) *Diffusion of Innovations*, 5th edition. New York: Simon and Schuster.

Rogers M.E. (1980) *An Introduction to a Theoretical Basis of Nursing*, 2nd edition. Philadelphia, PA: F.A. Davis & Co.

Roper N., Logan W. & Tierney A.J. (2000) *The Roper-Logan-Tierney Model of Nursing Based on Activities of Living*. Edinburgh: Churchill-Livingstone.

Roskoski, J. (2018). *Barriers to applying Nursing Theory*. https://careertrend.com/list-7429101-barriers-applying-nursing-theory.html

Roy C. (2019) Nursing knowledge in the 21st century: domain-derived and basic science practice-shaped. *Advances in Nursing Science*, **42**(1), 28–42. DOI: 10.1097/ANS.0000000000000240

Runquist J.J. & Reed P.G. (2007) Self-transcendence and well-being in homeless adults. *Journal of Holistic Nursing*, **25**(1), 5–13.

Schleur A.B. (2021) Wound care in the baby and young child. In Probst S. (ed.) *Wound Care Nursing E-Book: A Person-centred Approach*, 3rd edition, Ch 4. Oxford: Elsevier.

Silva M.C. (1986) Research testing nursing theory: state of the art. *Advances in Nursing Science*, **9**(1), 1–11.

Stephens Barnum B. (2004) *Nursing Theory: Analysis, Application, Evaluation*. New York: Lippincott Williams & Wilkins.

Sullivan H.S. (1953) The interpersonal theory of psychiatry. In Perry H.S. & Gawel M.L. (eds) *Psychiatry*, pp. 72–79. New York: W.W. Norton & Co. Inc.

Travelbee J. (1966) *Interpersonal Aspects of Nursing*. Philadelphia, PA: F.A. Davis.

Wiedenbach E. (1964) *Clinical Nursing: A Helping Art*. New York: Springer Publication Company.

Yip J.Y.C. (2021) Theory-based advanced nursing practice: a practice update on the application of Orem's self-care deficit nursing theory. *Sage Open Nursing.*, **20**, 7. DOI: 10.1177/23779608211011993

CHAPTER 8

Research and Theory: A Reciprocal Relationship

Outline of Content

From previous chapters you will have learned that there is a strong link between theory and research. We saw that the end product of theory + research was science. We also discussed the development of theory through induction, deduction and retroduction. In this chapter we will introduce you to how theory is generated by research, how research tests and evaluates theory and how a theory can simply be a framework from which to frame a research project. You will also be introduced to the meta-theorists Dickoff and James (1968), Fawcett (2017) and Meleis (2017), where we will demonstrate how their work is linked to research.

Learning Outcomes

At the end of this chapter, you should be able to:

1. Outline the relationship between research and theory

2. Show how theory is generated by research

3. Show how theory is tested by research

4. Show how theory is evaluated by research

5. Understand how theory can help guide or frame a research study

6. Link different levels of theory with different levels of research

7. Describe Meleis's five levels of research–theory linkages

Fundamentals of Nursing Models, Theories and Practice, Third Edition. Hugh P. McKenna, Majda Pajnkihar and Dominika Vrbnjak.
© 2025 John Wiley & Sons Ltd. Published 2025 by John Wiley & Sons Ltd.
Companion website: www.wiley.com/go/nursingmodels3e

Introduction

Building Theory Through Research: An Inductive Approach

Theories often emerge from what nurses experience in the real world of clinical practice, are tested by research and are then returned to practice. On their return, the theories may be unchanged, adapted or rejected. From earlier chapters you will recall that 'phenomena' are things, events or situations that we perceive through our senses. For example, clinical nurses notice phenomena through observing something as they undertake a procedure, hearing something a patient said or touch or smell. In fact, nurses continually come across a variety of phenomena in their daily work. Some of these are ignored because a nurse may see them as commonplace or unimportant, or simply because the nurse does not give them any attention. Alternatively, nurses may give considerable thought as to why some phenomenon has happened and what this means.

For example: John Smith, a nurse manager, noticed that two adjacent medical units had different lengths of patient stay, one being consistently shorter than the other. What puzzled him was that they were both medical assessment units where similar types of patient problems were treated. Furthermore, both wards were the responsibility of the same medical staff and nurse staffing levels and experience were identical. In fact, the only difference John could see was that one had open visiting and the other did not. In other words, one ward restricted visiting to one hour in the afternoon and one hour in the evening. In contrast, the other ward allowed visitors access at any time during the day. This seemed to be the only difference and he noticed this 'phenomenon' and was curious about it. His first thought was to check this out with other nurses in the ward to see if they too noticed this and if they agreed with his conclusion as to the possible cause of the difference. Few of his colleagues had noticed this phenomenon but once it was brought to their attention, they too found the phenomenon interesting.

John decided to investigate the phenomenon further and research it as part of a master's programme he was undertaking. He started by searching the literature but did not come up with any published papers or reports on open visiting being linked to shorter lengths of stay. This made him think that his conclusion may be incorrect.

Nonetheless, he then used a retrospective quantitative design to check for any statistically significant difference in discharge rates over the previous five years across both units. He took into account demographics and other patient and staff variables. For patients, these included gender, age, diagnosis and consultant, and for nurses this included gender, age, qualifications and length and type of clinical experience. He also used observation to check the number and types of visitors (e.g. family, friends, work colleagues) to both units. The results of these activities supported his hunch that this is a novel, and hitherto un-researched and largely unreported, phenomenon.

He then began to consider what concepts were linked to this phenomenon. The obvious ones were 'open visiting', 'age', 'medical condition', 'length of stay' and 'community support packages'. These were the building blocks for a new theory. From Chapter 1 you will remember that theory is developed when relationships are made between two or more concepts. Such relationships are called propositions and these are the links or associations that hold the concepts together. So, for John, a new theory was developing, which (for want of a better term) he called the *Open Visiting Length of Stay Theory*. It proposes that medical patients, regardless of age, gender or diagnosis, have significantly shorter lengths of stay on medical wards where open visiting is practised (see Reflective Exercises 8.1 and 8.2).

Reflective Exercise 8.1

Phenomena to Concepts to Propositions to Theory?

Having done the Reflexive Exercises in Chapter 1, you should now know how phenomena identified in a nurse's clinical work can be given attention and labelled as concepts, which can then be linked together to form theoretical propositions that can be tested through research.

Think of an event that you have noticed in your practice or in the clinical setting. Consider this phenomenon and, in a one-page account, take it through the same research process as that undertaken by John Smith.

In this example, the *Open Visiting Length of Stay Theory* emerged from clinical practice. We will expand later on how a phenomenon emerges and how it can be given a name to make it a concept, and how different concepts form propositions which, in turn, become a theory (see Key Concepts 8.1). John Smith and his master's supervisor decided to publish his research in a nursing journal. As a result of the publication, a nurse researcher in Canada tested the theory to see if it could be verified or refuted when applied to patients in medical wards in a large hospital in Toronto. Such testing is welcome and is crucial for the development of new knowledge and evidence-based practice. As more researchers across the globe confirm John's findings, open visiting practice and policy is introduced widely. Therefore, a change in visiting policy internationally started with one person giving a new phenomenon their attention.

However, it may be possible that researchers in various countries failed to replicate John's research. Their findings refuted his and they could not find a positive link between open visiting and early discharge. This too is important and adds to the body of existing knowledge. This refutation brings us back to Chapters 2 and 7 where we described Karl Popper and his paper boat!

Reflective Exercise 8.2

Extraneous Variables?

The example of the *Open Visiting Length of Stay Theory* is hypothetical.

Take a few moments to write down what else could have been making the difference in discharge rates between both units – remember, patients were assigned by the same medical staff to one or other unit, so there was no selection bias. Patients were controlled for age, gender and diagnosis. What else, from a nursing point of view, could have been different in one unit but not the other that could have caused the difference?

Key Concepts 8.1

When a phenomenon is named, it becomes a concept, when you link one or more concepts with others you get a proposition. This is the beginning of theory. So, research can be defined as a process of investigation where different methods can be used to study phenomena of interest. Linked to this, a theory can be described as a system of connected propositions that enable phenomena to be described, explained or predicted.

Popper's Boat

From Chapters 2 and 7, readers will recall that Popper (1989) was an Austrian philosopher who studied the development of knowledge and science. In his early days he was a hard-nosed quantitative positivist (see Chapter 2). In his later years, he mellowed and realized that things that could not be quantified or measured also contributed to knowledge. Here, he shifted his emphasis from trying to prove something to trying to refute (falsify) something. His analogy of the paper boat is worth re-emphasing here. Most children know how to make a paper boat and have probably done so at one time or another. Unfortunately, paper boats, like real boats, sink.

A child may make a paper boat to see if it floats in a pond, river or creek. The first time they push it out into the pond, it floats and so the boat has been well constructed and performs well. Maybe they then try putting small sticks or stones on the boat to see if it still floats and even try to make the water choppier. If the boat remains floating after all these challenging tests, it has done everything that was required of it. However, it is also possible that after two or three tests, the paper boat sinks. So, the boat has not done what it was supposed to do – in Popper's view, the theory has been refuted. However, all is not lost, and a great deal has been learned from its sinking (refutation), which could lead to the construction of a better and stronger boat (theory).

The same principle applies to the testing of John Smith's *Open Visiting Length of Stay Theory* theory. Nurse researchers in other countries try to replicate his study and see if it can be supported. Alternatively, they could test it to see if it can be refuted. If the former, the team of researchers would then publish the results showing that their research upheld Smith's theory (see Key Concepts 8.2). They would also make recommendations to strengthen the theory, such as doing a cost–benefit analysis to show how many more patients are treated on the ward with the shorter length of stay, and these could be taken up by other researchers in other parts of the world. Over time, the theory would become strengthened and established until, like Popper's boat, another study refuted it. However, as alluded to above, if it is never refuted, the theory would find its way into nursing textbooks and hospital management guidelines. In time it would become part of established practice. It may even, after a longer period of time, become the *Open Visiting Length of Stay Law*.

Key Concepts 8.2

Hypotheses: some propositions within existing theories are called hypotheses – these can be tested through research.

In summary, the *Open Visiting Length of Stay Theory* emerged from researching practice, was tested by others and returned to inform practice. This reciprocal relationship between theory, research and practice is how science can be developed in nursing and how theory can lead to improvements in patient care.

From the foregoing hypothetical example of the *Open Visiting Length of Stay Theory*, you can see that research does two main things. It generates theory inductively or it tests it deductively. John Smith, a very busy clinical nurse manager could easily have ignored the phenomenon that he observed and failed to see the propositional relationship between the concepts – 'open visiting', 'age', 'medical wards' and 'length of stay'. One wonders how many clinical phenomena are ignored by busy clinical nurses and how this slows down the development of nursing knowledge.

The best way to think of this is as a circular system; new theory generated from practice will stimulate the conduct of new research studies, which will lead to new knowledge for practice. In turn, new knowledge presents us with new facts, which encourage us to develop theories to explain these facts.

Meleis (2017) stated that researchers often view theorists as 'ivory tower' academics who dream up ideas unconnected with practice or research. Similarly, theorists view researchers as investigators who focus on small research projects to confirm, or not, disconnected propositions that do not add up to theory. Such research has limited usefulness. The end product of research is limited if it does not provide theory to help describe or explain phenomena or help practising nurses to predict outcomes and prescribe interventions.

You will recall from Chapter 3 that in 1968 the American philosophers James Dickoff and Patricia James made a major contribution to the generation and testing of nursing theory. While they were not nurses themselves, they worked closely with Ernestina Wiedenbach, who was a well-known early nurse theorist (Wiedenbach 1964). In 1968, Dickoff and James published a seminal paper in the American journal *Nursing Research*. It was entitled 'A theory of theories: a position paper'. They stated that research is for the sake of theory and theory is for the sake of practice and that theory produced without research has little hope of viability. Obviously, they were not fans of the Rationalist approach to knowledge development (see Chapter 2). Research, they argued, was pointless unless done (a) in the context of theory and (b) with a clear realisation of what it can contribute to theory. In other words, they believed that research was inextricably linked to theory – it either generates or tests theory.

What is the Link Between Theory and Research?

On the Current Nursing (2024) website, the link between research and theory is made clear. It is asserted that research without theory results in discreet information or data which do not add to the accumulated knowledge of the discipline. In recent years, nurses have become fascinated by evidence-based practice. This is where practice is informed by the best available research findings. It has led most nurses to view with suspicion any guideline, policy or intervention that is based on mere guesswork or hunch. The nursing care of patients is too important to be underpinned by speculation or untested rituals or routines.

Nursing has been criticised over the years for the large number of grand theories (nursing models) that have been generated by so called armchair theorists. These were nurse theorists who developed their models and theories through reasoning rather than rigorous and systematic investigation. Not only were these not generated through research, but most were not tested through research (see Reflective Exercise 8.3) You will remember from Chapter 5 that the concepts and propositions within grand theories are so broad in scope that it is not possible to test many of them. It is a fact that if nurses are taught theories that have no basis in research, then the nursing care based on these theories is unlikely to have the desired impact on patients. Those who support and push such theories must be aware of the ethical implications of doing so. Their implementation in practice with no research basis may do as much harm as the habitual carrying out of unproven routine tasks.

Hickman (2019) commented on the link between nursing theory and nursing research. He complained that grand nursing theories have stagnated, and that nursing research is in urgent need of the renovation of existing nursing theories and the development of new ones. He argued that the future of nursing research is dependent upon the development of mid-range and situation-specific theory (i.e. practice theory). In particular, he calls for sound theories that reflect phenomena that are relevant to nursing practice.

It was perhaps this lack of a sound research base that turned many clinical nurses off nursing theories. It may also be the reason why many contemporary educational programmes do not have much nursing theory content today or why curricula are not commonly supported by a nursing theory.

Reflective Exercise 8.3

Propositions from Grand Theory

By now you will know that all theories are made up of concepts and statements (propositions) linking them together in some way. Grand theories, such as those of Orem (1995), Roper et al. (2000) and Roy (2019), are also composed of these elements.

For this exercise, select one theory with which you are familiar or one from a textbook. Identify one or two propositions in that theory and write a short report on how you would go about testing whether the propositional relationship was valid.

Research in Nursing

For many years, research approaches in nursing have been divided into two main camps. There are hypothesis-testing studies where, through deductive testing, the object is to create explanatory and situation-specific theories (i.e. practice theories) from the top down. These are what Dickoff and James (1968) referred to as 'situation-relating' and 'situation-producing' theories. In the past, such research came from the philosophies of positivism or empiricism (see Chapter 2). By contrast, qualitative research approaches use induction where the emphasis is on creating descriptive and exploratory theories from the bottom up. As you should now be aware (see Chapter 2), these come from the philosophy of historicism.

Quantitative and qualitative research may be differentiated by where the theory lies in the research process. In qualitative research, the theory is the product and emerges (not always fully formed) at the end of the study. Sometimes this is referred to as the 'research-then-theory' approach. Conversely, in quantitative research, the theory is present at the beginning of the study and the researcher formulates testable hypotheses from its propositions, and tests these to see if the theory's propositions can be refuted or verified. This is sometimes referred to as the 'theory-then-research' approach.

In 'theory-generating research', the researcher identifies a phenomenon, discovers its conceptual characteristics and formulates testable propositions. In 'theory-testing research', the investigator seeks to develop evidence through researching hypotheses derived from the propositions of an existing theory.

A purist's view would be that research has to be linked in some way to theory, otherwise it is weak. The proponents of this perspective would assert that researchers either generate theory or test theory, the former mainly using qualitative methodologies and the later quantitative methodologies.

🔍 Key Concepts 8.3

Research–Theory Relationship

Research only does two things – it either generates or tests theory.

By contrast, Peggy Chinn and Maeona Kramer, two meta-theorists, who have been writing about nursing theories for decades, do identify research that has nothing to do with theory. In the latest edition of their textbook (Chinn et al. 2022), they argued that there are two main types of research: theory-linked research and theory-isolated research. They conceded that both can be of excellent quality and can contribute to new knowledge, but because the former is conducted within the framework of theory, it has greater potential for developing new understanding. Theory-linked research is related to the generation or the testing of theory while, by definition, theory-isolated research has no discernible theoretical connection. While it is possible to argue for or against Chinn et al.'s (2022) stance, we would assert that most useful research has strong links with theory (see Key Concepts 8.4).

While we assert that research either generates or tests theory, in our experience, we see four linkages between research and theory (McKenna et al. 2014):

- research generates theory inductively from practice – *theory-generating research* (TGR);
- research tests theory deductively in practice – *theory-testing research* (TTR);
- theory guides a research project – *theory-framed research* (TFR);
- research evaluates the use of theory in practice – *theory-evaluating research* (TER).

🔍 Key Concepts 8.4

There are four main linkages between research and theory. Research can generate, test or evaluate theory and theory can guide or provide a framework for a research study.

Theory-Generating Research (TGR)

Elsewhere in this book we have illustrated the difference between grand theory, mid-range theory and situation-specific theory (see Chapter 3). Grand theories are very broad and, in most cases, have not been generated through research. Many have been developed through reasoning based upon the experience of the theorist concerned or based upon non-nursing theories in other disciplines. This included the work of Peplau (1992), Orem (1995) and Henderson (1966). However, theory development based on experience or reasoning is not new. From previous chapters you will recall that Freud (1949) created his psychoanalytic theories without ever carrying out any empirical research. Most of his theory was developed from his experience seeing patients, and sometimes individual patients. It is also well known that the research methods and technology required to test Einstein's (1905) theory of relativity ($E = MC^2$) were not available until many years after it was developed!

In contrast to grand theories, mid-range and situation-specific theories have their origin in research. Therefore, the most useful outcome of nursing research is the number of meaningful theories that impact positively on the health and well-being of patients, their families and communities. TGR contributes significantly to the growth of such theories.

When little is known about existing clinical phenomena or new phenomena, TGR is conducted for the purpose of their discovery and exploration (remember nurse John Smith earlier in the chapter). The resultant theories are normally generated inductively by researchers who realise that within nursing practice there lies a large number of phenomena awaiting their attention, observation and description. Because the research eventually leads to inductively formulated theory, you will recall that TGR may be referred to as the 'research-then-theory' approach to knowledge development – simply because the research precedes the theory.

Dickoff and James (1992) claimed that since nursing practice predates nursing research, it creates a sound foundation for theorising. Furthermore, if nurse researchers are to be expert in TGR they must work in partnership with clinical staff who can provide them with researchable phenomena of specific interest to patient care.

Chinn et al. (2022) pointed out that, when attempting to generate theory, the researcher enters the research setting with as open a mind as possible in order to see new conceptual relationships within phenomena. This 'blank sheet' approach to knowledge creation is similar to what the empiricist John Locke referred to as the the blank slate or *tabula rasa* (Stokes 2015). However, we would question if this is really possible. No matter how much we try to clear our mind, we all enter a situation with our own conceptual baggage, so creating a *tabula rasa* (see Chapter 2) is not always an easy process. It is also possible that what a researcher sees as an 'extraordinary' researchable phenomenon could be perceived by experienced clinical nurses as 'ordinary'. Therefore, researchers and the clinical staff with whom they work should be acutely aware of the possibilities that phenomena may have for theory generation, but they should also be aware of their biases.

Research Approaches to Theory Generation

Theory generation research mainly employs qualitative methods where the theory is produced inductively from studying the phenomenon of interest. One of the most well-known research approaches to theory generation is Glaser and Strauss's (1999) work on *grounded theory*. The name itself suggests that theory can be built from the ground up. The approach involves the simultaneous collection of data, coding, categorising observations and forming concepts and relationships based on the data. Put simply, in grounded theory, researchers generate theory from analysing the data they collect.

Ethnography is another research approach to generating theory. Readers will be familiar with nature or documentary programmes on television where individuals travel to remote places to live with local tribes or communities. They question, observe and document cultural phenomena such as the hunting for and preparation of food and rites such as marriage and coming of age rituals. Here, the intent is to provide a detailed, in-depth description of such everyday life and practices (see Reflective Exercise 8.4).

Inevitably, the researcher seeks to get involved in the setting, experience the phenomenon firsthand and soak up the concepts that are important in describing and explaining a specific phenomenon. Only then do they feel that they really know the phenomenon and attempt to generate theory.

An example of ethnography would be where a nurse researcher goes to live in a migrant community, where people are leaving war and prosecution and seeking a new life in another country. The nurse would observe in a systematic and rigorous way how migrants live and what drives them to take their families on hazardous cross-border journeys. Phenomena are identified, concepts formed and relationships between concepts explored. In this way a new theory can be generated relating to the nursing needs of migrant communities.

Another approach to the generation of theory is *phenomenology* (see Chapter 2). This is also a qualitative research method used to identify phenomena through how they are perceived by the 'actors' in a situation. This normally takes the form of gathering 'deep' information and perceptions through interviews, discussions and participant observation, and representing it from the point of view of the research participant(s). Therefore, phenomenology is designed to describe the subjective 'lived experiences' of people and to comprehend the essence and meanings that they place on these experiences.

The word phenomenology means gaining an understanding of phenomena from the perspective of those who experience them. An example of phenomenology is where a nurse wants to gain insight into what it is like to receive a diagnosis of long Covid. What the researcher is seeking here is the 'lived experience' of the individuals and what that experience means to them. Therefore, the individuals would be interviewed to get their stories. The interviews will uncover new concepts and relationships between concepts and this forms the basis for a new theory.

Reflective Exercise 8.4

Types of Qualitative Research

In Chapter 2 you were introduced to historicism. This is the basis for qualitative research, and qualitative research methods are normally used in theory-generating research. Get a research methods textbook and look up qualitative research. Over the years different research approaches have been developed in qualitative research. Identify the main ones and write a paragraph on how you could use each to generate a theory.

Regardless of whether a researcher uses phenomenology, grounded theory or ethnography, the research findings are usually presented in the form of concepts and propositions that form the beginnings of a new theory. While the result of TGR is often mid-range theory, the following grand theories were developed using interpretative qualitative approaches: Paterson and Zderad (1976), Parse (1981) and Watson (1985).

The Research Process in TGR

In TGR, the clinical problem, the research questions and the research purpose need to be stated in advance (see Key Concepts 8.5). According to Chinn et al. (2022), research hypotheses may also be used. However, more commonly, research questions or problem statements are enough to guide the study.

In TGR the data are collected by direct (physical observation) or indirect (interviews/focus groups) approaches. Because of their existing theoretical bias, research instruments such as structured questionnaires or scales may not be very useful in TGR. Such structured research instruments are often based upon an existing conceptual understanding of the phenomena. In qualitative research the sample is carefully selected, and its size will be determined by data saturation or other robust means. Saturation means that no new information is being uncovered by subsequent interviews.

🔍 Key Concepts 8.5

Theory-generating research: this has been termed the research-then-theory approach to knowledge creation.

The TGR researcher approaches the study with the following mindset: there is some phenomenon or event happening in the world that will be become clear if I research it or this particular group of people. The results of TGR are often referred to as *posteriori* knowledge. This means it depends on evidence gathered from experiences, observations and questioning.

Strange as it may seem, a 'time series' with a comparison group could also be used for the qualitative generation of theory. For example, if researchers were studying the experiences of older people who have been hospitalized with COVID-19, they might take a longitudinal approach with qualitative data collected before, during and after their admission to hospital. At the same time. they might identify other groups of people with COVID-19 who were being treated in the community. The comparison would tell the researchers whether aspects of the phenomenon were unique to one care setting or another. These data could contribute to the development of theory related to the experiences of hospitalisation for this group of individuals.

TABLE 8.1   Types of propositional statements developed through theory-generating research.

Proposition	Relationship between concepts
Descriptive	There is a relationship between *x* and *y*
Directional	There is a positive relationship between *x* and *y*
Concurrent	If *x* occurs then *y* will also occur
Sequential	If *x* occurs then *y* will occur later
Deterministic	If *x* occurs then *y* will always occur, if there are no interfering conditions
Probabilistic (stochastic)	If *x* occurs then *y* will probably occur
Necessary	If *x* occurs, and only if *x*, then *y* will occur
Substitutional	If *x1* occurs but also *x2* then *y* will occur
Sufficient	If *x* then *y*, regardless of anything else
Contingent	If *x* then *y*, but only in the presence of *c*

In TGR the analysis of data involves identifying themes and categories that emerge from the data collected. The researcher identifies recurring concepts from these themes and categories and, how these concepts are related to one another. It is a good idea to try and define these concepts. For example, what is meant by 'older people with COVID-19'? As relationships between the concepts are identified, this will provide propositions, which form the structure of the theory.

It is possible that this theory could have immediate clinical impact because of its grounding in the experience or setting from which it was generated. Table 8.1 provides three different types of propositions that may arise from the concepts uncovered in TGR.

The next step in TGR is diagramming or putting the concepts and propositions into diagrammatic form. Diagramming is done after the concepts, definitions and propositions have been identified. Within the diagram, the existence of a rela-

tionship is denoted by an unbroken line. For connecting concepts, an arrowhead at one end indicates an asymmetrical relationship and an arrowhead at both ends indicates a symmetrical relationship. A positive relationship is denoted by a plus (+) sign and a negative relationship is denoted by a minus (−) sign (see Figure 8.1). A question mark may be used if the direction is unclear. A positive propositional relationship arising from the data could be 'As people get older the chance of getting COVID-19 increases'.

In a robust TGR report, there is a comprehensive literature review on the phenomenon being studied, the method employed is clearly described and the resultant concepts and propositional statements are stated accurately. Where possible, the researcher should also make clear what type of propositional statements have been generated and diagram the relationship in terms of existence, direction and symmetry. Some of the propositions discussed may also be stated as researchable hypotheses. In this way TGR is opening up an opportunity for future TTR to take place.

In TGR, the findings may:

- lead to the formulation of a new theory;
- lead to supporting an existing theory;
- lead to a rejection of an existing theory;
- lead to an existing theory being adapted or revised.

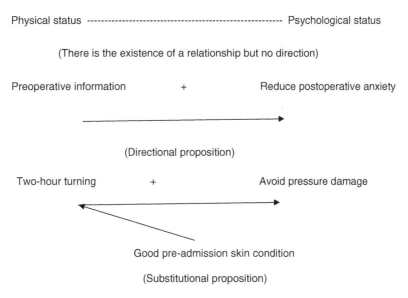

FIGURE 8.1 Examples of propositional diagramming.

Theory-Testing Research (TTR)

In contrast to the *a posteriori* knowledge created in TGR, TTR produces *a priori* knowledge. This means that it is independent of any experience. Here, hypotheses are derived from an existing theory and then verified or refuted through research. TTR can be referred to as the theory-then-research process – simply because the theory precedes the research that tests it (see Key Concepts 8.6).

It is a common view that in TTR a theory exists and research is undertaken to establish its validity. However, this is factually incorrect. A theory may have many propositions and some of these can be in the form of testable hypotheses. The researcher simply tests these hypotheses; but they may not test all the propositions. Therefore, it would probably be more correct to call this section proposition-testing research, but for the purposes of this chapter we will refer to this process as theory testing.

The research methods in theory-testing studies are designed to ascertain how accurately the theory depicts real-world phenomena and their relationships. For a theory to be testable you need:

- concepts that describe the phenomena of interest;
- theoretical and operational definitions of these concepts;
- propositional links between the concepts that describe, explain or predict phenomena.

Key Concepts 8.6

Theory-testing research: this has been termed the theory-then-research approach to knowledge creation.

Theory testing normally involves a quantitative deductive approach where propositions in the form of hypotheses are tested using randomised controlled trials, experimental or quasi-experimental approaches. Research questions can also be used to test a theory; this usually takes place within a correlational design. The concepts within the research questions or hypotheses are derived from the theory that is to be tested. Figure 8.2 shows one such theory-testing process. Please note that for ease of explanation the process illustrated is linear – but this may not necessarily be the case – it may be iterative. This figure shows how TGR is related to TTR. TGR uses induction to generate a theory and TTR uses

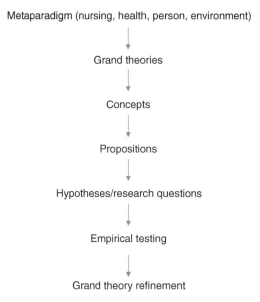

Metaparadigm (nursing, health, person, environment)

Grand theories

Concepts

Propositions

Hypotheses/research questions

Empirical testing

Grand theory refinement

FIGURE 8.2   A typical theory-testing process.

deduction to test the same theory. A study incorporating this would be using a mixed method – qualitative followed by quantitative.

Meleis (2017) reminded us that grand theories are the highest in abstraction and do not lend themselves to empirical testing. In contrast, mid-range theories lend themselves to empirical testing because the concepts are more specific and defined and can be readily operationalized.

The Research Process

In TTR, the research purpose, the research problem and the hypotheses/or research questions are formulated in advance of conducting the study. Previous research that studied the theory or its propositions forms a substantial part of the literature review. The review also includes a critique of alternative theories shown to be relevant to the study's central purpose. Furthermore, the literature review should indicate how the study was conceived and why the specific propositional relationships within the theory are being tested, and not others. There should also be a critical review of existing research that relates to the phenomena.

In TTR the data are collected by direct (physical observation) or indirect means (interviews and self-completion tools such as questionnaires and scales). Psychometric properties of the data collection tools, such as reliability and validity, should be described. The sample and population must be carefully considered, and statistical power analysis is invariably used in deciding sample size. In TTR, the analysis focuses on whether the data provide sufficient evidence to support or reject the hypotheses or answer the research questions. Conclusions are then made regarding the validity of the theory.

The reasons why a theory is verified or refuted may not always be obvious, but knowledge and understanding will have been increased and possible false leads eradicated. Strange as it may seem, TTR can lead to theory generation. Because of the insight gained through the research, the basis for a new theory may be formed.

As with Popper's (1989) paper boat analogy, the theory is a description or explanation of the phenomenon unless it is refuted or until a better one comes along. However, because of ethical considerations, some theories are not testable. For instance, while theories may be formulated on sleep deprivation in children or on the starvation of pregnant women, it would be unethical to test them in practice.

To conclude this section, there has been a great deal written about the necessity to test theories of relevance to nursing to provide evidence of the validity and accuracy of their concepts and propositions. Some progress has been made towards this goal by the theorists themselves, researchers or those nurses who use them in practice. This has to be welcome, as not to test theory would have consequences for the quality of care and evidence-based practice. The negative implications of nurses using a theory of dubious validity to underpin the care of patients are obvious. In TTR, the findings may:

- confirm the validity of the theory;
- refute the validity of the theory;
- lead to the theory being adapted or revised;
- lead to the formulation of a new theory.

Theory-Framed Research (TFR)

In TFR, researchers may not necessarily be generating theory or testing theoretical propositions. Rather, the theory is used to guide a research study and provide it with a focus. So important is the theoretical framework to a study that researchers could more easily dispense with the physical operations of a study than the framework which gives meaning to the research's objectives. The same methods could be used in a different study and give different outcomes if the theoretical framework was changed.

Littzen-Brown (2021) pointed out that theory-guided research is the application or use of a theory, whether developed, applied, borrowed or adapted, to support a research project. She maintained that it should not be about simply 'fitting' a theory to your research. Rather, it should be using theory in a way that helps you see, describe, explore, explain or test the phenomena in which you are interested. She concluded that using theory to guide research is important because it connects and builds upon previously developed nursing knowledge. Theory guides the research process, forms the research questions and aids in design, analysis and interpretation. So, using a theory to frame a research project enables the researcher to prepare the research questions, informs the design, analysis and interpretation and helps to weave these parts together. However, nurses were slow to see the connection and between 1928 and 1959 only 2 out of 152 studies reported a theoretical basis for the research design (Current Nursing 2024).

When used as a framework to structure a study, a theory can:

- give direction to the research project;
- give structure to a thesis, publication or report;
- summarise and order research findings;
- relate the study to previous research and theory.

More specifically, a theoretical framework for a project provides parameters for the study, guides data collection and provides a perspective for interpreting the data so that the researcher can weave together the findings in a meaningful pattern (see Key Concepts 8.7). In other words, when a study is placed within such a theoretical context, the theory guides the research process from the research questions through design, analysis and interpretation to the conclusions. It is like a 'red thread' weaved through the study from the beginning to the end. This means that researchers should identify the theoretical framework at the beginning of the study, however tentative it may seem.

Lor et al. (2017) stated that theory offers a set of concepts and propositions that can be applied consistently and examined systematically across studies of clinical problems. They believed that when researchers communicate clearly about how they have applied a theory in their studies, others can synthesize evidence more readily across studies where the same theory was used. By doing so, researchers can build scientific knowledge more efficiently than if they were not theory-guided. However, they admit that research reports often do not provide adequate information about whether, and how, researchers applied theory when conducting their studies. They suggested that such an absence impedes development of knowledge to guide nursing practice. Furthermore, they assert that if nurses improve their understanding of theory-framed research, they could better assess, select and apply theory-guided interventions in their practices.

Key Concepts 8.7

Theory can provide a guiding framework to a research study that helps to bring coherence, structure and credibility to the investigation.

For example, if you were investigating how nursing students' examination results are affected by the introduction of an e-learning course, you could use John Dewey's Social Learning Theory to frame your study. Dewey's theory (1904) is based on the premise that human beings learn through a 'hands-on' approach. Similarly, if the research topic is how families cope when their loved one has a stroke, you could use Roy's adaptation theory (Roy 2019). Another example would be using Orem's (1995) self-care theory when investigating the discharge of patients from hospital to home (Hartweg & Metcalfe 2022).

However, the selected theory must be relevant and used in a meaningful way. Too often we have seen nurses introduce a theoretical framework at the beginning of a study simply to lend the research report some theoretical credibility, after which the theory is not referred to again; it was, in reality, merely 'theoretical window dressing'. A potentially more serious problem relates to the inappropriate selection of a theory to frame the study. Such a choice may lead to premature commitment to a particular theory with the result that the researcher's theoretical and research vision is restricted. For instance, an elderly care support theory developed in sub-Saharan Africa by a social anthropologist may not be appropriate when applied to research into the effects of engagement with older people in inner-city Paris. Similarly, a theory that focuses on self-care may disregard patients who do not want to be self-caring or who cannot be independent.

It might also be the case that a theoretical framework used to structure a research study could take on an agenda-setting role, bringing with it inherent biases. In other words, do not select a theory because you think it will provide you with the answers you want. Like all good investigators, nurse researchers should ask 'why' when they start a study, and the answer should contain a relevance to nursing. Controversially, Fawcett (2012) argued that in research that pertains to nursing practice, the theory framing the study should be a nursing one. This seems like premature theoretical closure. Also, because of the relatively short history of nursing theories, this might result in a focus that is too narrow. A better suggestion would be that nurse researchers identify the best possible theory they can to frame the study, and are able to justify their choice.

As mentioned earlier, a theoretical framework links the various parts of a study together in a coherent fashion. If applied correctly, such a theory will mean that the literature review, methodology, findings and conclusions come together in an aesthetically pleasing way. For instance, if a study was focusing on the development of advanced practitioners in nursing, the researcher could use role theory (Anglin et al. 2022) to frame the research (see Chapter 4). In such a TFR study, one would expect to see reference in the literature review to role conflict, role overlap, role norms, role set, role stress and role confusion. The questions asked in the questionnaire or interview schedule would also reflect these concepts. The findings and discussion sections could also be structured using subheadings from role theory. Remember in this research study, role theory is not being generate or tested; rather it is being used almost as a theoretical skeleton to hang the research upon (Anglin et al. 2022).

Afaf Meleis's Transitions Theory deals with the various transitions that people make in their lives. It informs us how people can be helped and supported during the transition from one role to another and how they can better understand what is happening during a transition (Zhan et al. 2022). A nurse researcher who wants to understand the transition for a man who has had an amputation and how this will change how he lives and works could use Meleis's Transitions Theory as a theoretical framework to guide the research study.

In TFR, the findings may:

- establish the worth of the theory as a template for the study;
- ensure that the study is focused;
- lead to a rejection of an existing theory as a guide for a research study;
- lead to an existing theory being adapted or revised as a guide for a research study.

Theory-Evaluating Research (TER)

While there is the potential for confusion between TER and TTR, there are significant differences. We have already stated that some grand theories, because of their broad scope, cannot easily be tested and the best we can do is to evaluate their application in practice to see if they have any noticeable effect on patient care. Therefore, while it may not be possible to research the underlying assumptions and propositions of some of the grand nursing theories, it is possible to analyse certain aspects of nursing care that are affected by their introduction. Their impact could also be evaluated in nurse management or nurse education situations.

Why would a nurse researcher wish to evaluate the effects of using a theory in clinical practice. You will recall that nursing theories can bring a great deal of benefit to patient care. Current Nursing (2024) maintained that they can assist nurses to describe, explain and predict everyday experiences, serve as a guide for the assessment, intervention and evaluation of nursing care and identify criteria that could be used to assess the quality of nursing care. Furthermore, theories can provide a common nursing terminology to use in communicating with other clinical nurses. It is not surprising that it is important to select the correct theory to suit a clinical situation (see Chapter 7). However, once a theory is selected, it is crucial to evaluate its impact on clinical decision-making and clinical interventions.

You will recall from Chapter 7 that at one time many senior nurse managers and educators were dictating what grand theories nurses should use in their practice. This order came 'from on high' and meant that theories such as those of Orem (1995), Henderson (1966) and Roy (1970) were being shoehorned into practice without taking account of their suitability and without a sound knowledge of the theories by clinical nurses. In most cases, the theory was used to structure the admission paperwork for the assessment of patients, and it had no further application thereafter. In some less common instances, it was used to assess, plan, guide and evaluate nursing actions.

Many of the theories that busy clinical nurses had to use were not evaluated to see if they had a positive, negative or neutral effect on patient care. In other words, no TER was undertaken. Unlike TTR, TER does not attempt to test the propositional hypotheses; rather, it focuses on what impact the theory can have when applied in clinical practice (see Key Concepts 8.8). We will discuss the evaluation of theories in greater detail in Chapter 9. In the meantime, a short overview here will suffice.

Even though nursing theories were introduced into curricula across the US and the UK many decades ago, the amount of empirical research regarding their impact on nurse learning is conspicuous by its scarcity.

Key Concepts 8.8

Theories for their own sake are unimportant. What is crucial in a practice discipline like nursing is that they have a positive effect on nurses' thinking and actions and that this improves patient care.

After undertaking a comprehensive trawl of the literature, McKenna (1994) identified three major assumptions. You will recall that assumptions are held to be true until tested:

1. Nursing theories lead to better quality of care.
2. Nursing theories have an uncertain effect on quality of care.
3. Nursing theories lower the quality of care.

He undertook an action research approach to implement a nursing theory in a long-stay psychiatric setting. The theory concerned was the human needs theory, previously selected by a population of ward managers ($n = 95$). Within a broader quasi-experimental design, quality-of-care indicators were appraised before and after the implementation of the theory. These dependent variables were also monitored on a control ward and data were collected on both wards at one pre-test and two post-test points. Planned change theory (Lewin 1946) was used as a guiding framework for the implementation of the theory (TFR).

Results showed that on the experimental ward there were statistically significant improvements in care quality, patient and nurses' perception of ward atmosphere, client satisfaction, nurses' views about nursing theories and client dependency levels. No significant changes were noted in practitioner satisfaction levels or practitioners' perception of patients' behaviour. These findings suggested that when implemented through an action research approach, where practitioners were involved as partners in the change process, a nursing theory has positive influences on quality of care (see Reflective Exercise 8.5).

But will such findings be adopted by others and create positive differences to future practice? It is reasonable to suggest that nurses are no different from anyone else and research evidence is not a good enough reason in many instances for changing established behaviour.

In TER, the findings may:

- contribute to establishing the worth of the theory in practice or education;
- contribute to the generation of ideas for new theory;
- lead to a rejection of an existing theory as a guide for practice or curricula;
- lead to an existing theory being adapted or revised within practice or education.

Reflective Exercise 8.5

Theory Evaluation

The evaluation of theory focuses on the impact or effect of that theory on nursing processes and outcomes of practice.

Think specifically about your clinical setting and what processes and outcomes you would expect to see improve after the introduction of a nursing theory. Examples could include improved patient satisfaction, earlier discharge or improved staff satisfaction.

Outline research approaches that you could use to assess whether the changes in processes and outcomes had really happened (e.g. a patient satisfaction questionnaire).

The Relationship Between Theory and Research

In Chapter 3, it was noted that the philosophers Dickoff and James (1968) had identified four levels of theory. Table 8.2 shows how, a decade later, Diers (1979) linked these to research approaches.

Building on this hierarchy of theories, it is possible to identify three main types of theory and their related research methods. Although these were mentioned in Chapter 3, the following descriptions are more in-depth and research-oriented:

- *Descriptive theory.* There are two types of descriptive theories: naming theories and taxonomies (classification theories). Descriptive theories are generated and tested by descriptive research – generally called descriptive/exploratory research. The sorts of research questions asked within descriptive studies are: What is this? Or, What are the characteristics of . . .? Descriptive studies involve the observation of phenomena in their natural setting. Data collection can

TABLE 8.2   **The relationship between levels of theory and levels of research.**

Dickoff and James (1968)	Diers (1979)
Factor-isolating theory – describes and names concepts	Factor-naming or factor-searching research – describes, names a phenomenon, situation or event in order to gain new insights (also called descriptive or exploratory research), e.g. patient dependency.
Factor-relating theory – relates named concepts to one another	Factor-relating or relation or searching research – develops links among variables and describe the relationships that are discovered after factor searching research (may be qualitative or grounded theory), e.g. the relationship between age and patient dependency.
Situation-relating theory – forms interrelationships among concepts or propositions	Explanatory/correlational research – aims to determine factors that occur or vary together (no attempt is made to experiment), e.g. as age increases, dependency also increases.
Situation-producing theory – prescribes actions to reach certain outcomes	Causal-hypothesis testing – research addresses causal relationships between variables in an attempt to predict events, e.g. encouraging healthy aging will reduce dependency.

be qualitative (e.g. case studies, ethnography, phenomenology, grounded theory) or quantitative (surveys of attitudes, attributes, knowledge, opinions).

- *Explanatory theory*. This type of theory focuses on relationships between the dimensions or characteristics of individuals, groups, situations or events. They explain how the parts of the phenomena under study relate to each other. These theories can only be formulated once phenomena have been identified through the previous development of descriptive theories. Explanatory theories are developed through explanatory (qualitative) or correlational (quantitative) studies. An example of a research question would be: to what extent is age related to dependency?

   Data for explanatory theories can be collected through surveys (observations, interviews, questionnaires) yielding quantitative or qualitative data. Closed-ended instruments may also be employed because the parts of the phenomena are believed to be already known (as a result of the existence of descriptive theories). To prove a correlation, qualitative data may be transformed into quantitative data and statistical tests applied, such as Pearson's product–moment coefficient (parametric) or Spearman's rho (non-parametric). Other more sophisticated tests, such as multiple regression and path analysis, may also be used.

- *Predictive theory*. This type of theory goes beyond whether one thing is related to another and seeks to identify cause-and-effect relationships. Predictive theories may build on explanatory theories and are generated and tested by experimental research. Questions addressed include: What will the effect be post operatively if you give specific information to patients before surgery? Or, Will hospitalised children recover better if their parents are closely involved in their care? Quantitative data are required so as to check for statistical significance. Tests include Mann–Whitney *U*-test (non-parametric) and *t*-test, ANOVA and MANOVA (parametric) (see Key Concepts 8.9).

To recap, if little is known about the phenomena, descriptive (descriptive theory) research is required, but if the phenomena have been adequately described, correlational (explanatory theory) research may be carried out. If phenomena have been adequately described and relationships are well known, then experimental (predictive theory) research may be carried out. Table 8.3 shows the relationship between these types of theories and the research approaches.

Key Concepts 8.9

The best type of theory for a practice profession is predictive theory. From elsewhere in this book, you will recall that it can help nurses to prescribe care. For instance, in the above-mentioned example, if research showed that exercise by older people reduces patient dependency, then nurses can prescribe these interventions. While such predictive theory is the best for clinical nurses, we will continue to have theories at all three levels.

Quantitative and qualitative methods are mutually supportive and can provide the researcher with binocular vision of the phenomena under investigation, which neither can provide when used in isolation. This is probably the reason why many nurse researchers are using mixed methods in their studies.

TABLE 8.3   Relationships between types of theory and research methods.

Theory	Research
Descriptive	Qualitative descriptive Quantitative descriptive
Explanatory	Qualitative explanatory Quantitative correlational
Predictive	Quantitative experimental

TABLE 8.4   Ways of knowing as related to research approach.

Way of knowing	Mode of enquiry
Empirics	Scientific research
Ethics	Dialogue about justice and fairness
Personal knowing	Reflection on the congruity between the authentic and disclosed selves
Aesthetics	Critique of the act of nursing

Adapted from Carper (1978) and Chinn et al. (2022).

Readers will recall from Chapter 2 that Carper (1978) identified four different ways of knowing in nursing. These were empirics, ethics, aesthetics and personal knowing. Chinn et al. (2022) outlined how these are produced by a specific research approach (Table 8.4).

Strategies for Theory Development Through Research

Meleis (2017) identified five major strategies for theory development:

- theory–practice–theory;
- practice–theory;
- research–theory;
- theory–research–theory;
- practice–theory–research–theory.

You will recognise some of these strategies from what has already been described in this chapter. In particular, you will see how these strategies are linked to theory-generating and theory-testing approaches, with which you are already familiar.

Theory–Practice–Theory Strategy

Here theory from other disciplines is introduced into nursing and becomes shared knowledge. For example, the application from Helson's (1964) physiology of adaptation theory led to the formulation of Roy's (1970) theory. Similarly, Von Bertalanffy's (1951) systems theory, when applied in nursing, led to the development of Neuman's (1995) theory. Therefore, a non-nursing theory exists and knowledge of it has enabled a nurse to apply the theory to nursing and in doing so produce a new nursing theory.

Practice–Theory Strategy

The discerning reader will note the relationship of this strategy to TGR. In this strategy, theory emanates from clinical experience. The process usually starts when the nurse has a nagging hunch about some phenomena they experienced in practice. They develop concepts and identify definitions, boundaries and examples of these concepts. This strategy has similarities to Glaser and Strauss's (1999) grounded theory approach, where the theorist keeps diaries, observes, analyses similarities and differences, develops concepts and then conceptual linkages in the form of propositions.

Nurse theorists such as Orlando (1961), Wiedenbach (1964) and Travelbee (1966) used these methods. They became immersed in the clinical area, either giving care themselves or observing other nurses doing so. They collected data using case studies, interviews and observations and formulated their theories.

Research–Theory Strategy

This strategy is also related to TGR and is an inductive approach using four steps:

1. Select a phenomenon that occurs frequently – list all its characteristics.
2. Measure characteristics in a variety of settings.
3. Analyse resultant data to determine systematic patterns worthy of further attention.
4. Formalise these patterns as theoretical statements (axioms).

Proponents of this strategy believe that truth exists in the world and it can be captured through the senses and verified or refuted. Repeated verification or refutation are indicative of truth and prompts the development of scientific theories.

Theory–Research–Theory Strategy

This strategy shows similarities with the TTR approache. The following four steps are followed:

1. A theory is selected that explains the phenomena of interest.
2. Concepts or propositions of the theory are redefined and operationalised for research.
3. Findings are synthesised and used to modify or refine the original theory.
4. In some instances, the result may be a new theory.

Practice–Theory–Research–Theory Strategy

There are seven stages in this strategy, as follows:

1. taking in;
2. description of the phenomenon;
3. labelling;
4. concept development;
5. proposition development;
6. explicating assumptions;
7. sharing and communicating.

These seven steps may not occur linearly; rather they may occur simultaneously or out of sequence (see Key Concepts 8.10).

Key Concepts 8.10

The practice–theory–research–theory strategy is a very robust approach to generating theory for practice.

Taking In

A clinical situation has attracted a nurse's attention and she develops a hunch about it. She may have observed this event not only through her eyes but also through her other senses and through mental activity (remember John Smith's experience earlier). The result is 'attention grabbing', which may occur concurrently or retrospectively. The 'attention-grabbing' phase is followed by the 'attention-giving' phase, a more deliberate process. She may ask the following questions:

- What has attracted my attention?
- Why does it happen?
- Is it similar to or different from similar things that happen under different sets of circumstances?
- Under what conditions do I observe it, see it, hear it, touch it?
- Can I describe it?
- Can I document it with theory cases and prototype situations?

Description of the Phenomenon

At this second stage the nurse should attempt to answer a further set of questions:

- What is the phenomenon?
- When does it occur?
- What are its boundaries?
- Does it vary? If so, under what circumstances?
- Does it have a function?
- It is related to disease, age, time or place?

   Another way to begin the description of a phenomenon is by asking questions that start with:

- Why do patients . . .?
- How do patients behave when . . ..?
- What is it that happens when . . .?
- What are the properties of . . .?

   To ensure that the phenomena are of specific interest to nurses and nursing, it is a good idea to attempt answers to some further questions:

- In what way is the phenomenon related to nursing's knowledge base?
- In what way would understanding the phenomenon contribute to understanding some aspect of nursing care?
- Can I think of some questions relating to the phenomenon, the answers to which would be significant to nursing?
- How is the phenomenon related to the definition of nursing?

   For instance, a nurse may observe that cancer patients get nausea and vomiting when it is coming near the time for their chemotherapy but before it is provided. This is a beginning observation of a phenomenon. As similar observations occur, the nurse can ask questions of other staff, and read and reflect. The result would be an in-depth description of a phenomenon.

Labelling

In the example in the preceding section, the nurse labels the phenomenon with a word or a short phrase. What she is doing is identifying a concept that best describes the phenomenon. These labels should be concise and precise, they should be used consistently when referring to the phenomenon, contain one cardinal idea and be fundamental to the definition/description of the phenomenon. In this particular case, the nurse may label the observed phenomenon 'Pre Chemo Sickness'.

Concept Development

The techniques shown in Table 8.5 are similar to the steps taken in concept analysis (Cutciffe & McKenna 2008) as an appropriate way of developing concepts from phenomena.

TABLE 8.5   Developing concepts.

Activity	Rationale
Defining	Seek definitions/synonyms of the concept
Differentiating	Ask the question: How does this concept differ from similar concepts? If so how?
Delineating antecedents	Define the context – part of this relates to identifying what precedes the occurrence of the concept
Delineating consequences	Identify what results from, or follows, the occurrence of the concept – positive as well as negative consequences should be identified
Modelling	Identify model cases – contrasting and similar – to help depict what the concept is and what it is not
Analogising	Compare the concept with similar concepts that have been studied more extensively – this may help to shed more light on the new concept
Synthesising	Bring together the findings, meanings and properties that have been amplified by the previous processes

Propositional Development

As you are now aware, propositions are simply statements of relationships between concepts. The identification of propositional statements is a further step in the process of theory development. As outlined in Table 8.1, there are different types of propositions and the more developed the propositions, the better they are able to define, explain and predict the nature of the relationship between concepts.

Explicating Assumptions

The observer reflects on the concepts and propositions and identifies both explicit and implicit assumptions. Assumptions are statements that we accept as true even though they have not been tested. For example, 'humans are biopsychosocial beings' or 'young children need help with self-care'. Reflections on one's own views, values and beliefs will help to delineate assumptions. Assumptions were also dealt with in Chapters 1 and 5.

Sharing and Communication

This step goes beyond publishing and presenting at conferences. It involves seminars, journal clubs and other fora where theoretical issues are presented and discussed.

Role of the Study

It is important that nurse researchers are aware of the part their study will play in the generation, testing, or evaluation of theory (see Key Concepts 8.11). One way of checking this is to answer the following questions:

- What are the nature and scope of the research aims? Are the aims exploratory, descriptive, explanatory or predictive?
- Did an existing theory provide the initial idea for the research?
- Is the aim of the study to test existing concepts or propositions from an existing theory?
- Were study concepts or propositions derived from practice?
- Is the purpose of the study to describe or understand phenomena and from these phenomena develop descriptive or explanatory theory?
- What predominant world view is reflected in the nature of the research questions?
- Has there been much theoretical progress undertaken on this particular topic?

🔍 Key Concepts 8.11

It is important that nurse researchers are aware of the part their study will play in the generation, testing or evaluation of theory.

Conclusions

This chapter has provided particular emphasis on the linkages between research and theory. Four links were identified, theory-generating research, theory-testing research, theory-framed research and theory-evaluating research. All four were discussed and their contribution to the knowledge base of nursing was explored.

According to Wayne (2023), to improve the nursing profession's ability to meet societal duties and responsibilities, there needs to be a continuous reciprocal and cyclical connection with theory, practice and research. McKenna et al. (2014) asked us to imagine that theory, practice and research are three dancers. This is a useful metaphor. The dancers interact to produce a systematic and aesthetic beauty, grace and elegance. One weak dancer who stumbles or does not undertake the appropriate movements would cause problems for all three and such a passenger can only be 'carried' for so long. Therefore, all three partners need to be performing at their best. Similarly, research with weak theory or practice with weak research can damage nursing as a discipline. It is in the profession's best interest to keep these three performing at their best, that they are strong and that they interact appropriately.

Revision Points

- Research does one of two things – it either tests or generations theory.

- There are four links between research and theory: theory-generating research (TGR), theory-testing research (TTR), theory-framed research (TFR) and theory-evaluating research (TER).

- TGR inductively develops theory from clinical phenomena.

- TTR empirically tests the validity of the theory's propositions.

- TER does not test propositions for truth; rather it assesses the effects of implementing a grand theory in a practice setting.

- TFR is where a theory acts as an organising structure for a research investigation.

- Dickoff and James identified four levels of theory and Donna Diers linked these to four levels of research.

Additional Reading

Hickman R.L. (2019) Nursing theory and research: the path forward. *Advanced in Nursing Science.*, **42**(1), 85–86. DOI: 10.1097/ANS.0000000000000255

Littzen-Brown, C. (2021).Theory-guided Research: What, Why, and How? Nursology. https://nursology.net/nurse-theories/

Useful Web Links

http://currentnursing.com/nursing_theory/research_and_nursing_theories.html
http://en.wikipedia.org/wiki/Nursing_theory
https://nursekey.com/outline-of-nursing-theories-and-frameworks-of-care/
https://nursology.net/
https://www.wgu.edu/blog/understanding-nursing-theories2109.html
www.wileyfundamentalseries.com/nursingmodels

References

Anglin A.H., Kincaid P.A. & Allen D.G. (2022) Role theory perspectives: past, present, and future applications of role theories in management research. *Journal of Management*, **48**(6). DOI: 10.1177/01492063221081442

Carper B.A. (1978) Fundamental patterns of knowing in nursing. *Advances in Nursing Science*, **1**(1), 13–23.

Chinn P.L., Kramer M.K. & Sitzman K. (2022) *Knowledge Development in Nursing: Theory and Process*, 11th edition. St. Louis, MO: Elsevier.

Current Nursing (2024). Nursing theories: open access articles on nursing theories and models. https://currentnursing.com/nursing_theory/research_and_nursing_theories.html

Cutciffe J.R. & McKenna H.P. (2008) *Essential Concepts in Nursing*. London: Elsevier.

Dewey J. (1904) *The Relation of Theory to Practice in the Education of Teachers*. Chicago: University of Chicago.

Dickoff J. & James P. (1968) A theory of theories: a position paper. *Nursing Research*, **17**(3), 197–203.

Dickoff J. & James P. (1992) Correspondence. In Nicholl L. (ed.) *Perspectives on Nursing Theory*, 2nd edition. New York: J.B. Lippincott.

Diers D. (1979) *Research in Nursing Practice*. Philadelphia, PA: J.B. Lippincott.

Einstein A. (1905) On the electrodynamics of moving bodies. *Annalen der Physik*, **17**(10), 891–921.

Fawcett J. (2012) Thoughts about evidence-based nursing practice. *Nursing Science Quarterly*, **25**(2), 199–200.

Fawcett J. (2017) *Applying Conceptual Models of Nursing: Quality Improvement, Research, and Practice*. New York: Springer Publishing Company.

Freud S. (1949) *An Outline of Psychoanalysis*. New York: W.W. Norton.

Glaser B.G. & Strauss A.L. (1999) *The Discovery of Grounded Theory: Strategies for Qualitative Research*. New York: Aldine de Gruyter.

Hartweg D.L. & Metcalfe S.A. (2022) Orem's self-care deficit nursing theory: relevance and need for refinement. *Nursing Science Quarterly*, **35**(1), 70–76. DOI: 10.1177/08943184211051369

Helson H. (1964) *Adaptation Level Theory*. New York: Harper and Row.

Henderson V. (1966) *The Nature of Nursing: A Definition and its Implications for Practice, Education and Research*. London: Collier Macmillan.

Hickman R.L. (2019) Nursing theory and research: the path forward. *Advanced in Nursing Science*, **42**(1), 85–86. DOI: 10.1097/ANS.0000000000000255

Lewin K. (1946) Action research and minority problems. *Journal of Social Issues*, **2**(4), 34–46.

Littzen-Brown, C. (2021).Theory-guided Research: What, Why, and How? Nursology. https://nursology.net/nurse-theories/

Lor M., Backonja U. & Lauver D.R. (2017) How could nurse researchers apply theory to generate knowledge more efficiently? *Journal of Nursing Scholarship.*, **49**(5), 580–589. DOI: 10.1111/jnu.12316

McKenna H.P. (1994) *Nursing Theories and Quality of Care*. Aldershot: Avebury Press.

McKenna H.P., Pajnkihar M. & Murphy F.A. (2014) *Fundamentals of Nursing Models Theories and Practice*. London: Wiley Blackwell.

Meleis A.I. (2017) *Theoretical Nursing: Development and Progress*. Philadelphia, PA: Walters Kluwer Publishers.

Neuman B. (1995) *The Neuman Systems Model*, 3rd edition. Norwalk, CT: Appleton and Lange.

Orem D.E. (1995) *Nursing Concepts of Practice*, 5th edition. St. Louis, MO: Mosby, Inc.

Orlando I. (1961) *The Dynamic Nurse Patient Relationship. Function, Process, and Principles*. New York: G.P. Putnam & Sons.

Parse R.R. (1981) *Man-Living-Health: A Theory of Nursing*. New York: John Wiley & Sons.

Paterson J.G. & Zderad L.T. (1976) *Humanistic Nursing*. New York: John Wiley & Sons.

Peplau H.E. (1992) Interpersonal relations: a theoretical framework for application in nursing practice. *Nursing Science Quarterly*, **5**, 13–18.

Popper K. (1989) *Conjectures and Refutations: the Growth of Scientific Knowledge*, revised edition. London: Routledge.

Roper N., Logan W. & Tierney A.J. (2000) *The Roper-Logan-Tierney Model of Nursing Based on Activities of Living*. Edinburgh: Churchill Livingstone.

Roy C. (1970) Adaptation: a conceptual framework for nursing. *Nursing Outlook*, **18**(3), 42–45.

Roy C. (2019) Nursing knowledge in the 21st century: domain-derived and basic science practice-shaped. *Advances in Nursing Science*, **42**(1), 28–42. DOI: 10.1097/ANS.0000000000000240

Stokes P. (2015) *Philosophy: 100 Essential Thinkers*. London: Arcturus Publishing Ltd.

Travelbee J. (1966) *Interpersonal Aspects of Nursing*. Philadelphia, PA: F.A. Davis.

Von Bertalanffy L. (1951) General system theory, a new approach to unity of science. 6. Towards a physical theory of organic teleology, feedback and dynamics. *Human Biology*, **23**(4), 346–361.

Watson J. (1985) *Nursing: Human Science and Care*. New York: Appleton Century Crofts.

Wayne G. (2023). Nursing theories and theorists: the definitive guide for nurses. Nurseslabs. https://nurseslabs.com/nursing-theories/

Wiedenbach E. (1964) *Clinical Nursing: A Helping Art*. New York: Springer Publication Company.

Zhan L.J., He Y.C., Liu Q.J., Pei M.Y., Yu L.X. & Liu X.Y. (2022) Progress in the application of Meleis transition theory in the nursing field. *Nurs Commun*, **6**, e2022016. DOI: 10.53388/IN2022016

CHAPTER 9

Criteria for Theory Description, Analysis and Evaluation

Outline of Content

This chapter begins with the assertion that theories are still uncritically accepted to support practice and education. The development of theories is a dynamic and never-ending process in relation to the emergence of phenomena in the discipline of nursing and represents a continuous evolution of science. They describe, explain or predict the unique core of knowledge that nurses apply to caring for patients and the development of a science that distinguishes nursing from other disciplines. They need to be continually evaluated and tested so that they can systematically underpin theory-based practice or education.

In this chapter, theory analysis is described in relation to scope, context and content. In contrast, theory evaluation involves the consideration of terminology, including a discussion of clarity, simplicity/complexity, importance/ significance, adequacy, testability and acceptance. Theory evaluation is a multifaceted process that delves into the core of theoretical development, emphasising critical examination to ensure the robustness and applicability of a theory. Problems arising from theory that was analysed or evaluated and found not to be useful, adequate or significant are addressed. The place of theory testing in nursing is considered, and the relationship between theory evaluation and theory testing is clarified. The usability criterion is presented as an important consideration, in respect of the theory–practice relationship, and is proposed together with others as a core evaluation criterion. Finally, acceptance by the scholarly community reflects the theory's resonance with existing knowledge and its potential to advance understanding in its field. Together, these criteria form the bedrock of theory evaluation, guiding students in the rigorous examination and refinement of theoretical knowledge.

Fundamentals of Nursing Models, Theories and Practice, Third Edition. Hugh P. McKenna, Majda Pajnkihar and Dominika Vrbnjak.
© 2025 John Wiley & Sons Ltd. Published 2025 by John Wiley & Sons Ltd.
Companion website: www.wiley.com/go/nursingmodels3e

Learning Outcomes

At the end of this chapter, you should be able to:

1. Discuss theory description

2. Define theory analysis and evaluation

3. Identify criteria for concept analysis

4. Determine the scope, context and content of theory analysis

5. Discuss important criteria for theory evaluation

Introduction

Over the decades, many approaches to theory analysis and evaluation have been published. The criteria to do this are constantly changing and developing, possibly confusing students and clinical staff who often have to assess the worth of a nursing theory. No reasonable reader will deny that before theories can be used in practice, they need to be reviewed for their usefulness and fitness for practice. You have seen elsewhere in this book that nurses have frequently selected theories for education, practice and research in an uncritical way.

Each discipline has a unique orientation for knowledge development (Smith 2018a). Nursing is a professional discipline that needs knowledge to guide practice based on theory. However, nursing theories change and develop over time because there are always new demands from patients and new technologies are being introduced. You will recall from Chapter 1 that all theorists try to describe, explain and predict the important phenomena for nursing. Many of the more recent nursing theories that were developed in the mid- to late twentieth century have been revised. Therefore, we need to embrace change and remain open to the potential growth of theoretical evolution for better nursing outcomes (Im 2021: 64).

As you have seen, the nursing literature contains many grand, mid-range, situation-specific theories (often called practice theories). While they may all be useful for practice, education or research, each needs to be analysed and evaluated before its usefulness in practice is ascertained (Pajnkihar 2011; Pajnkihar & Vrbnjak 2020a, 2020b).

It is important to distinguish the essence and content of nursing from other disciplines, to describe what nurses do and to define the outcomes of nursing activities (Meleis 2021: 9). Theories developed in other disciplines have also proved relevant to nursing, helping to solve problems in practice for which there were no obvious solutions (Chinn, Kramer & Sitzman 2022). Evaluating a theory is therefore the process by which we arrive at an insight into its worth or value (Smith 2018b: 34). The chapter is based on the steps outlined in Figure 9.1 and refers to 'evaluators' as a generic term for any student of theory.

The Evaluator of a Nursing Theory

Any educator, researcher, student or clinical nurse may want or need to evaluate a theory in order to assess the significance of the theory. They need to understand how the theory is internally constructed and how its components interrelate. The process of theory description, analysis and evaluation depends on the evaluator's experience, knowledge, professional commitment and confidence. In a theory evaluation approach, it is relevant that the evaluator starts as Smith (2018b: 36) suggested, from a position of empathy, curiosity, honesty and accountability.

For postgraduate students wishing to assess the strengths, weaknesses and applicability of a theory to practice or to select a theory as a theoretical framework for research, it is essential that the criteria are clear and not excessive.

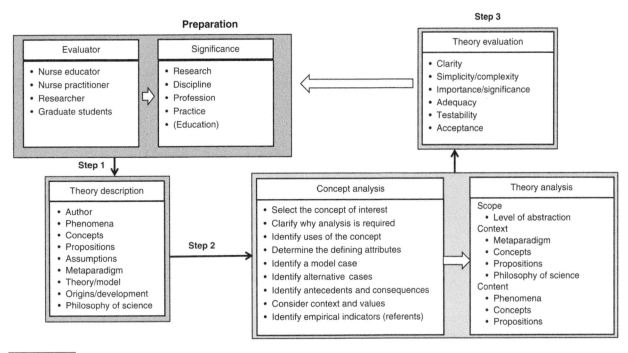

FIGURE 9.1 Theory description, analysis and evaluation.

Pajnkihar's (2012) criteria for theory analysis and evaluation (in Table 9.3) were based on a study conducted among full-time and part-time nursing master's students in Slovenia and Croatia using the approach described by Smith (2018b).

Significance of the Theory

The evaluator has to be aware of the significance of a theory (see Key Concepts 9.1). It must be clear what a theory can bring to nursing practice, education or research. The best theories are those that have repeatedly withstood challenges sufficiently well so that we can have a high degree of confidence when it is applied to practice (remember Popper's boat analogy in Chapter 2). The evaluator must be convinced that the knowledge contained within the theory is accurate or presents the best available knowledge under the circumstances, even though we accept that absolute truth or rightness is not always possible.

Meleis (2018) asked whether the theory will make a difference in the lives of people using it and if it has a positive effect on the quality of care. She further elaborates that theories help in identifying the core of nursing practice by delineating specific boundaries of nursing and providing a rationale for what constitutes nursing actions. In this sense, Alligood (2018) maintained that the historical background also provides a context and perspective for nursing theories and highlights their relevance to the discipline and the profession of nursing.

Key Concepts 9.1

Significance of a theory: a theory is significant if it addresses the essential issues of nursing and contributes to the development of nursing knowledge.

It is important to ask if a theory will improve patients' situations so that they can retain their 'personality' with self-respect and dignity and improve their health and well-being. So it needs to have the flexibility and ease of application to respond quickly to the changing demands of different healthcare systems. In addition, Chinn, Kramer and Sitzman (2022) pointed out the importance of being able to modify the theory. Using description and critical reflection to examine a theory helps determine its usefulness and potential modification. A theory may not perfectly fit your situation, but it can still guide care. The key is understanding how the theory aligns with your needs so that informed decisions can be made on its application.

Step 1: Theory Description

It is vital that students have a basic understanding of the structure and function of nursing theory and the relationships between its concepts, only then can they understand its most important features and its theoretical and practical utility. Meleis (2018) suggested that this is an important first step to a proper understanding before heading to the next stage of the evaluation. Chinn, Kramer and Sitzman (2022) asserted that describing a theory is a process of asking questions about its structure.

The Theorist

Several writers (Alligood 2018; Meleis 2018; Chinn, Kramer & Sitzman 2022) begin their description of a theory by introducing the author's personal, theoretical and practical background. Why did he or she develop the theory and for what purpose? This gives an evaluator first-hand information about the context in which the theory was developed and provides a specific language and a perspective from where the theory was developed. In the following section, we learn about the theorist's practical, educational and research experience.

Chinn, Kramer and Sitzman (2022) emphasised the role of theorists in fostering critical thinking and reflective practice among nurses. Meleis (2018) added that the theorist's professional and academic backgrounds are also important because this environmental context is affected by internal and external factors, which will influence the theorist. Therefore, the evaluator needs to know who the author of the theory is and what the author's academic and practical experiences are.

In essence, it is very important that the evaluator knows the *phenomena*, *concepts*, metaparadigm concepts, *propositions* and *assumptions* of the theory and its core parts (see Reflective Exercise 9.1).

Reflective Exercise 9.1

Core Parts of a Theory

Take a blank sheet of paper and draw a diagram of the link between phenomena, concepts, metaparadigm concepts, propositions and assumptions. If you are having difficulty, refer back to Chapters 1 and 5 and refresh your memory about these.

The identification of phenomena occupies the lowest point in the hierarchy of theoretical conception. A phenomenon is the foundation from which the theorist starts to develop or refine a theory. Therefore, an evaluator will think about how the phenomenon or phenomena are described in the theory. The evaluator should also check what the basic concepts are within a theory, and understand their meanings. Remember from Chapter 1 that theorists use concepts to give a unique abstract name or label to the phenomenon or phenomena that are observed in everyday practice. It is generally accepted that concepts are the basic building blocks of the theory and need to be recognised and described within the content and context of the theory. Propositions are statements of relationships between concepts, and the nature of propositions depends on the nature of the concepts they link within the theory. For the evaluator, it is also critically important to understand the assumptions that describe the values and beliefs underpinning the theory. McKenna (1997: 217) suggested asking yourself the question: Can the stated assumption be accepted as true?

In addition, it is very important to know what the theory says about the metaparadigm (see Chapter 5). Theorists should explicitly describe the four elements of the metaparadigm and make their relationship clear. McKenna (1997: 228) believed that the evaluator should closely examine the metaparadigm concepts within the theory (see Appendix A). What does the theorist have to say about the nature of people, the environment, health and nursing? Are these components and the assumptions relating to them made explicit? Does the theorist emphasise one to the detriment of the others? Evaluators need to check whether the relationships between the metaparadigm elements of a theory are stated clearly and if there is a transparent presentation or explanation of the beliefs, values and goals associated with them (Pajnkihar 2003).

If a theorist refers to 'persons', is he or she referring to patients, potential patients, communities or societies at large? When 'nursing' is described in the theory, is it the profession or the art or science of nursing that is being alluded to, or is it the nursing act? Does 'environment' mean external environment or internal environment (e.g. inside the body)? Is 'health' a state of well-being, a physical status or a psycho-social feeling? It is important that the evaluator is clear as to what theorists mean when they refer either implicitly or explicitly to the metaparadigm. In defining nursology, Fawcett (2023) has broadened the concepts of the metaparadigm from a global and cultural perspective to give a contemporary focus in countries on the planet for understanding human beings, global health and the environment. Are these components highlighted in the theory?

King's theory is very clear in how it describes the basic concepts and the metaparadigm elements (Harih & Pajnkihar 2009; Pajnkihar & Vrbnjak 2020c). Watson (1985a) excluded 'nursing' in her metaparadigm and referred instead to 'transpersonal caring'. By contrast, while Swanson (1991, 2015) saw caring as a basic building block of her mid-range theory, she also described nursing, environment, health and person as elements of the metaparadigm.

Chinn, Kramer and Sitzman (2022) elucidated that the description of a theory involves probing its components through questions and interpreting these elements based on one's understanding. Moreover, they highlighted the significance of understanding a theory's purpose, which is often tailored to clinical nursing practice. In addition, they described the key points regarding the significance of the metaparadigm concepts, and they used of the term 'Metalanguage' to describe these concepts.

Students usually have problems differentiating between basic concepts coming from the phenomena (content) and metaparadigm concepts (context) within the theory and their relationships. Furthermore, they often have problems identifying propositions that enable the theory to work. Hopefully, this will be easier once you read this book.

In previous chapters, we outlined how the level of abstraction and scope decrease as you move from grand theory to mid-range theory, to a situation-specific theory. For evaluators, the level of abstraction and scope of the theory has to be clear (see Reflective Exercise 9.2).

Reflective Exercise 9.2

Levels of Abstraction and Scope

Open Google Earth on your computer. Zoom out until you can see the Earth. Consider this to represent a grand theory. Zoom in to Spain. Consider this to represent a mid-range theory. Zoom in further to the city of Madrid. Consider this to be a practice theory. You will agree that the view of the Earth is very general with a broad scope. As you zoom in, the view becomes more specific and the scope much narrower.

Origins and Logical Development of a Theory

For a key question was: What was the origin of the theory? Previously, Walker and Avant (2011: 195) believed that the origins of a theory refer to its initial development, what prompted its development, whether it is inductive, deductive or retroductive in its formation (see Chapter 2) and whether there is any evidence to support or refute it. Meleis (2018) situated nursing theory within a wide-ranging framework that recognises the significance of multiple philosophical and theoretical foundations, arguing for a synthesis of diverse theoretical viewpoints to encapsulate the complexity and richness of the nursing profession. Further, McKenna (1997) wrote of the need to take account of socio-cultural factors and political issues and uncover which philosophy the theorist prefers (see Reflective Exercise 9.3). Philosophies influencing theory development are described in Chapters 2 and 5.

Reflective Exercise 9.3

Philosophies and Their Influence on Nurse Theorists

Everyone's thoughts, attitudes and actions are influenced by their belief systems. Belief systems are influenced by different philosophies. The same goes for nurse theorists. They have beliefs about what is important for nurses and patients and their beliefs are influenced by various philosophies (e.g. rationalism, empiricism and historicism). Think about the philosophies that influence your views and behaviour. Write these down. If you need to, refer back to Chapter 2 to review philosophies and their influence on the development of nursing theories.

Step 2: Theory Analysis

An evaluator should recognise the structure and meaning of a theory, its content and context, its concepts and their relationships and be able to determine its strengths and weaknesses (see Key Concepts 9.2). Alligood (2018) highlighted that analysis is the initial step in understanding theoretical adequacy, crucial for incorporating nursing theories into education, research, administration or practice. She emphasised that comprehending and critically reflecting on theories are fundamental for their practical application and for advancing nursing science.

This should be an objective process where the evaluator tries to understand how concepts are related without judging them. This also involves putting aside our own beliefs and biases as much as possible so that we do not impose our own views of the world on the theory (remember *tabula rasa* in Chapter 2).

While this section is related to theory analysis, an important aspect of this is concept analysis. Alligood (2018) underscores the importance of analysis as the foundational phase in assessing the adequacy of theoretical concepts. Furthermore, she accentuated the necessity of a deep understanding and critical examination of theories, seeing these activities as essential for the onward development of nursing science.

Key Concepts 9.2

Theory analysis: the process of recognising the content and context of a theory (Meleis 2018).

Concept Analysis

Several authors have described the process of concept analysis (Meleis 2018; Walker & Avant 2019) and there are similarities and differences in the steps and techniques.

It is generally accepted that concepts are mental constructions of the basic building blocks of the theory and need to be recognised and described within the content and context of the theory.

Walker and Avant (2019) suggested that concept analysis has to be rigorous and precise, but the end product is always tentative because knowledge changes very quickly.

The purpose of concept analysis can be described as follows (Walker & Avant 2019):

- a useful process in the cycle of theory development, as well as in theory evaluation (Meleis 2012, 2018);
- to make theory solid and strong because concepts are the basic building blocks of theory;
- to determine a concept's structure;
- to refine ambiguous concepts within the theory;
- to distinguish one concept from another;
- to examine the language used and to develop standardised language.

The procedure relevant to concept analysis is as follows (see also Table 9.1):

- Select the concept of interest; the evaluator should be clear about what the concept of interest is for practice or theory analysis.
- Clarify why a concept analysis is required. It is mostly to gain an in-depth understanding of a concept within a theory.
- Identify the uses of the concept: to search for its meanings until no more new meanings are uncovered.
- Determine the defining attributes; these attributes distinguish the concept from similar or related concepts.
- Identify a 'model case' that describes the concept perfectly. The best model cases should be drawn from real-life examples.
- Identify alternative cases that are not model cases. These include borderline cases, related cases, contrary cases, invented cases and illegitimate cases. These can all be used to enhance the identification and clarification of the concept.
- Identify antecedents (the events or situations that prompt or stimulate a concept) and consequences (those that happen after as a result of a concept). (See Reflective Exercise 9.4.)
- Consider context and values. Concepts alter depending on the context within which they occur, and values have different meanings for different people in different settings.
- Identify empirical indicators (referents). These are for defining the attributes of the concept; they are a means by which it is possible to recognise or measure the defining characteristics or attributes (Walker & Avant 2011, 2019).

TABLE 9.1 Concept analysis.

	McKenna (1997)	Cutcliffe and McKenna (2005)	Walker and Avant (2011, 2019)
Select the concept of interest	✓	✓	✓
Clarify why analysis is required	✓	✓	✓
Identify uses of the concept	✓	✓	✓
Determine the defining attributes	✓	✓	✓
Identify a model case	✓	✓	✓
Identify alternative cases	✓	✓	✓
Identify antecedents and consequences	✓	✓	✓
Consider context and values	✓	✓	
Identify empirical indicators (referents)	✓	✓	✓

Reflective Exercise 9.4

Antecedents and Consequences

Consider a concept that interests you – it could be 'hope', 'empathy', 'sorrow' or 'compassion'. Think of what led up to the concept or what happened before the concept appeared (its antecedents). Consider also what happened as a result of the concept appearing (its consequences). For instance, if the concept was 'loss', the antecedents might be a death in the family or unemployment. The consequences of loss might be sadness or depression.

Think of three different concepts and identify antecedents and consequences.

Concept analysis advances the knowledge needed in practice and informs theory-based practice (see Reflective Exercise 9.5). Together with the phenomena, the main concepts within a theory may enhance and develop the constantly changing knowledge in healthcare and nursing.

Although theory analysis and theory evaluation will be treated separately in this chapter, in some books, they are mentioned together. Table 9.2 offers an overview and comparison of different approaches to theory description, analysis and evaluation taken from Stevens Barnum (1998), Fawcett (2005), McKenna and Slevin (2008), Chinn and Kramer (2008, 2011), Alligood (2010a, Alligood 2018), Walker and Avant (2011, 2019), Meleis (2012, 2018), Pajnkihar (2012) and Chinn, Kramer and Sitzman (2022). Only Fawcett (2005) has a set of criteria for analysis and evaluation of nursing models (grand theories) and theories (mid-range theories). Parse (1987) and McKenna (1997) used criteria for evaluating theories that were developed from quantitative and qualitative research.

Reflective Exercise 9.5

Analysis of a Concept

Concepts are the basic building blocks of a theory. Select a concept and use the criteria outlined to undertake concept analysis. If you need further help, refer to Table 8.5 in Chapter 8 or Chapter 1 in where the process and criteria for concept analysis are described and various concepts are analysed.

Internal and External Criteria

Table 9.2 demonstrates that the criteria for theory analysis and evaluation can be broadly divided into internal and external factors.

Internal evaluative criteria refer to philosophical and theoretical issues. This means that they are concerned with the philosophical ideas of the theorist (his or her background, education, experience, worldview and reasons for developing a theory, i.e. his or her personal contribution to the development of a theory). They also include the characteristics of a theory, such as clarity, consistency, simplicity and adequacy.

External evaluative criteria refer to societal and practical issues. This means that they are concerned with social significance, social utility, social acceptance/congruence, simplicity, testability and so on, that is, those aspects of evaluative criteria that are connected with the cultural, political and environmental issues of society.

McKenna (1997) referred to 'internal' and 'external' structures; Stevens-Barnum (1998) to 'internal' and 'external' criticism; and Meleis (2018) and Chinn, Kramer and Sitzman (2022), though not explicitly stating a difference, implicitly indicated the use of individual criteria. Alligood (2018) used the criteria for theory analysis described by Chinn, Kramer and Sitzman (2022). Even Marriner Tomey (1998), although not giving any internal criteria apart from the theory description, represents the theories' authors in terms of their background, education, etc., thus implicitly including them as factors to consider.

TABLE 9.2 Analysis and evaluation of theories by various authors.

	Analysis and critique	Internal criticism	External criticism	Theory analysis	Evaluation	Description of theory	Critical reflection	Theory critique
McKenna (1997)	How the theory: – was developed – is internally structured – may be used – influences knowledge development – stands up to testing							
Stevens-Barnum (1998)		Clarity Consistency Adequacy Logic development Level of theory	Reality convergence Utility Significance discrimination Scope of theory Complexity					
Fawcett (2005) and Fawcett and DeSanto-Madeya (2013)				Scope Context Content	Significance Internal consistency Parsimony Testability Empirical adequacy Pragmatic adequacy			
Chinn and Kramer (2008, 2011), Chinn, Kramer and Sitzman (2022)						Purpose Concepts Definitions Relationships Structure Assumptions	Clarity Simplicity Generalisability Accessibility Importance	

(Continued)

TABLE 9.2   (Continued)

Analysis and critique	Internal criticism	External criticism	Theory analysis	Evaluation	Description of theory	Critical reflection	Theory critique
McKenna and Slevin (2008)			Parsimony and testability Defeasibility Evidence and justified true belief Coherence and consistency	Relevance and utility Prescriptive value Quality enhancement Meaningfulness Dynamism Originality Reflection of stakeholder interests Scope and range			
Alligood (2010a, 2018)			History of nursing theory Significance	Clarity Simplicity Generality Empirical precision Derivable consequences			
Walker and Avant (2011, 2019)			Origins Meaning	Logical adequacy Usefulness Generalisability/ transferability Parsimony Testability			
Meleis (2012, 2018)			The theorist Paradigmatic origins Internal dimensions				Relationship between structure and function Diagram of theory Circle of contagiousness Usefulness Personal values Congruence with other professional values Congruence with social values Social significance
Pajnkihar (2012)			Scope Context Content	Clarity Simplicity/ complexity Importance/ significance Adequacy Testability Acceptance			

188

Both internal and external criteria exert an influence on theorists. This is one reason why individual categories, though sometimes seemingly very similar, do not allow researchers to draw parallels among them. To do so would curtail or expand their original formulation, meaning and scope.

Other common evaluation criteria used by different authors are as follows:

- adequacy, empirical and pragmatic (McKenna 1997; Walker & Avant 2011, 2019; Pajnkihar 2012);
- clarity (Stevens-Barnum 1998; Chinn & Kramer 2008, 2011; Alligood 2010a, 2018; Pajnkihar 2012; Chinn, Kramer & Sitzman 2022);
- simplicity–complexity (Stevens-Barnum 1998; Chinn & Kramer 2008, 2011; Alligood 2010a, 2018; Walker & Avant 2011, 2019; Pajnkihar 2012; Chinn, Kramer & Sitzman 2022);
- scope (Stevens-Barnum 1998; Fawcett 2005a; Chinn & Kramer 2008, 2011; Alligood 2010a, 2018; Pajnkihar 2012; Chinn, Kramer & Sitzman 2022);
- significance (McKenna 1997; Stevens-Barnum 1998; Fawcett 2005a; Chinn & Kramer 2008, 2011; Pajnkihar 2012; Chinn, Kramer & Sitzman 2022);
- testability (McKenna 1997; Fawcett 2005a; Walker & Avant 2011 2019; Pajnkihar 2012) (Table 9.3).

According to Fawcett (2012a), theory evaluation and analysis frameworks are helpful because analysis involves the objective and non-judgemental description of theories. It needs to be explicitly pointed out that the theory has to be described and analysed in the words and terminology of the theory's author. Although this is difficult when translated into other languages, exotic words used by the author, such as 'holarchy' or 'negatropic', can be learned and understood.

TABLE 9.3   Theory evaluation.

	McKenna (1997)	Stevens-Barnum (1998)	Fawcett (2005); Fawcett and DeSanto-Madeya (2013)	Chinn and Kramer (2008, 2011); Chinn, Kramer and Sitzman (2022)	Alligood (2010a, 2018)	Walker and Avant (2011, 2019)	Meleis (2012, 2018)	Pajnkihar (2012)
Adequacy	✓	✓				✓		✓
Clarity	✓	✓		✓	✓		✓	✓
Consistency	✓	✓		✓				
Complexity/ simplicity	✓	✓		✓	✓		✓	✓
Generality/ scope of theory	✓	✓		✓	✓	✓		
Significance/ importance		✓	✓	✓				✓
Usefulness	✓	✓						
Congruence	✓							
Testability	✓	✓	✓	✓	✓	✓	✓	✓
Acceptance								✓

Fawcett (2005); Fawcett & DeSanto-Madeya 2013) pointed out that analysis is accomplished by a systematic examination of exactly what the author has written about the theory.

Relying on references about what might have been meant or referring to other people's interpretations of the theory is not sufficient. When the theory's author is unclear about a point or has not presented some information, it may be necessary to make inferences to or look up other reviews of the theory. That, however, must be noted explicitly, so that the distinction between the words of the theory's author and those of others is clear. Theory analysis follows a clear pattern and includes theory scope, context and content. Understanding theory and its role, as well as analysing, evaluating and taking a critical view of it, can help to develop a body of knowledge that nurses need for everyday work, for the competent and efficient implementation of their actions and for the creative and significant further development of knowledge that encompasses real nursing situations (Pajnkihar 2003).

Meleis (2018) suggested that the description of theory consists of structural and functional components. Within the structural components of the theory, she described assumptions, concepts and propositions; as functional components, she included focus, patient, nursing, health, nurse–patient interactions, environment, nursing problems and nursing therapeutics. Last of all, a critical examination of the relations between structural and functional elements is needed.

For theory analysis, Meleis (2018) suggested the following components established by theorists as external dimensions: 'references, citations, assumptions, concepts, propositions, hypotheses, laws'. For internal dimensions she suggested 'rationale, system of relations, content, beginnings, scope, goal, context, abstractness and method'. These topics have been addressed in the previous chapters (see Chapter 5).

In the theory analysis of Fawcett and DeSanto-Madeya (2013), the structure is that of theory scope, context and content. These will now be explained.

Scope of the Theory

The evaluator needs to determine the level and scope of the theory, that is, if it is a grand theory, a mid-range theory or a specific situation theory (see Step 1 in Figure 9.1).

Theory Context

Theory context includes descriptions of:

- metaparadigms: concepts and propositions;
- philosophical claims on which a theory is based; its values and beliefs about nursing; and the world views of the relationships between nursing, human beings, health and the environment;
- the contribution of knowledge from nursing and adjunctive disciplines (see Chapter 5).

Theory Content

Theory content includes the concepts and propositions of the theory (see Step 2 in Figure 9.1). Fawcett and DeSanto-Madeya (2013) and Meleis (2018) introduced theory analysis and evaluation as a two-in-one-step process. At the end of the theory analysis, the evaluator should know the scope and context of a theory, especially how it deals with the metaparadigm, concepts, propositions and description of the relationships between metaparadigm concepts. It is also important to determine the philosophy of science and paradigm (e.g. systems, interactional, developmental and behavioural) that influence the theory's development. It should also be clear if the theory was developed inductively, deductively or retroductively. Figure 9.2 shows the difference between induction and deduction.

Step 3: Theory Evaluation

Clarity

The analysis of the criterion 'clarity' means that the selected theory is expressed simply and consistently. If the theory is also introduced in diagram form, this should make it even clearer and lead to a better understanding of its consequent usefulness in practice. Although the criterion simplicity is treated separately in the following section, it is also very important for clarity.

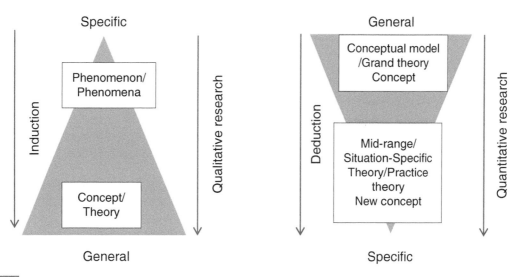

FIGURE 9.2 Difference between inductive and deductive development of theory.

Meleis (2018: 186) asserted that clarity 'denotes precision of boundaries, a communication of a sense of orderliness, vividness of meaning and consistency'. Clarity is:

> demonstrated in assumptions, concepts and propositions as well as in domain concepts ... To have clarity in concepts is to have theoretical and operational definitions that are consistent throughout the theory, are represented in a parsimonious [simple, straightforward] way and are consistent with the theory's assumptions and propositions ... Propositional clarity is manifested in a coherent and logical presentation of propositions and systematic linkages between the theory's concepts ... The degree to which a congruency exists between the different components of a theory describes its consistency ... The fit between different components of a theory describes its consistency. The fit between assumptions and concept definitions, between concepts as defined and their use in propositions, and between concepts and clinical exemplars can all be considered as consistency.

Clarity and consistency are often used as a single criterion. Alligood (2018) also described clarity with respect to semantics and structure. Within the criterion of 'internal consistency' used by Fawcett (2005a: 443), she described the evaluation of the context and content of the theory where she included semantic clarity and consistency:

> This criterion requires all elements of the theorists' work, including the philosophical claims, ... and the theory concepts and propositions to be clear ... the semantic clarity requirement is more likely to be met when a constitutive definition is given for each concept than when no explicit definitions are given ... the semantic consistency requirement is met when the same terms and the same definitions are used for each concept in all authors' discussions about the theory.

Both Alligood (2018) and Chinn, Kramer and Sitzman (2022) also highlighted semantic clarity and semantic consistency. In addition, Walker and Avant (2019) included semantic clarity and consistency to try to explain the theoretic meanings of concepts, whereas structural clarity and consistency focus on understanding the intended connections between concepts within the theory (i.e. propositions). McKenna (1997: 227) asserted that 'all components within a theory should support each other and be free from contradictions'.

Therefore, the clear link between components of the theory (concepts, their definitions, assumptions and propositions) focuses on structural clarity and consistency (congruency between the different components). They represent the functions of the theory and theoretical explanations. Furthermore, semantic clarity and consistency (language, method and explanations) help in understanding the meaning of the concepts within a theory. They make the presentation of the theory understandable to potential users.

Simplicity and Complexity

The criterion 'simplicity' demands that a theory is written in short affirmative sentences. Simplicity and complexity complement each other in their interrelationships. Concepts that describe a particular phenomenon within a theory have features of complexity, but simplicity of expression assists in clarifying the phenomenon. Also, the simpler the explanation of the relationship between the concepts, the more understandable they are.

The principle of simplicity is paramount for ensuring coherence, with descriptive simplicity enabling the concise articulation of the theory's complex ideas. Similarly, inductive simplicity pertains to the theory's depiction of phenomena, suggesting that a theory should contain a limited number of concepts to remain effective and avoid overwhelming its ability to offer a comprehensive framework for understanding (Smith 2018b).

McKenna (1997) asserted that the theory should be simple and elegant and that the theoretical message should be in the simplest possible format. For Walker and Avant (2011: 195, 2019: 210), 'parsimony refers to how simply and briefly a theory can be stated while still being complete in its explanation of the phenomenon in question'. In addition, Chinn and Kramer (2008, 2011) and Chinn, Kramer and Sitzman (2022) connected parsimony with theoretical simplicity and the idea of generality. This is similar to the principle of Occam's razor, which we came across in Chapter 8. The generality of the theory is based on the scope of its concepts and purposes. Broad concepts contain more ideas in fewer words than narrow concepts. Meleis (2018: 186) stated that the:

> simplicity of a theory is more desirable if it focuses on fewer concepts and a few relationships that may enhance its utility [and the] complexity of a theory may be a desirable criterion if the complexity enhances the number of explanations and predictions the theory offers.

Chinn, Kramer and Sitzman's (2022) evaluation criteria included the minimum number of elements within each descriptive category, particularly concepts and their interrelationships within propositions. Complexity implies many theoretical relationships between and among numerous concepts in a theory.

McKenna (1997) stated that the reason for simplicity is to gain the attention of practising nurses so as to create a link with practice. However, he accepts that due to the complexity of nursing, not all theories can be presented in a simple manner. Also, Walker and Avant (2019) suggested that theory can be simple and broad to guide practice or simple but more empirically accessible to guide research. Stevens-Barnum (1998) noted that a narrower theory has more potential for guidance, and McKenna (1997) added that the narrower the scope of a theory, the higher its social utility (i.e. usefulness). Similarly, he said that the broader the scope of a theory, the greater the possibility that it will be more socially congruent. There is a possibility that broad theories have low social congruence because they are not easy to test (see Reflective Exercise 9.6).

Reflective Exercise 9.6

Clarity, Simplicity and Complexity

These three criteria are important in denoting harmonisation between the context and the content of the theory and the clarification of the phenomenon. The criteria complement each other in their relationships.

Describe in 200 words the importance of clarity and simplicity for practising nurses. Outline, too, why you think complexity is important in a nursing theory.

Importance and Significance

The importance of a theory in nursing is closely tied to its clinical significance or practical value. More precisely it 'addresses the extent to which a theory leads to valued nursing goals in practice, research, and education' (Chinn, Kramer & Sitzman 2022: 176). Fawcett (2012a: 352) stated that significance refers to the importance of the theory for the discipline of nursing. Alligood (2018) believed that the broader the scope of the theory, the higher its significance. Significance is also achieved when the metaparadigmatic, philosophical and conceptual origins of a theory are made explicit, when earlier supportive nursing literature is cited (Fawcett 2012a), and when the special contributions of the theory are acknowledged.

Chinn, Kramer and Sitzman (2022) considered that if a theory contains concepts, definitions, purposes and assumptions that are grounded in practice, it will have practical value for clinical nurses. Conversely, if the underlying assumptions are unsound, the importance of the theory is minimised. However, a theory that has extremely broad purposes may have limited value in creating useful clinical outcomes.

The importance of a theory also depends on the personal and professional values contained within it. For evaluators, it is imperative to ask, as McKenna (1997) does, whether the theory leads to actions that make important differences for patients. This is a difficult question to answer, especially if the theory has not been tested or applied in practice. It can accomplish this if positive patient outcomes are achieved through the use of interventions suggested by the theory. This can include the effect the theory has on the quality and safety of patient care. Although this includes outcomes of the theory, it also includes the interventions carried out and the resources needed to undertake best practice.

As we have seen consistently throughout this textbook, theories can be used to guide practice, research, education and administration (Meleis 2018). But, most importantly, they need to prove their contributions to knowledge development and to patients' and nurses' benefits (see Reflective Exercise 9.7). It is important to remember that what is significant for one person may not be significant for another.

Reflective Exercise 9.7

The Criteria of Importance and Significance

There is a very thin line between the importance and the significance of nursing theories for clinical practice. Select a nursing theory with which you are familiar and make a list of why it is important for nursing or why it is significant for nursing.

Adequacy

A theory needs to be useful in practice, to acknowledge the complexity of nursing practice and to guide research on the basis of sound evidence and empirical adequacy. The complexity of a theory must correspond to the complexity of practice, thus increasing practical and empirical adequacy. However, Stevens-Barnum (1998: 174) noted that 'a nursing theory is adequate if its prescriptions are extensive enough to cover the scope claimed by its author'. McKenna (1997) noted that most of the grand theories are not accessible, because they lack empirical indicators that reflect their concepts. In this respect, Chinn, Kramer and Sitzman (2022) suggested that the theory that is used in practice for explaining some aspect of practice needs to have theoretic concepts linked to empirical indicators of practice (see Key Concepts 9.3). This can be achieved, according to Fawcett and DeSanto-Madeya (2013), by reviewing all descriptions of the use of the theory in practice and by means of a systematic review of the findings of all studies that have been guided by the theory.

193

Key Concepts 9.3

Empirical Indicators

You were made aware in earlier chapters that concepts were really named phenomena and as such they were the building blocks of theory. Furthermore, concepts form relationships with each other to form propositions. Some of these propositions are written as hypotheses and so are testable. However, the concepts that make up hypotheses should be expressed in ways that can be measured. Such measurable concepts are called empirical indicators.

Fawcett and DeSanto-Madeya (2013) believed that the evaluation of empirical adequacy helps to determine the degree of confidence, given the best empirical evidence. Research testing requires evidence of empiric accessibility because accessibility and adequacy for research and practice of a chosen theory should be considered in the widest possible context.

A point to consider is that the theory can have empirical accessibility and adequacy for practice, but the conditions in nursing do not allow for the theory to be successful because of an inadequate number of nurses to care for patients. As with Karl Popper's paper boat, there is no final or absolute theory because it is always possible that subsequent studies will undermine the theory by producing different findings or that another theory will better fit the data (Fawcett 2005a).

McKenna (1997) gave the following example: If the theory is written specifically for the United Kingdom, and specifically for some nursing field, and the theorist claims that its propositions could apply transculturally to all nursing fields, this cannot represent adequacy. Achieving a profound comprehension of the theory necessitates the examination of foundational documents pivotal to its conceptualisation. An exhaustive evaluation entails the scrutiny of questions and feedback generated by the theory throughout the analytical review (Smith 2018b).

Chinn, Kramer and Sitzman (2022) highlighted that while the nursing field has traditionally relied on empirical methods, new knowledge structures are emerging that do not fit within this empirical framework. Additionally, they acknowledge the rise of knowledge forms and methods based on alternative assumptions, expanding beyond empirical confines.

Testability

As we saw in Chapter 8, testing can be seen as the end or the beginning of a never-ending circle of development, use, redefining, and improvement of theory. The following authors suggest that theory testing should focus on concepts, propositions and empirical indicators. Meleis (2018: 191) pointed out that theory testing 'presumes the complete cyclical relationship between theory, research, and theory' (Figure 9.3). Assessing the empirical validity of the theory can be impeded by lack of clarity about what constitutes sound theory-testing research.

Fawcett and DeSanto-Madeya (2013) described that the evaluation of a grand theory, which is abstract and general in nature, can lack operational definitions, the concepts may not be measurable and their propositions may not be easily amenable to direct empirical testing. Evaluating the testability of grand theory includes determining its mid-range theory-generating capacity (Figure 9.4). In addition, Fawcett (2021) described advances in nursology knowledge about the importance and relevance of empirical indicators as measures of people's health-related experiences. She presented the links between the concepts of the conceptual model, mid-range theory and situation-specific theory and the way they are measured, that is, empirical indicators. She introduces three types of empirical indicators – instruments, assessment

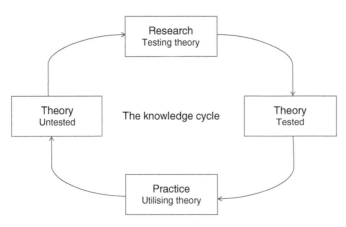

FIGURE 9.3   Testing theory.

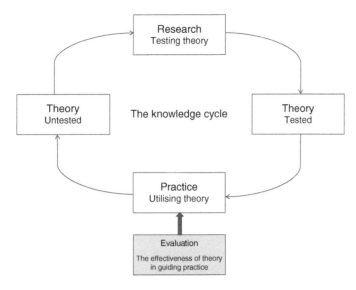

FIGURE 9.4 Evaluating theory.

tools and interventions. However, Walker and Avant (2019) suggested that a valid theory must be testable, at least in principle, which means that hypotheses (testable propositions) can be generated from the theory, research can be carried out and the theory is supported by the evidence or modified because of it. When testing hypotheses, Walker and Avant (2019) suggested that the measures and indicators of concepts should be selected with great care because conclusions can be drawn about the credibility of a hypothesis or the validity of measures when these are still in the testing process. Theories that generate hypotheses are useful to scientists and add to the body of knowledge. A theory that, by its nature, is untestable in its entirety may still yield testable hypotheses and statements that support the total theory. On the other hand, Chinn, Kramer and Sitzman (2022) emphasised that for a theory to be effectively applied in practice, its concepts must be linked to empirical indicators – observable experiences that can be measured or assessed within practice settings. These indicators are crucial for evaluating whether the theoretical aims are achieved as proposed. However, they caution that only certain aspects of highly abstract concepts might be empirically accessible. If a theory's concepts lack empirical dimensions or these dimensions are not clearly defined, the concepts may remain theoretical and untestable in practical contexts.

The final goal of theory development in any professional discipline is empirical testing of interventions that are specified in the form of prescriptive mid-range theories. The testability of descriptive, explanatory and prescriptive mid-range theories means that they should have operational definitions and their propositions must be amenable to empirical testing. Fawcett (2005a: 444) described traditional empiricism as an approach to test mid-range theories that require the concepts to be observable and the propositions measurable:

> *Concepts are empirically observable when operational definitions identify the empirical indicators that are used to measure the concepts. Propositions are measurable when empirical indicators can be substituted for concepts named in each proposition and when statistical procedures can provide evidence regarding the assertions made.*

Specific instruments or experimental protocols are needed to observe the theory concepts and statistical techniques to measure the propositions. As (Fawcett 2005a: 445) wrote:

> *The evaluation or testability for a middle-range theory is therefore facilitated by a thorough review of the research methodology literature associated with the theory, including descriptions of questionnaires and other instruments designed to measure concepts, research designs that will elicit the required data, and statistical or other data management techniques that yield evidence about the theory.*

Acceptance

When nurses are asked what theory would be appropriate for their specific practice, they should be aware that there is no simple and straightforward answer, and that an answer, to a great extent, depends on the nature and characteristics of their work and circumstances. You saw in Chapter 7 that the acceptance of a theory is greatest when the basic principles of the theory match the values and beliefs of nurses, their wishes and abilities. In the research carried out by Pajnkihar (2003) and Pajnkihar and Butterworth (2005), nurses recognised the essential need for theory in practice and they acknowledged that nursing theories currently applied in education offer little help in this respect. The study respondents suggested that the theories were widely incomprehensible and hard to apply; therefore, the workforce did not accept them. In recent decades, the landscape of nurse education has undergone a significant transition, notably with its incorporation into university settings. This shift has been instrumental in advancing the scope and depth of knowledge within the nursing profession and discipline. Specifically, advancements in postgraduate education, Advanced Nursing Practice (ANP) and, notably, doctoral education have catalysed a profound evolution in the profession's approach to the selection, evaluation, testing and practical application of knowledge. This development underscores a pivotal shift towards a more rigorous and scholarly framework in nursing education, reflecting its increasing complexity and the growing demands of healthcare delivery. However, the respondents called for a theory that is clear and simple to apply and use (see Key Concepts 9.4).

Key Concepts 9.4

Set or Model of Criteria for Evaluation

We can examine the chosen theory according to its clarity, simplicity/complexity, importance/significance, adequacy, testability and acceptance.

Conclusion

In theory-based practice, nursing science and nursing art come together. Therefore, for theory-based practice, nurses need robust and reliable knowledge and skills to be able to describe, analyse and evaluate a theory and justify its application to enhance practice and patient care.

The progression of nursing as a discipline is reliant on the ongoing application of this knowledge in both practice and research. However, the evaluation of nursing theories necessitates a balance between identifying theoretical weaknesses and appreciating their strengths. This evaluative process is not about establishing the absolute truth of a theory but rather assessing its value for further exploration within the scientific community (Smith 2018b).

Essentially, a theory must be simple and useful and have a connection to real practice. Students need a simple description of theoretical knowledge that is understandable and connects with everyday practice and life. In our long experience of working with postgraduate students, we would point out that the most important thing is to understand the theory and to be convinced of the benefits that an evaluated theory can bring in its application.

Revision Points

- Theory, which needs to be useful in practice, needs to be analysed and evaluated.
- Concept analysis is important because concepts are the basic building blocks of a theory.
- Theory analysis is undertaken in relation to scope, context and content of a theory.
- We can examine the chosen theory according to its clarity, simplicity/complexity, importance/significance, adequacy, testability and acceptance.
- The process of theory evaluation should be rigorous and objective.

Additional Reading

Kim E., Baek G., Jo H., Kim J., Cho A. & Byun M. (2024) Nurses' media competency: a concept analysis. *Nurse Education Today*, **139**, 106232.

Krel C., Vrbnjak D., Bevc S., Štiglic G. & Pajnkihar M. (2022) Technological competency as caring in nursing: a description, analysis and evaluation of the theory. *Zdravstveno Varstvo*, **61**(2), 115–123.

Pajnkihar M., McKenna H.P., Štiglic G. & Vrbnjak D. (2017) Fit for practice: analysis and evaluation of Watson's theory of human caring. *Nursing Science Quarterly*, **30**(3), 243–252.

Park S. & Shin H. (2021) An analysis and evaluation of the theory of planned behavior using Fawcett and DeSanto-Madeya's framework. *Advances in Nursing Science*, **44**(4), E141–E154.

References

Alligood M.R. (2010a) Introduction to nursing theory: its history, significance, and analysis. In Alligood M.R. & Marriner Tomey A. (eds) *Nursing Theorists and Their Work*, 7th edition, pp. 3–15. St. Louis, MO: Mosby, Inc.

Alligood M.R. (2018) *Nursing Theorists and Their Work*, 9th edition. St. Louis, MO: Elsevier.

Chinn P.L. & Kramer M.K. (2008) *Integrated Theory and Knowledge Development in Nursing*, 7th edition. St. Louis: Mosby, Inc.

Chinn P.L. & Kramer M.K. (2011) *Integrated Theory & Knowledge Development in Nursing*, 8th edition. New York: Elesvier-Mosby.

Chinn P.L., Kramer M.K. & Sitzman K. (2022) *Knowledge Development in Nursing: Theory and Process*, 10th edition. St. Louis: Elsevier.

Cutcliffe J.R. & McKenna H. (2005) *The Essential Concepts of Nursing: A Critical Review*. Edinburgh: Elsevier.

Fawcett J. (2005) *Contemporary Nursing Knowledge: Analysis and Evaluation of Nursing Models and Theories*, 3rd edition. Philadelphia, PA: F.A. Davis.

Fawcett J. (2012a) Criteria for evaluation of theory. In Redd P.G. & Crawford Shearer N.B. (eds) *Perspectives on Nursing Theory*, 6th edition, pp. 352–357. Philadelphia, PA: Wolters Kluwer/Lippincott.

Fawcett J. (2021) Empirical indicators: conceptual and theoretical origins. *Aquichan*, **21**(4), e2144. DOI: 10.5294/aqui.2021.21.4.4

Fawcett, J. (2023) Evolution of one version of our disciplinary metaparadigm. Blog. https://nursology.net/2023/01/17/evolution-of-one-version-of-our-disciplinary-metaparadigm/

Fawcett J. & DeSanto-Madeya S. (2013) *Contemporary Nursing Knowledge: Analysis and Evaluation of Nursing Models and Theories*, 3rd edition. Philadelphia, PA: F.A. Davis.

Harih M. & Pajnkihar M. (2009) Aplikacija teoretičnega modela Imogene M. King pri obravnavi starostnika s sladkorno boleznijo. Application of Imogen M. King's nursing model in the treatment of elderly diabetes patients. *Obzornik Zdravstvene Nege*, **43**(3), 201–208. (in Slovene)

Im E.O. (2021) Historical background for theories: revisiting the past to create the future. In Im E.O. & Meleis A.I. (eds) *Situation Specific Theories: Development, Utilization, and Evaluation in Nursing*, pp. 3–11. Cham: Springer.

Marriner Tomey A. (1998) Introduction to analysis of nursing theories. In Marriner Tomey A. & Alligood M.R. (eds) *Nursing Theorists and Their Work*, 4th edition. St Louis, MO: Mosby Year Book.

McKenna H.P. (1997) *Nursing Theories and Models*. London: Routledge.

McKenna H.P. & Slevin O.D. (2008) *Nursing Models, Theories and Practice. Vital Notes for Nurses*. Oxford: Blackwell Publishing.

Meleis A.I. (ed.) (2012) *Theoretical Nursing: Development and Progress*, 5th edition. Philadelphia, PA: Wolters Kluwer/Lippincott Williams & Wilkins.

Meleis A.I. (2018) *Theoretical Nursing: Development and Progress*, 6th edition. Philadelphia, PA: Wolters Kluwer/Lippincott Williams & Wilkins.

Meleis A.I. (2021) Development of situation-specific theories: an integrative approach. In Im E.O. & Meleis A.I. (eds) *Situation Specific Theories: Development, Utilization, and Evaluation in Nursing*, pp. 49–65. Cham: Springer.

Pajnkihar M. (2003) Theory development for nursing in Slovenia. PhD thesis. Manchester: University of Manchester, Faculty of Medicine, Dentistry, Nursing and Pharmacy.

Pajnkihar M. (2011) Teorija v praksi zdravstvene nege. Theory in nursing practice. *Utrip*, **19**(2), 4–5. (in Slovene)

Pajnkihar M. (2012) Models and criteria for theory analysis and evaluation. In: Skela Savič B. et al. (eds) 5th International Scientific Conference Quality Health Care Treatment in the Framework of Education, Research and Multiprofessional Collaboration – Towards the Health of Individuals and the Society, Proceedings of Lectures with Peer Review, pp. 77–84. Jesenice: College of Nursing.

Pajnkihar M. & Butterworth T. (2005) Nursing in Slovenia: a consideration of the value of nursing theories. *Journal of Research in Nursing*, **10**(1), 45–56.

Pajnkihar M. & Vrbnjak D. (2020a) *Teorije, koncepti in praksa zdravstvene nege: (zbrano učno gradivo): podiplomski študijski program 2. stopnje Zdravstvena nega*. Maribor: Univerza v Mariboru, Fakulteta za zdravstvene vede (in Slovene).

Pajnkihar M. & Vrbnjak D. (2020b) *Teorije, koncepti in praksa zdravstvene nege: (zbrano učno gradivo): podiplomski študijski program 3. stopnje Zdravstvena nega*. Maribor: Univerza v Mariboru, Fakulteta za zdravstvene vede (in Slovene).

Pajnkihar M. & Vrbnjak D. (2020c) *Zdravstvena nega: (zbrano učno gradivo): (2020–2021)*. Maribor: Univerza v Mariboru, Fakulteta za zdravstvene vede (in Slovene).

Parse R.R. (1987) *Nursing Science: Major Paradigms, Theories, and Critiques*. Philadelphia, PA: Saunders.

Smith M.C. (2018a) Disciplinary perspectives linked to middle range theory. In Smith M.J. & Liehr P.R. (eds) *Middle Range Theory for Nursing*, 4th edition, pp. 3–13. New York: Springer Publications.

Smith M.C. (2018b) Evaluation of middle range theories for the discipline of nursing. In Smith M.J. & Liehr P.R. (eds) *Middle Range Theory for Nursing*, 4th edition, pp. 33–45. New York: Springer Publications.

Stevens-Barnum B. (1998) *Nursing Theory: Analysis, Application, Evaluation*, 5th edition. New York: Lippincott Williams & Wilkins.

Swanson K.M. (1991) Empirical development of a middle range theory of caring. *Nursing Research*, **40**(3), 161–166.

Swanson K.M. (2015) Kristen Swanson's theory of caring. In Smith M.C. & Parker M.E. (eds) *Nursing Theories and Nursing Practice*, 4th edition, pp. 521–531. New York: Springer Publications.

Walker L.O. & Avant K.C. (2011) *Strategies for Theory Construction in Nursing*, 5th edition. Boston, MA: Prentice Hall.

Walker L.O. & Avant K.C. (2019) *Strategies for Theory Construction in Nursing*, 6th edition. Boston, MA: Pearson.

Watson J. (1985a) *Nursing: The Philosophy and Science of Caring*. Colorado, CO: Colorado Associated University Press.

The Metaparadigm Elements as Outlined in Twenty Nursing Grand Theories

	APPENDIX A			
Theorist	**'Person'**	**'Nursing'**	**'Health'**	**'Environment'**
Roper, Logan and Tierney (1980) [UK]	Unfragmented whole who carries out or is assisted in carrying out activities which contribute to the process of living.	A profession whose focus is to help the patient prevent solve, alleviate or cope with problems associated with the activities of living.	The optimum level of independence in each activity of living, which enables the individual to function at his or her maximum capacity.	Circumstances that may impinge upon people as they travel along the life-span and cause movement towards dependence or independence.
Wiedenbach (1964) [USA]	A functionally competent being, able to determine if a need for help is being experienced.	A helping art that uses a unique blend of thoughts and feelings and overt actions in relation to an individual who is in need of help.	A nurse's concern for the patient is related to his or her health.	That which may produce an obstacle, which may result in the need for help.
Orem (1995) [USA]	Functional integrated whole with a motivation to achieve self-care.	A human service related to the patient's need and ability to undertake self-care and to help him or her sustain health, recover from disease and injury or cope with their effects.	A state of wholeness or integrity of the individual, his or her parts and modes of functioning.	A subcomponent of the person, and with the person forms an integrated system related to self-care.
Minshull, Ross and Turner (1986) [UK]	A holistic individual having interdependent physical, psychosocial, spiritual and social needs.	Supports, enables or helps the individual, either directly or indirectly, to meet their need to achieve maximum wellness and independence.	A relatively stable state of maximum wellness, which equates with independence.	That area in which the individual functions.

(Continued)

Fundamentals of Nursing Models, Theories and Practice, Third Edition. Hugh P. McKenna, Majda Pajnkihar and Dominika Vrbnjak.
© 2025 John Wiley & Sons Ltd. Published 2025 by John Wiley & Sons Ltd.
Companion website: www.wiley.com/go/nursingmodels3e

APPENDIX A				
Theorist	**'Person'**	**'Nursing'**	**'Health'**	**'Environment'**
Rogers (1980) [USA]	A unique whole: a unique unitary field of energy that manifests characteristics that are more than and different from the sum of their parts.	A learned profession with compassionate concern for maintaining and promoting health, preventing illness, caring for and rehabilitating the sick and disabled.	Defined by cultures and individuals to denote behaviours that are of high value and low value.	A four-dimensional negatrophic energy field identified by pattern and organisation, and encompassing all that is outside any given field.
Henderson (1966) [USA]	Biological human beings with inseparable mind and body who share certain fundamental human needs.	A profession that assists the person, sick or well, in the performance of those activities contributing to health or its recovery (or to a peaceful death), that the person would perform if she or he had the strength, will or knowledge.	The ability to function independently regarding 14 activities of daily living.	That which may act in a positive or negative way upon the person.
Johnson (1959) [USA]	A behavioural system having 8 subsystems, which are interrelated and interdependent.	A professional discipline giving a socially valued service, which focuses on the individual who is attempting to maintain or re-establish equilibrium.	An elusive state determined by psychological, social and physiological factors, which is held as a desired value by all the health professions.	That which is external to the person, but from which he or she received sustenal needs.
Roy (1970) [USA]	A biopsychosocial being, who presents as an integral whole.	A socially valued service, whose goal is to promote a positive adaptation to the stimuli and stresses encountered by the patient.	The adaptation of the person to stimuli on a continuous line between wellness and illness.	Both internal and external, from the environment the person is subject to stresses.
Neuman (1982) [USA]	A total person having physiological, psychological, socio-cultural and developmental influences.	A unique profession that can purposefully intervene at primary, secondary or tertiary prevention levels.	A varying state of wellness and illness, which is influenced by physiological, psychological sociocultural and developmental factors.	Both internal and external, with the person maintaining varying degrees of harmony between both.
Fitzpatrick (1982) [USA]	An open system, a unified whole, characterised by basic human rhythms.	A science and a profession that has as its central concern the meaning attached to life and health.	A continuously developing characteristic of humans; awareness and meaningfulness of life and full life potential.	An open systemin continuous interaction with the person.
Parse (1981) [USA]	A synergistic open being coextensive with the universe and free to choose in situations.	Science and an art focusing on man as a living unit.	A process of becoming, as experienced by the person.	Co-constituted becoming in mutual simultaneous energy exchange with the person.
Newman (1979) [USA]	An energy filed that is part of the life process.	Nursing assists individuals to utilise their own resources to attain higher levels of consciousness.	A fusion of disease and non-disease that is a basic patter unique to the personas he or she evolves towards expanded consciousness.	An energy field that is part of life process, which is outside any given human field.

APPENDIX A				
Theorist	**'Person'**	**'Nursing'**	**'Health'**	**'Environment'**
Travelbee (1966) [USA]	Unique irreplaceable individuals who are always in the process of learning, evolving or changing.	An interpersonal process that assists the individual, family or community to prevent, or cope with illness/suffering and find meaning and hope in these experiences.	A subjective state that is determined in accord with each person's appraisal of his or her physical, emotional or spiritual status.	The arena where humans experience the full range of the human condition.
Peplau (1952) [USA]	A unique self-system composed of biochemical, physiological and interpersonal characteristics.	A significant therapeutic interpersonal process, which acts as a maturing force and an educative instrument.	Forward movements of personality and other ongoing human processes in the direction of creative, constructive, productive personal and community living.	Microcosms of significant others and interpersonal situations with whom the person interacts.
Levine (1966) [USA]	A living being who interacts with his or her environment and responds to change by means of adapting.	A process of human interaction, which incorporates scientific principles in the use of the nursing process.	A pattern of adaptive change.	Both internal (physiological) and external (perceptual, operational and conceptual) components.
Patterson and Zderad (1976) [USA]	An incarnate being always becoming in relation to persons and things in a world of time and space.	An intersubjective transaction between patient and nurse related to the health-illness quality of living.	More than just freedom from disease.	The person's inner world (a biased and shaded reality) and the real world (persons and things in time and space).
King (1971) [USA]	An open system interacting with the environment, each permitting and exchange of matter, energy and information through permeable boundaries.	A process of interaction between nurse and client whereby each perceives the other and the situation and through communication they set goals, explore means and agree on means to achieve goals.	A dynamic state in the life cycle, which implies continuous adaptation to stresses through optimal use of one's resources to achieve maximum potential for daily living.	An open system permitting an exchange of matter, energy and information with human beings through permeable boundaries.
Orlando (1961) [USA]	A behaving human organism.	Interaction with a patient with a need, which involves patient validation with the needed and the help provided in order to improve the patient's heath.	Mental and physical comfort, a sense of adequacy and wellbeing.	Time and place – the context of the nursing situation.
Riehl (1974) [USA]	One who has intrinsic value and who is constantly striving to make sense of the situation in which her finds himself.	A professional service involving direct and personal ministrations to individuals, families and groups wherever they are when health needs arise.	An optimum state of health is considered as a state of wholeness.	Environment is dynamic with many interesting forces serving as a constraint impinging on and influencing the person's state of health.
Watson (2008) [USA]	A being in the world who holds three speres of being – mind, body and spirit that are influenced by the concept of self and who is unique and free to make choices.	Nursing is concerned with promoting health, preventing illness, caring for the sick and restoring health.	A high level of overall physical, mental and social functioning. A general adaptive-maintenance level of daily functioning. The absence of illness or the presence of efforts that leads to its absence.	The internal and external factors that can help a person actualise his or her inner power of self-healing.

Index

Page numbers followed by 'f' refer to figures. Page numbers followed by 't' refer to tables.

Fundamentals of Nursing Models, Theories and Practice, Third Edition. Hugh P. McKenna, Majda Pajnkihar and Dominika Vrbnjak.
© 2025 John Wiley & Sons Ltd. Published 2025 by John Wiley & Sons Ltd.
Companion website: www.wiley.com/go/nursingmodels3e